Obesity Medicine
Board Review Questions

Obesity Medicine Board Review Questions

Kevin B. Smith, DO, FACP
ABOM Diplomate

270+ Board Style Review Questions to Prepare for the American Board of Obesity Medicine Certification

2024 Edition

ISBN: 9798874146467

Independently published

Disclaimer: All efforts have been made to ensure accuracy and that the most up-to-date information is provided. Information in this review book should be used for study, not as a reference for patient care. It is up to the provider to ensure all information is accurate, and the author will not be held liable for inadvertent errors.

The item domains and rubrics for the Certification Examination for Obesity Medicine Physicians are available without charge on the ABOM website to facilitate individual study as well as review course development. The author of this review book has not been provided information regarding examination questions, nor does the author have preferential knowledge regarding actual questions included in the examination.

Copy editing performed by Kelly Smith

For correspondence, including questions, concerns, or errata, please contact: obesitymedicinereview@gmail.com

Free weekly study blogs, book updates, and discounts can be found at obesitymedicinereview.com or by scanning QR code.

To maximize study potential,
use with the companion book:

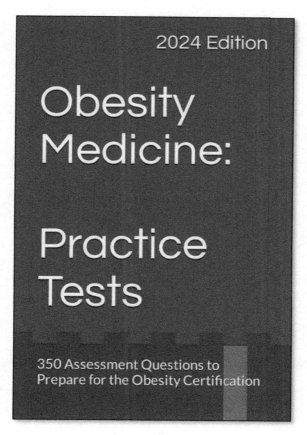

2024 Edition

Obesity
Medicine:

Practice
Tests

350 Assessment Questions to
Prepare for the Obesity Certification

Free study blogs, discounts,
resources, and book updates at
obesitymedicinereview.com

I. Basic Concepts

1. A 41-year-old male is seen in the hospital on postoperative day one status post Roux-en-Y gastric bypass. Home medications include glargine 30 units nightly and aspart sliding scale with meals. Since surgery, he has not required any insulin to maintain normal glucose levels and has plans to be discharged on a low dose of immediate-release metformin. The increased endogenous hormone responsible for this diabetic medication adjustment

A. is only secreted in the small intestine
B. is secreted in response to fat and protein ingestion
C. reduces hepatic gluconeogenesis
D. has the same quantitative effects as seen after sleeve gastrectomy
E. causes gallbladder contraction

2. A 24-year-old female presents for genetic counseling regarding obesity. She is frustrated by the lack of ability to lose weight and being classified as "overweight" at a very young age despite her tall stature. She admits to wanting to give up regarding weight loss since obesity "is a family curse." She has diabetes and is on metformin. Previous testing indicated that she had significantly elevated circulating insulin levels. Which of the following genetic abnormalities is most likely present?

A. MC4R
B. POMC
C. FTO
D. PCSK1
E. LEPR

3. A 51-year-old female presents to the health clinic with questions about a diet she heard about through a health magazine. Although she cannot remember the name of the diet, it promoted a higher intake of omega fat than other diets she has researched. Benefits included lowering cardiovascular disease and preventing type 2 diabetes, both of which run in her family. In addition, she will still be able to consume seafood, an important component given her fishing hobby. What is the most likely diet that this patient is referencing?

    A. Vegan
    B. Pescatarian
    C. Lacto-ovo
    D. Mediterranean
    E. Low carbohydrate

4. A 31-year-old female wants to know her total energy expenditure. She estimates her non-exercise activity thermogenesis to be 300 kcal/day, her thermic effect of meals to be 10% of her total expenditure, and her calories from exercise to be 400 kcal/day. What other testing is necessary to determine her total energy expenditure accurately?

    A. Indirect calorimeter
    B. Skinfold calipers
    C. Duke's treadmill score
    D. Bioelectric impedance analyses
    E. Basal body temperature

5. A research team is developing a thesis regarding intrauterine predisposition to factors, such as how maternal obesity affects the developing fetus through adulthood. So far, the longitudinal study has shown that a mother's body mass index correlates with comorbidities of cognitive deficits and autism spectrum disorders. This type of research is best associated with which of the following?

    A. Neurohormonal physiology
    B. Epigenetics and environment
    C. Behavioral determinants
    D. Mutations of genetic DNA
    E. Socioeconomic and culture

6. A longitudinal study was completed looking at the effects of sleep on weight. Both weight and the time of quality sleep, measured through a smartwatch device, were documented over 10 years. At the end of the study, what hormones or receptor levels would be expected to be increased in those who received 5 hours of sleep compared to those who received 8 hours?

    A. Leptin and neuropeptide Y
    B. α-MSH and peptide YY
    C. POMC receptors and ghrelin
    D. Cortisol and leptin
    E. Ghrelin and orexin A

7. A 65-year-old male is following up with his dietician after starting a low-fat diet six weeks ago. He has increased his exercise to 250 minutes/week and has noticed a 1% total body weight loss since initiating these lifestyle changes. He comments that he has always had to work hard to maintain or lose weight, and it seems that if he stops dieting for a few weeks, he regains weight rapidly. In contrast, he states that his wife can eat whatever she likes, has always remained thin, and seldomly exercises. Compared to his wife, this patient most likely has which of the following?

    A. Decreased energy harvest from food
    B. Higher fasting-induced adipose factor expression
    C. Increased levels of Firmicutes in his gut
    D. Higher AMPK

8. A research study is underway in which patients fast for 8 hours, followed by consuming a meal of 500 kcal. Several hormones are monitored every 2 hours during the fasting and postprandial period for 12 hours. Six hours into the fast, ghrelin hormone levels are at their peak. What other finding would most likely be present during this time?

    A. Y1 and Y5 receptor stimulation
    B. Leptin hormone elevation
    C. Suppressed agouti-related peptide hormone levels
    D. Activation of the POMC/CART pathway
    E. Orexin A and B hormone suppression

9. A 31-year-old female presents to her primary care physician for follow-up regarding weight-gain. Over the past three months, she has noticed a weight gain of approximately 10 pounds (4.5 kg), which is discouraging because she has been trying to get healthy and lose weight before her wedding in 2 months. She quit smoking with the help of bupropion and has been walking daily. She had a copper intrauterine device inserted four months ago. Although she goes to bed later due to wedding planning, she states she still sleeps 8 hours nightly. Which of the following is most likely playing a role in her weight gain?

A. Bupropion
B. Intrauterine device
C. Decreased tobacco
D. Sleep habits

10. Several medical students are trying to create a project to determine the best way to impact childhood obesity rates, as this rate has nearly tripled in the past 30 years. They begin to review epidemiologic data on a national level to see who is most affected by obesity prevalence, focusing on children 2-19 years old. They compare age, race, gender, and financial status. During their research, what are they most likely to find?

A. The highest prevalence of obesity is in Hispanic female children
B. Class 3 obesity in children has declined over the past decade
C. Asian adolescents had higher obesity rates than Hispanics
D. The highest income class had the lowest obesity rates
E. The prevalence of obesity was nearly 40% in all children

11. A 19-year-old female presents to her family practice practitioner to request a referral to a lymphedema clinic. She states that since she was 15 years old, she has gained excessive weight, predominantly in her lower extremities. She says her grandmother had similar findings on her upper extremities after undergoing a mastectomy, and she was treated at a lymphedema clinic with good results. She has a normal waist circumference and a BMI of 26 kg/m². Her lower extremities have a sensation of round peas when the fatty tissue is palpated. What other findings would be expected in this patient?

    A. Decreased lymphatic flow
    B. Positive cuff sign
    C. Marked pitting edema
    D. Eventual progression to arms
    E. Positive Stemmer's sign

12. A 33-year-old female recently underwent a sleeve gastrectomy and is losing weight appropriately. She is most impressed by her decreased appetite, irrespective of meals, which has helped maintain a significant calorie deficit. The hormone most likely responsible for her decreased appetite initially acts on what area of the brain?

    A. Dorsal vagal complex
    B. Amygdala
    C. Nucleus of the tractus solitarius
    D. Arcuate nucleus
    E. Lateral hypothalamus

13. A dietician is reviewing terminology with one of her students. She discusses a term that describes the value of the amount of a nutrient estimated to meet the requirement of half of all healthy individuals in a population. What term is she defining?

    A. Estimated average requirement
    B. Adequate intake
    C. Recommended daily allowance
    D. Tolerable upper intake level
    E. Daily value

14. A human research study is ongoing and is recruiting patients with a body mass index > 30 kg/m^2 who have not previously been diagnosed with thyroid disease and do not have symptoms of overt hypothyroidism. Inclusion criteria requires a thyroid-stimulating hormone (TSH) level > 5 mcU/mL (reference range 0.4-4.2 mcU/mL). At the end of the study, 130 patients met the above criteria. The patients were then provided resources to assist in losing 5% of their total body weight. Which lab finding would be expected after they achieved their weight-loss goal?

    A. Increased thyroid-releasing hormone
    B. Increased T_4 (thyroxine) levels
    C. Decreased T_3 (triiodothyronine) levels
    D. Unchanged thyroid levels

15. A 49-year-old male presents to the office to discuss weight-related complications. He states he was recently promoted to chief operating officer of a Fortune 500 company and the fear of messing up and losing the associated lifestyle, prestige, and salary is "driving me mad." Per chart review, it is noted that since starting this new position, he has gained nearly 45 lbs (20.4 kg). Compared to before the promotion and now, which hormonal change is most likely?

A. Insulin sensitivity increase with glucagon suppression
B. Activation of α-MSH and increased levels of leptin
C. Poor quality of sleeping activating the POMC/CART pathway
D. NPY activation related to excess cortisol section
E. Suppressed ghrelin levels due to vagal nerve suppression

16. A researcher is looking to evaluate different climates' effects on obesity rates. He believes warmer temperatures should allow more outdoor activity, thus lowering obesity rates. He wants to begin his research in the state with the lowest obesity rates. Which state should he start his research?

A. Colorado
B. Mississippi
C. Oklahoma
D. Florida
E. West Virginia

17. An endocrinologist is discussing with a medical student the vast number of hormones that play a role in obesity and satiety. In particular, one hormone is an insulin sensitizer, in which levels are inversely related to body fat mass. In addition, the endogenous levels of this hormone decrease in the setting of type 2 diabetes. The hormone described above most likely originates from which of the following structures?

    A. Adipose tissue
    B. Gastric fundus
    C. Duodenum
    D. Beta cells of the pancreas
    E. Alpha cells of the pancreas

18. A grandmother brings her 9-year-old granddaughter for a wellness visit. The grandmother gained full custody when the child's parents were incarcerated for child neglect and physical abuse. The child is reserved and demonstrates poor eye contact. The child's growth chart is in the 87th percentile for weight based on age and gender. Which of the following is the most appropriate advice to provide to the grandmother?

    A. Now that the homelife is stabilized, her weight should improve
    B. The child should be monitored for anorexia given life stressors
    C. The child is at risk for developing obesity given her parent's actions
    D. Enrollment in social sports like basketball will be beneficial
    E. Trazodone may help with depression symptoms and improve sleep

19. A pediatric patient presents for genetic testing regarding an abnormal appetite. The patient is described as having a small head size with narrow hands and feet. The patient's mouth is open and eyebrows are thickened. Which of the following is the most likely etiology of his findings?

A. Prader-Willi syndrome
B. Borjeson-Forssman-Lehmann syndrome
C. MC4R deficiency
D. Trisomy of chromosome 21
E. Cohen syndrome

20. A 44-year-old male with a past medical history of insomnia presents for an annual wellness exam. He denies any current complaints but does admit to right knee pain that is worsened with prolonged walking. He has a moderate score on the Epworth sleepiness scale. His body mass index is 31 kg/m^2, his waist circumference is 81.3 cm (32 inches), and his body fat composition is 24%. Laboratory work, including a hemoglobin A1c, complete metabolic panel, and lipid panel, is unremarkable. An x-ray of his right knee shows moderate osteophytes and joint space narrowing. Which of the following best describes his condition?

A. Sick fat disease
B. Obesity class II
C. Obesity based on % body fat
D. Fat mass disease
E. Abdominal obesity

21. A 6-year-old male is being seen by a pediatric endocrinologist for severe obesity. The mother states that the patient had a normal birth weight and even required nutrient supplementation due to failure to thrive early on. However, since age three, he has had extreme hunger, which has led to progressive weight gain. The child currently weighs 178 lbs (80.7 kg). A genetic mutation is discovered, and subsequent treatment with hormone replacement is initiated with impressive results. Which of the following neuromodulators was most likely activated with the hormone replacement?

A. Orexin A and B
B. Alpha melanocyte-stimulating hormone
C. Agouti-related peptide
D. Melanin-concentrating hormone

22. Researchers are looking at potential intravenous medications to assist with weight loss. One treatment that has shown promise is a synthetic form of a gastrointestinal hormone produced in both the large and small intestines and rectum and is found to be elevated within 1 hour after meals. Its contributions to weight loss are due to its potent appetite suppressant effect and ability to delay gastric emptying and intestinal transit time. The hormone level increases irrespective of macronutrient intake. What is the hormone most likely being studied?

A. Ghrelin
B. Cholecystokinin
C. Glucagon-like peptide 1
D. Oxyntomodulin
E. Peptide YY

23. A previously healthy 9-year-old female presents to her pediatrician for a well-child check. Her growth chart is shown below. Her percentile BMI has steadily increased over the last four visits despite lifestyle changes incorporated within her family. She has breast bud development. Which of the following conditions may be contributing to these findings?

A. Excessive caloric intake
B. Precocious puberty
C. Bulimia
D. Achondroplasia
E. Hypothyroidism

24. A 7-year-old female presents with her mother for a dietician evaluation and education session. The family drinks a lot of sweetened tea in the home and inquires about changing from sugar to nonnutritive sweeteners (NNS). The best response to her inquiry would be that NNS

A. are a preferred alternative to sucrose
B. increase the risk of ADHD in children
C. may help with weight loss, as they are calorie-neutral
D. can cause a dysregulation in appetite
E. are regarded as "not safe for children" by the FDA

25. A 5-year-old male with the disease of obesity is seen in the pediatric clinic for follow-up after meeting with a childhood obesity specialist. The patient has had many difficulties, including significant intellectual disability, retinal dystrophy, and polydactyly. Renal malformations have led to polyuria and polydipsia, requiring a percutaneous endoscopic gastrostomy tube to be placed to keep up with fluid replenishment. Given these findings, the patient most likely carries which of the following diagnoses?

A. Prader-Willi syndrome
B. Cohen syndrome
C. Borjeson-Forssman-Lehmann syndrome
D. Albright hereditary osteodystrophy
E. Bardet-Biedl syndrome

26. A research lab is performing studies on hormonally active tissue. In the study, tissue is obtained from pathological specimens upon autopsy. One tissue biopsy displays resistin, interleukin 6, and estrogen. Which of the following tissues did this biopsy most likely come from?

A. Ovaries
B. Lymph nodes
C. Adrenal glands
D. Adipose
E. Intestines

27. A 26-year-old patient is frustrated that they have been diagnosed with obesity based on a body mass index (BMI) of 31 kg/m². She is an active bodybuilder and has competed in several national championships. Which of the following is the best response to her concerns?

A. You meet the diagnostic criteria for obesity
B. I want to order a CT scan to see if you meet criteria for obesity
C. The BMI is a useful screening test for most patients
D. Body mass index has been determined to be an inaccurate tool
E. Would it be alright if I discussed some ways to improve your health?

28. A previously healthy 29-year-old male with a diagnosis of obesity presents to the clinic for a physical examination. He is an accountant and thus is relatively inactive during the day. Vital signs are within normal limits. His BMI is 35 kg/m². He is frustrated that despite exercising and eating similarly to his identical twin brother, he is nearly 40 lbs (18.1 kg) heavier than his brother, who is a mail carrier. Which of the following best explains the weight difference between him and his twin brother?

A. Basal metabolic rate
B. Non-exercise activity thermogenesis
C. Intentional exercise
D. Resting energy expenditure
E. Dietary thermogenesis

29. On a medical mission trip, a 7-year-old patient is being seen in the clinic. He appears very malnourished, but he seems unphased by his lack of nutrition. His abdomen is distended, and anasarca is present. He is supplemented with low doses of protein in incremental amounts to prevent refeeding syndrome. Which of the following must be consumed in his diet, as his body cannot produce it?

A. Alanine
B. Aspartate
C. Glycine
D. Leucine
E. Proline

30. A researcher is trying to create a calculator that will take into account epigenetic factors contributing to childhood obesity rates to predict which children are most prone to obesity. He plans to have a smartphone application that contains a checklist of risk factors for childhood obesity, thus providing a percent risk of obesity based on current risk factors. Practitioners would then be able to discuss with the parents how reducing certain risk factors could improve the odds of a healthy weight in their children. Which of the following should be taken into account for his predictive calculator?

A. Kids have similar obesity rates whether one/both parents have obesity
B. A cesarean delivery increases the child's risk of obesity
C. Maternal smoking leads to decreased childhood obesity rates
D. Breastfed infants have fewer infections but increased obesity rates
E. Insufficient gestational weight gain is protective against obesity

31. A 36-year-old female status post sleeve gastrectomy six years prior presents to her primary care physician complaining of numbness in her lower extremities. She has lost 120 lbs (54.4 kg) postoperatively. She is currently taking prenatal vitamins. Physical examination reveals diminished vibratory sense bilaterally in her lower extremities and a positive Romberg test. What is the most likely underlying cause of this patient's clinical presentation?

A. Decreased intrinsic factor production
B. Anti-parietal antibodies
C. Tissue transglutaminase antibodies
D. Impaired terminal ileum absorption
E. Decreased dietary intake

32. A 29-year-old professional bull rider sustained a significant head injury during one of his performances. He is intubated and undergoes imaging showing a right frontal head injury with cerebral edema. After a prolonged recovery period he is finally discharged from an inpatient rehab facility. His wife notices that he no longer enjoys her cooking, but rather wishes to discuss gourmet dishes and their intricacies from different television shows he now watches. Which of the following conditions is most consistent with his presentation?

A. Gilbert's syndrome
B. Gourmand syndrome
C. Gorlin syndrome
D. Gardner syndrome
E. Gilles de la Tourette syndrome

33. A patient is enrolled in a research study determining which variables have the strongest alterations on resting energy expenditure. Indirect calorimetry is performed weekly, with different variables changed prior to undergoing the study. The initial baseline calorimetry reading the week prior at rest, supine, and in a dark room showed a resting energy expenditure of 1750 kcal/day. Today, it showed 2300 kcal/day. Which of the following performed prior to testing caused this discrepancy?

A. Fasting for 48 hours
B. Taking sodium bicarbonate tablets
C. Exercise
D. Ice bath

34. A patient presents to an exercise physiologist to discuss different workout routines. The physiologist discusses different exercise options and their effect on excess post-exercise oxygen consumption (EPOC). Which of the following would have the highest levels of EPOC?

A. Bicep curls
B. Aerobic exercise
C. Muscle strengthening
D. High-intensity interval training
E. Yoga

35. A 15-year-old male presents for an annual physical exam. The patient has hearing loss requiring a cochlear implant and visual impairment. In addition, the patient has type 2 diabetes mellitus. A recent echocardiogram displayed worsening dilated cardiomyopathy. His younger brother has similar findings. The patient's growth chart reveals severe obesity. The condition is most likely due to which of the following genetic abnormalities?

A. ALMS 1 mutation
B. Chromosome 11p15.5 dysregulation
C. X-linked inheritance
D. Genetic imprinting
E. MC4R mutation

36. A 31-year-old female presents to her dietician's office five months after undergoing a sleeve gastrectomy. During this period, she has lost 43 lbs (19.5 kg) and is encouraged and motivated to continue working toward weight loss. She has followed all dietary recommendations and vitamin replacement. What is the most accurate statement regarding the hormone most affected by this surgery, contributing to her weight loss?

A. Patients with Prader-Willi syndrome have normal levels
B. Those with a vagotomy would have similar qualitative levels
C. Glucose suppresses the hormone for extended periods
D. Sleep deprivation reduces this hormone, while stress increases it
E. Leptin levels are directly proportionate to this hormone

37. A pathophysiologist is lecturing medical students on the hormones that regulate appetite. In particular, one of these hormones plays a role in energy balance and is directly proportionate to the amount of adipose tissue in the body. As adiposity increases, this hormone increases, signaling satiety and increasing the rate of energy expenditure. Which of the following is most likely being discussed?

A. Pancreatic polypeptide
B. Cholecystokinin
C. Leptin
D. Glucagon-like peptide 1
E. Ghrelin

38. A 39-year-old female presents to the emergency department for dyspnea on exertion and chest pain. She states she flew in from Europe to go skiing with friends in Colorado. She had a duodenal jejunal bypass liner placed 9 months prior and has lost 43 lbs (19.5 kg) and wanted to celebrate with her friends. A CT scan is negative for pulmonary embolism and shows no pulmonary edema. Lab work is shown below:

Lab	Patient's Value	Reference Range
Hemoglobin	8.4 g/dL	12.0–16.0 g/dL
MCV	78 μm^3	80–100 μm^3
Platelets	490,000/mm^3	150,000–400,000/mm^3

Which of the following deficiencies is most likely contributing to her presentation?

A. Folic acid
B. B$_{12}$
C. Pyridoxine
D. Iron
E. Thiamine

39. A 7-year-old patient presents to his family medicine physician with his father for ongoing obesity management. Physical examination reveals a broad forehead with large earlobes and strabismus. Upon record review, a loss of function mutation to the FMR1 gene (Xq27.3) is noted. Which of the following other findings is most likely present in this patient?

    A. Polydactyly
    B. Decreased testicular size
    C. Organomegaly
    D. Hypertonia
    E. Elongated face

40. A 9-year-old male presents to a geneticist as the patient has had a speech delay and learning difficulties including dyslexia. On review of his growth chart, he has remained persistently in the 97th percentile for weight. On examination, a scar is noted on the hand which his mother states is related to the removal of a "sixth digit" as a neonate. Which of the following cellular structures is likely involved in this patient's underlying syndromic condition?

    A. Endoplasmic reticulum
    B. Lysosomes
    C. Golgi apparatus
    D. Cilia
    E. Cell wall

41. A 26-year-old female presents to the emergency department via ambulance in cardiac arrest with the following rhythm strip:

Per her husband, she was planning to lose a significant amount of weight before a friend's wedding next month and started over-the-counter supplements and a new diet. She has congenital long QT syndrome and class III obesity (BMI 54 kg/m²). Which of the following dietary plans most likely contributed to this patient's presentation?

A. Ketogenic diet
B. Intermittent fasting
C. Very low-calorie diet
D. Mediterranean diet
E. Meal-replacement plan

42. A 33-year-old female presents to her primary care physician for follow-up regarding her polysomnography results. Her results reveal her apnea-hypopnea index was > 30, indicating severe obstructive sleep apnea; the test was split with continuous positive airway pressure (CPAP) titration. She has a prescription for a CPAP machine but has not picked it up yet. Given these findings, which neurohumoral hormone would be expected to be decreased?

A. Ghrelin
B. Orexin
C. Leptin
D. Neuropeptide Y

43. A physician is discussing with a medical student the ethnic disparities within obesity. Of the following ethnicity and gender combinations in adults, which would likely have the most significant disparity of increased obesity (based on percentage)?

A. Asian males
B. Hispanic males
C. White females
D. Black females

44. A patient is presenting to discuss weight loss options. He has tried several dietary plans without success and has trouble maintaining a persistent exercise schedule. Which of the following statements would be most accurate?

A. Caloric absorption is similar amongst individuals with identical intake
B. For every 3500 kcal you decrease in your diet, you will lose 1 lb
C. Losing weight is all about willpower and motivation
D. It is easier to maintain weight loss, rather than lose it
E. Both subcutaneous and visceral fat can negatively affect health

45. A 46-year-old female presents for an annual follow-up with her obesity medicine specialist. She underwent a successful biliopancreatic diversion and duodenal switch seven years ago. She has been adherent with all nutritional visits and supplemental vitamin intake. She had lost 162 lbs (73.5 kg), but has regained 10 lbs (4.5 kg) in the past year. She denies any new symptoms. Laboratory work reveals a microcytic anemia with a decreased ferritin level. Which gastrointestinal area is most likely responsible for this patient's laboratory abnormalities?

A. Stomach
B. Duodenum
C. Jejunum
D. Ileum
E. Colon

46. A 6-year-old male presents to an obesity management center for evaluation and treatment of severe obesity. His parents state that he has always had unquenchable hunger and they feel guilty for restricting food. Laboratory work reviews normal cortisol levels, undetectable leptin, and a hemoglobin A1c of 5.8% (reference range < 5.7%). He has normal mentation and flesh-colored striae on the abdomen. The most likely cause of this patient's findings is a mutation in the

A. leptin gene
B. leptin receptor
C. pro-opiomelanocortin gene
D. MC4R receptor
E. prohormone gene

47. A PhD candidate is working with a pediatric infectious disease physician to determine if there is an association between a prior upper respiratory infection and the development of obesity. She looks for serum antibodies and finds a correlation between a positive viral assay and an increased body mass index and waist circumference. Which of the following viruses most likely correlated with her findings?

    A. Parvo B19
    B. HPV-16
    C. Covid-23
    D. Pneumonia serotype 15B
    E. Adenovirus-36

48. A nutritionist is discussing how energy relates to food intake and nutrition labels. How much energy would it take to raise 1 kilogram of water by 1 °C?

    A. 1 Calorie
    B. 10 kilocalories
    C. 100 Calories
    D. 1,000 Calories
    E. 10,000 calories

49. A 23-year-old male presents to his family practice physician after he read an article on high-dose calcium intake related to weight loss. He is currently taking twice the recommended daily allowance, but hasn't noticed a significant weight loss at this point. He asks if this is an effective obesity treatment. His current BMI is 27 kg/m². His only complaint is constipation. Given his current status, which of the following is most likely increased in this patient?

A. Parathyroid hormone activity
B. Vitamin D levels
C. Lipogenesis
D. Lipolysis
E. Fat storage levels

50. A group of physicians are developing a program to address patients with coronary artery disease who are at the highest risk of mortality within the next five years. To simplify the program, they only evaluate the body mass index and waist circumference. Those with the highest mortality risk will be entered into an intensive physical, dietary, and behavioral modification program. Which of the following parameters of patients should receive priority entrance into this class?

A. BMI 22 kg/m²; Waist circumference 85 cm
B. BMI 22 kg/m²; Waist circumference 101 cm
C. BMI 26 kg/m²; Waist circumference 85 cm
D. BMI 30 kg/m²; Waist circumference 85 cm
E. BMI 30 kg/m²; Waist circumference 101 cm

51. A 49-year-old female is discussing a recent incident with her health coach. She states that she recently dropped off her only child at college. A week later, she walked by a bakery and the smell brought back memories of her and her child baking bread on the weekends. Despite recently finishing up lunch and not being hungry, she indulged in two large pieces of bread. Which area of activation played the largest role in this incident?

    A. Amygdala
    B. Hippocampus
    C. Pre-frontal cortex
    D. Hypothalamus
    E. Occipital lobe

52. A 4-year-old male with weight and height consistently in the 95th percentile presents to his pediatrician for follow-up regarding tumor surveillance. He recently underwent an abdominal ultrasound showing hepatosplenomegaly without concerning findings for malignancy. What genetic characteristic is most likely associated with this condition?

    A. Autosomal recessive inheritance
    B. Chromosome 15q deletion
    C. Chromosome 8q22 mutation
    D. Chromosome 11p15.5 dysregulation
    E. ALMS 1 mutation

53. A 24-year-old pregnant female is considering breastfeeding her child. However, she works a full-time job and is concerned about the logistics of pumping while at work. Which of the following statements is most accurate as it relates to breastfeeding?

A. Breastfed infants will initially gain weight more rapidly
B. The risk of childhood obesity is increased with breastfeeding
C. Guidelines recommend exclusive breastfeeding for 12 months
D. Non-breastfed infants are placed at an undue risk of obesity
E. Complimentary food should be introduced at 4 months of age

54. A 37-year-old female presents to her surgeon for a 12-month follow-up after a successful sleeve gastrectomy. She has followed all diet and exercise regimens as prescribed by her dietician and electrophysiologist. However, she has noticed that even though she has increased her exercise time to 220 minutes weekly, she has not seen a significant decrease in weight as expected. She has lost 95 lbs (43 kg) postoperatively but has plateaued. Which of the following most likely explains this plateau effect?

A. Increased total energy expenditure
B. Increased muscle efficiency
C. Adaptive thermogenesis
D. Modified set-point
E. Increased leptin levels

55. A 29-year-old male plans to run a marathon in the next four months. He has been training daily and can run nearly 18 miles without stopping. What is true of the muscle fibers he predominantly utilizes to prepare for this marathon?

A. Energy is from glycolysis
B. Creates forceful contractions
C. Fatigue susceptible
D. Increased mitochondria are present

56. A 66-year-old female presents to the clinic for worsening vision. She states that this has been progressing for the past six months, but recently nearly caused a car accident. She has also had daily headaches, which she attributes to the vision changes, and reports she always feels hungry. Her vital signs are normal except for her BMI, which has increased from 31 to 33 kg/m^2 since last year. Physical exam reveals bilateral loss of the lower peripheral visual fields. Laboratory work reveals a TSH is 0.1 µU/mL (reference range: 0.5–5.0 µU/mL) and a T$_4$ is 2 µg/dL (reference range: 5–12 µg/dL). Prolactin levels are normal. Which of the following is the most appropriate next step?

A. Brain imaging
B. Levothyroxine replacement
C. Ophthalmology referral
D. Radioactive iodine scan of the thyroid
E. Growth hormone and ACTH levels

57. A double-blinded study is performed with patients who have a body mass index between 25-30 kg/m². They receive either a placebo or an intravenous medication theorized to increase brown adipose tissue (BAT) activation. At the end of the infusion, patients undergo a positron emission tomography (PET) scan to evaluate the presence of BAT. After the trial, there was an 11% increased tracer uptake, as evidenced by the PET scan, in those receiving the medication compared to the placebo group. Which of the following most accurately describes the studied adipose tissue?

A. Its brown color is due to increased lysosomes
B. It couples oxidative phosphorylation, increasing ATP production
C. It is stimulated by acetylcholine of the parasympathetic system
D. Resting metabolic rate is inversely proportional to BAT levels
E. It utilizes glucose and free fatty acids to increase lipolysis

58. A 29-year-old health-conscious female is discussing her diet with a nutritionist. Although not focused on weight loss, she is interested to see if her diet matches the recommendations based on the acceptable macronutrient distribution range, as set forth by the United States Department of Agriculture (USDA). Which of the following would meet that criteria if the macronutrient was listed as a percentage of her total calories?

A. Protein 45%
B. Carbohydrate 60%
C. Fat 40%
D. Linoleic acid (Ω -6 fatty acid) 15%
E. α-Linolenic acid (Ω-3 fatty acid) 5%

59. A 29-year-old female presents for a follow-up appointment with her primary care physician. Over the past year, she has lost 40 lbs (18.1 kg), which she attributes to meal replacements and an effective exercise regimen. A recent body composition scan revealed a 3% reduction in adipose tissue. However, she has regained 5 lbs (2.3 kg) over the past two months. She denies changing her diet or exercise regimen but admits to "sneaking a few extra snacks here and there," as she states her hunger has increased. Which of the following neurohormonal changes is most likely contributing to her increased weight gain?

A. Increased leptin levels
B. Loss of inhibition of the NPY/AgRP pathway
C. Melanocortin 4 receptor activation
D. Orexin A and B hormone suppression
E. Inhibition of neurotrophic factor

60. A poster presentation by medical students compares different exposures that occur both in utero and childhood that may affect weight in order to promote healthy habits and reduce risk factors for children. Which of the following is protective for developing childhood obesity?

A. Authoritative parenting style
B. Treatment of recurrent ear infections
C. Low birth weight
D. In utero exposure to tobacco
E. Untreated attention deficit disorder

61. A 26-year-old entered a hot dog-eating contest at the fair. In preparation for this event, he has fasted since the night prior. If hormone levels were checked at the completion of the event, which of the following would be suppressed the most?

A. Glucagon
B. Cholecystokinin
C. Glucagon-like peptide 1
D. Peptide-YY
E. Growth hormone-releasing peptide

II. Diagnosis and Evaluation

62. A 34-year-old female with a BMI of 29 kg/m² presents to her primary care physician with overeating concerns. She states that she often eats a large amount of food and lacks control while eating during these episodes. She hides this behavior from her roommate as she feels intense embarrassment and guilt. What other finding would most likely be expected?

A. Eating more rapidly than normal
B. Compensatory purging
C. Consuming > 25% of calories after dinner
D. Repetitive behaviors
E. Eating small, unplanned amounts of food

63. A 43-year-old female is presenting with increased thirst and urination. She states that over the past 2-3 months, she has woken up multiple times in the night to urinate and feels like she cannot "drink enough water." She has a past medical history of autoimmune hemolytic anemia and obesity class II. In addition to other age-appropriate screenings, which laboratory test is most sensitive to diagnose her with the most likely condition?

A. Hemoglobin A1c
B. Fasting glucose levels
C. HOMA-IR levels
D. Oral glucose tolerance test
E. Fructosamine levels

64. A 3-year-old male is brought into the pediatric office, as the mother has recently noticed increased weight gain and an insatiable appetite that was not previously present. After reviewing the growth chart, it is noted that his height has maintained the 60th percentile. However, his weight has increased from the 50th percentile to the 90th percentile in the past 1.5 years. A speech therapist has seen him for delayed speech, and he is scheduled to see a therapist for late motor development. Which of the following would most likely be seen on physical examination?

A. Short 4th and 5th metacarpals
B. Hepatosplenomegaly
C. Polydactyly
D. Macroglossia
E. Almond-shaped eyes

65. A 33-year-old Caucasian female is presenting to her primary care physician for an annual exam. She is up to date on her preventative screenings and immunizations. Although she exercises and avoids eating at fast-food restaurants, she is concerned about her cardiovascular risk, as her father had a heart attack at age 42. At what BMI is it recommended to measure waist circumference for additional cardiovascular risk stratification?

A. 18 kg/m^2
B. 24 kg/m^2
C. 33 kg/m^2
D. 40 kg/m^2

66. Researchers are performing a study on obesity and the effects on the associated comorbidities as weight fluctuates over two years. They desire the most accurate fat composition measurements at a molecular level, regardless of cost. Which of the following measurement modalities would meet these criteria?

A. Skinfold calipers
B. Deuterium dilution hydrometry
C. Bioelectric impedance analysis
D. Dual-energy x-ray absorptiometry
E. Body mass index

67. A 23-year-old healthy female presents for an annual examination at her family practice physician's clinic. She has decided to pursue a vegan diet in place of the pescatarian diet she had previously consumed. She wants to ensure she does not become malnourished and asks about vitamin supplementation. What deficiency will most likely be present if supplementation is not initiated within the next year?

A. Vitamin C
B. Cyanocobalamin
C. Vitamin D
D. Folate
E. Vitamin K

68. A 61-year-old male diagnosed with hypertension and obesity class II presents to his sleep specialist to discuss his overnight polysomnography results. His primary care physician referred him after he was experiencing unrefreshing sleep and waking up holding his breath. His spouse also had concerns about loud snoring with pauses in his breathing. Given this patient's history, what is the minimal apnea-hypopnea index (AHI) needed to diagnose obstructive sleep apnea?

A. 5 per hour
B. 15 per hour
C. 30 per hour
D. 60 per hour

69. A physician is working in an obesity medicine clinic and seeing a patient with inadequate insurance coverage. The patient meets criteria for pharmacologic therapy and is interested but cannot afford name-brand combination medications. Therefore, the physician discusses the off-label use of medications, including emulating the newer combination medications by prescribing the two medications separately. The patient comes back one month later with no weight loss. He explains that he lost one of the two prescriptions. Which medications did he most likely take for the past month?

A. Topiramate
B. Phentermine
C. Bupropion
D. Liraglutide
E. Naltrexone

70. A 9-year-old female is brought to her pediatrician for a well-child check. A few years ago, she was diagnosed with depression. Although the medications prescribed have helped with her mood symptoms, her appetite has significantly increased. She eats approximately 3500 kcal/day and admits to playing on the computer and watching more television than previously. Lab work including thyroid hormone levels are normal. Her weight is displayed on the growth chart below. Which stature curve would best correlate with her height?

A. Line A
B. Line B
C. Line C

71. A 27-year-old female with a history of hypertension and recently diagnosed obstructive sleep apnea (OSA) presents for evaluation after having failed many name-brand diets. She states she has always been "on the heavier side," but needing a CPAP machine for OSA motivated her to lose weight. Physical examination reveals a rounded face and truncal obesity with widened abdominal striae. Laboratory work reveals a hemoglobin A1c in the pre-diabetes range. What other finding would most likely be present on physical exam?

A. Scalloped tongue
B. Hirsutism
C. Decreased deep tendon reflexes
D. Periumbilical hernia
E. Superficial ecchymosis

72. A female sprinter undergoes indirect calorimetry to determine her respiratory quotient (RQ), which is obtained by measuring carbon dioxide eliminated divided by oxygen consumed. When the athlete is slowly jogging, it is determined that her body mostly utilizes lipids for energy. However, during sustained sprinting, her RQ would be expected to be near which of the following values?

A. 0.5
B. 0.7
C. 1.0
D. 1.3

73. A 44-year-old female presents for a follow-up three years after undergoing a Roux-en-Y gastric bypass. She is pleased with her results, having lost nearly 55% of her total body weight, and she states she continues to lose weight despite no longer following the dietician's recommendations or exercising. She denies depression and says she feels well but admits to diarrhea. Preoperative BMI was 47.3 kg/m^2, and today it is 22.7 kg/m^2. Physical exam is normal except for excess skin in the abdomen and arms. She has not followed up with her surgeon after the first year. Which of the following may explain her weight loss?

A. Vitamin deficiency
B. Anastomotic stricture
C. Small intestinal bowel overgrowth
D. A shorter common intestinal channel
E. Expected post-surgical weight loss

74. A 14-year-old female with a BMI of 39 kg/m² presents to her family practitioner for recurrent headaches. She states the headaches are pulsatile and occasionally cause loss of appetite. In addition, she now has difficulty seeing the board during school and must sit toward the front of her class. She has intermittent loss of vision and diplopia when standing up. Which of the following would be the best test to determine the cause of her headaches?

A. Orthostatic vital signs
B. Overnight sleep study
C. Ophthalmologic evaluation
D. Brain imaging
E. Cerebral spinal fluid studies

75. A mother brings her 9-year-old son to his pediatrician for evaluation, as is concerned that his height and weight are increased in comparison to his peers. The mother states that her son does tend to watch 4-5 hours of television daily and is "constantly snacking." The son has no known health concerns, and overall appears happy. Physical examination reveals a BMI of 19.75 kg/m², which is the 86th percentile for his age and gender. Which of the following most accurately describes his weight categorization?

A. Underweight
B. Healthy weight
C. Overweight
D. Class 1 obesity
E. Class 2 obesity

76. A 19-year-old male presents to his primary care physician for an annual physical evaluation. He admits to eating significantly more since he started college. He relates this to stress and a change in sleep habits since moving to the dormitories. He states he has gained approximately 20 lbs (9.1 kg) over the past five months. His BMI is 29 kg/m². Laboratory findings include a hemoglobin A1c of 5.9% (reference range: < 5.7%), and his fasting cholesterol panel is consistent with dyslipidemia. To diagnose him with metabolic syndrome, what additional finding is necessary?

A. Abdominal circumference of 100 cm (39 inches)
B. Diagnosis of obstructive sleep apnea
C. Diastolic blood pressure of 82 mmHg
D. Being treated with amlodipine

77. A 14-year-old female presents to her pediatrician's office for an annual examination. She denies any concerns but appears withdrawn. She states school is "going okay." When asked about diet, she says she hardly eats because she is "fat and ugly." Physical examination reveals a BMI of 17 kg/m², with a global cachectic appearance. Which of the following is most associated with her underlying condition?

A. Tachycardia
B. Urinary phosphate wasting
C. Increased osteoblast activity
D. Decreased luteinizing hormone
E. Respiratory alkalosis

78. A 4-year-old child experiences a decline in BMI during the first few years of life, reaching a minimum point. However, instead of a gradual increase in BMI typical for this age, there is an early onset of BMI increase before the age of 5. This phenomenon places the patient at risk for an

A. early growth spurt
B. adiposity nadir shift
C. early adiposity rebound
D. accelerated BMI normalization

79. A 22-year-old female presents to the emergency department with persistent nausea, vomiting, and lack of nutrition for the past week since her discharge from the hospital after undergoing a Roux-en-Y gastric bypass. She has skin tenting and dry mucous membranes. Which of the following physical exam findings is most likely to be present?

A. Night blindness
B. Positive Romberg sign
C. Jaundice
D. Nystagmus

80. A 13-year-old male presents to urgent care with hip and knee pain. His weight is in the 95th percentile and his height is in the 80th percentile. He takes no multivitamins and avoids meat. Imaging is completed, as shown below.

Which of the following is the most appropriate recommendation at this time?

    A. Encourage increased vitamin D supplementation
    B. Urgent surgical evaluation
    C. Discuss weight loss options
    D. Rest, ice, compression, and elevation
    E. Endocrinopathy testing

81. A researcher is planning to initiate a study evaluating the effectiveness of four different dietary plans compared to an unrestricted eating plan. There are 100 volunteers that will be split into each of the five study arms and will be followed for six months. Prior to being placed into their groups, the dietician overseeing the study discusses her personal success with intermittent fasting. Which research bias is being demonstrated?

    A. Measurement bias
    B. Recall bias
    C. Response bias
    D. Sampling bias
    E. Observer bias

82. A sports medicine physician is working with athletes to optimize their performance. He has them undergo testing to determine the VO_2 maximum, in order to calculate their cardiorespiratory fitness level. Which of the following statements is most accurate regarding VO_2 max?

A. VO_2 max increases with age
B. Professional athletes have low levels of VO_2 max
C. Decreasing body fat percentage improves VO_2 max
D. VO_2 max is similar among genders

83. A 34-year-old male presents to the clinic after attending a bariatric seminar. He is interested in weight loss surgery. He takes amlodipine for hypertension and is adherent with continuous positive airway pressure (CPAP) for his obstructive sleep apnea. He denies any tobacco or alcohol history. Which of the following would be the most appropriate initial screening test for metabolic-associated fatty liver disease at this time?

A. History
B. Physical exam findings
C. Laboratory work
D. Right upper quadrant ultrasound
E. Liver biopsy

84. A 22-year-old male is frustrated by his recent diagnosis of "overweight," which was made at an insurance screening exam. He weight-lifts for 3-4 hours daily and competes at the state and national level for body-building. Prior testing reveals an 18% body fat composition. What other condition would act similarly to this patient in terms of an increased BMI with a discordant obesity-related risk association?

A. Congestive heart failure
B. Increased age
C. Southeast Asian ethnicity
D. Sarcopenia
E. Osteoporosis

85. A 63-year-old female presents to her primary care physician's office for follow-up after starting methotrexate with complaints of a sore tongue and irritability. She was diagnosed with polymyalgia rheumatica two years ago and was placed on 15 mg of prednisone daily. However, she had gained nearly 60 lbs (27.2 kg) while on prednisone. Eight months ago, she was transitioned to methotrexate for glucocorticoid-sparing therapy. Her BMI is 35 kg/m². Which of the following is most responsible for her current condition?

A. Vitamin B_1
B. Vitamin B_2
C. Vitamin B_3
D. Vitamin B_9
E. Vitamin B_{12}

86. A 14-year-old male presents to his family practice physician for his annual physical examination. He is in the 105th percentile for weight and the 65th percentile for height. His upper arm circumference is 37 cm. Which of the following would likely cause an inaccurately elevated systolic blood pressure?

A. Using a large adult-sized cuff (16x36 cm)
B. Sitting in a chair with back support
C. Having the patient rest his arm by his side
D. Telling the patient not to talk during inflation
E. Deflating the cuff at 5-10 mmHg per second

87. A 44-year-old female presents to the office with concerns about weight gain. She rarely eats breakfast but instead eats from the time she gets home from work until bedtime. She occasionally awakens and consumes calories at night. The only medication she takes is zolpidem for insomnia. Which of the following questions would be most helpful to determine if the nocturnal caloric intake is caused by zolpidem versus night eating syndrome?

A. Are you aware during your nocturnal eating episodes?
B. What is the dose of your zolpidem?
C. Do you have a prior history of sleep walking?
D. Do you take any other over-the-counter medications?
E. Are you drowsy in the mornings after taking zolpidem?

88. A university hospital is working with the Centers for Medicare and Medicaid Services (CMS) regarding billing and repayments. The current system allows for an increased hospital length of stay based on body mass index alone. The new proposal is to establish repayments and recommended appropriate length of stay on obesity-related comorbidities and functional limitations. Which of the following would be the best categorization method to initiate?

A. New York Heart Association Classification
B. Edmonton Obesity Staging System
C. Epworth Sleepiness Score
D. World Health Organization Obesity Classification
E. King's Obesity Staging Criteria

89. A physician is discussing the different terminology used in body composition to a rotating internal medicine resident. She describes a term that encompasses muscles, organs, water, bones, ligaments, tendons, and essential fat, but does not include nonessential adipose tissue. Which of the following terms is she most likely describing?

A. Fat mass
B. Fat-free mass
C. Lean body mass
D. Total body mass
E. Percent body fat

90. A 21-year-old female with class II obesity presents to urgent care for periodic headaches and recent vision changes. She states that the vision changes have started to interfere with her collegiate studies. Physical exam shows the following findings on fundoscopic examination. What is the next best step in management for this patient?

A. Request an ophthalmology referral
B. Order a lumbar puncture
C. Initiate therapy with topiramate
D. Order brain imaging
E. Discuss weight loss medications

91. A 7-year-old female presents to her pediatrician for a follow-up regarding her blood pressure. On three separate office visits, her blood pressure has averaged in the 90th percentile. She has occasional headaches after reading for long periods of time but otherwise has no complaints. She is performing well at school. Which of the following blood pressure categories for her age does this fall into?

A. Normal
B. Elevated blood pressure
C. Stage 1 hypertension
D. Stage 2 hypertension
E. Hypertensive urgency

92. A 37-year-old mother of two presents to her primary care physician's office for follow-up after recently being diagnosed with binge-eating disorder (BED). She has started cognitive behavioral therapy and has noticed improvements. She states that upon researching BED, she has seen a lot of the same tendencies and characteristics of her condition in her 11-year-old daughter. Her daughter is scheduled to meet with her pediatrician and will likely be diagnosed with which of the following?

A. Grazing
B. Anorexia nervosa
C. Loss of control eating disorder
D. Night eating syndrome
E. Bulimia nervosa

93. A patient is discussing a news story that was heard earlier in the day with a physician. The report stated patients who have a BMI ≥ 25 kg/m^2 have a longer life expectancy than those with a BMI < 25 kg/m^2. The patient now questions the utility of obtaining a BMI at each visit. Which is a true statement regarding the correlation between BMI and obesity-related comorbidities?

A. A BMI of 35 kg/m^2 decreases life expectancy the same as smoking
B. BMI is the best indicator of cardiovascular disease
C. 50% of those with type 2 diabetes have a BMI ≥ 25 kg/m^2
D. A 5-unit increase in BMI increases ischemic stroke risk by 20%

94. A 3-year-old female is referred to a geneticist for evaluation after persistent milestone delays and a recent seizure. The child appears very happy, smiling and laughing frequently during the examination. Her movements are spastic and she is only able to pull herself up to a seated position and stand with assistance. She does not talk and only babbles intermittently. What would the genetic workup most likely reveal?

A. Angelman syndrome
B. Turner syndrome
C. Borjeson-Forssman-Lehmann syndrome
D. Albright hereditary osteodystrophy
E. Fragile-X syndrome

95. A 68-year-old female with a history of type 2 diabetes presents to the clinic following a bariatric seminar. Although she understands there is no definitive age limit to surgery, she elects to undergo medical management. Her current diabetic medication regimen includes a maximum dose of metformin. Her hemoglobin A1c is 9.6%. The risks and benefits of a daily FDA-approved injectable, anti-obesity medication for long-term use is discussed. What medical history would be necessary for the physician to inquire about before starting this medication?

A. Papillary thyroid carcinoma
B. Suicidal ideation
C. History of cholelithiasis
D. Diabetic gastroparesis

96. An 11-year-old male presents to his pediatrician with right lower extremity pain. He states the pain has worsened over the past month, describing it as a dull ache. There was no preceding trauma. His mother brought him in after she noticed him walking with a limp. His BMI is in the 120th percentile for his age and gender. Physical examination reveals limited internal rotation of his right hip and an antalgic gait. Which of the following is most likely the culprit of his presenting condition?

A. Blount disease
B. Slipped capital femoral epiphysis
C. Osgood-Schlatter disease
D. Legg-Calve-Perthes disease
E. Aseptic necrosis

97. A mother of three children presents to her family practitioner for well-child examinations. Two of the children have been diagnosed with obesity. The mother has not followed up with the dietician as recommended, and the children are still consuming high-caloric density packaged food. Which of the following would be the most appropriate question to ask now?

A. Do you run out of food towards the end of the month?
B. Is your transportation adequate for making appointments?
C. Do you feel like you are suited to take care of your children?
D. What sweets could be eliminated from your children's diets?
E. How can we incorporate physical activity?

98. An 11-year-old male is presenting for a well-child check with his growth chart below. What is the most accurate criteria this patient met on their first documented visit?

A. Overweight
B. Obesity
C. Obesity class I
D. Obesity class II
E. Obesity class III

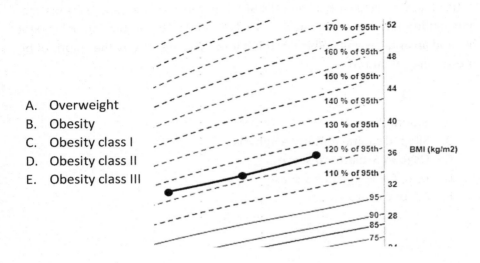

99. A 14-year-old male is being evaluated for excess weight at a family medicine visit. After undergoing a comprehensive physical examination with appropriate testing, he is diagnosed with metabolic syndrome. Which of the following diagnostic criteria is most likely present in this patient?

A. Diagnosis of obstructive sleep apnea
B. Low HDL levels
C. Treatment of hypercholesterolemia
D. Left ventricular hypertrophy
E. Family history of coronary artery disease

100. A 27-year-old female was recently diagnosed with polycystic ovarian syndrome after a workup for infertility. The patient is educated on complications and the physiology of this condition. Her chief concern is the development of diabetes, which her mother has. Which is the best test to determine early insulin intolerance in this patient?

A. Hemoglobin A1c
B. Fasting glucose level
C. Oral glucose tolerance test
D. Homeostasis model assessment of insulin resistance

101. A 30-year-old male is being seen in an obesity medicine clinic with a nutritionist who wants to determine his basal metabolic rate. The clinic has no access to indirect calorimetry. He weighs 100 kg and is 5' 11" (180 cm). Which of the following is closest to his resting metabolic rate utilizing the Mifflin – St. Jeor formula?

A. 1600
B. 1800
C. 2000
D. 2200

102. A 25-year-old male presents to his primary care physician's office with the complaint of weight gain. Over the past two years, he has gained nearly 35 lbs (15.9 kg). He states that he first noticed the weight gain once he began to work the night shift. He says he still exercises 30 minutes daily before work but does admit to increased hunger and snacking throughout his shift. Compared to 4 years ago, which of the following would most likely be observed in the patient at this visit?

A. Decreased orexin
B. Increased cortisol
C. Suppressed ghrelin
D. Increased melatonin
E. Increased adiponectin

103. A 31-year-old male presents as a 2-week follow-up to his weight management clinic. Since being seen previously, he has decreased his soda consumption and has reduced the number of times he eats fast food from three times weekly to once. Also, he has started to briskly walk around his neighborhood for approximately 30 minutes three times weekly. He has lost 4 lbs (1.8 kg) since his last appointment. According to current minimum recommendations, what goal should be set regarding his 30-minute exercise sessions?

A. Increase to daily sessions
B. Increase to 5 sessions weekly
C. Change from walking to jogging
D. Set a goal in terms of miles, not minutes
E. No changes necessary

104. A 16-year-old female presents to her family practitioner at the request of her mother after being found to be self-inducing vomiting. The patient states this is something she has done for the past few months, often after she eats more than she intends to, saying it helps with the guilt. She is active in sports, has several close friends, and is getting good grades. Given the underlying diagnosis, which abnormality is most likely to develop in this patient if left untreated?

A. Anion gap metabolic acidosis
B. Shortened corrected QT interval
C. Mallory-Weiss tear
D. Melanosis coli
E. Keratoconjunctivitis sicca

105. A 26-year-old female is presenting to her family practitioner for an infertility evaluation. She states that although she has unprotected sex approximately three times weekly, she has not become pregnant for the past two years. She says she averages one heavy menstrual cycle every three months. Her BMI is 34 kg/m². Physical examination reveals facial hair stubble. Pelvic examination is unremarkable; however, clitoromegaly is noted. An ovarian ultrasound is unrevealing. Given these findings, which lab test would most likely be present?

A. Increased luteinizing hormone
B. Decreased free thyroxine levels
C. Decreased androgen levels
D. Elevated cortisol levels
E. Elevated vitamin D (25-OH) levels

106. A 45-year-old female presents to her internist with concerns of bleeding within her mouth. She states that she has been utterly frustrated with her weight and has decided to go on an "extreme diet" for the past three months. She has been consuming water and only small amounts of protein and carbohydrates. She lost nearly 45 lbs (20.4 kg) during this time. A physical exam shows dried blood on her gums and spiral hair on her arms. Given her most likely deficiency, which of the following is a potential complication?

A. Peripheral neuropathy
B. Hallucinations
C. High-output cardiac failure
D. Dermatitis
E. Poor wound healing

107. A 63-year-old female presents to her primary care office for a routine evaluation. Her lab results reveal a TSH level of 11.1 mU/L (reference range: 0.4-4.5 mU/L) with a normal T$_4$ level. She had similar lab values two months prior, completed for insurance screening purposes. She feels well overall and denies fatigue, constipation, or cold intolerance. Which of the following would be the next best step?

A. Start levothyroxine if the patient begins having symptoms
B. Order thyroid peroxidase antibodies
C. Initiate weight-based synthetic thyroxine replacement
D. Repeat TSH, T$_3$, and T$_4$ levels in 3 months
E. Discuss desiccated thyroid replacement therapy

108. A 15-year-old male is presenting to a dietician to discuss healthy eating patterns. To get a better idea of what foods the patient is consuming, she had him fill out a 5-day food record prior to this appointment. She noticed more intake of fruits and vegetables on the food record than what the primary care physician had documented. What is the most likely cause of this discrepancy?

A. Altered eating behaviors
B. Fraudulent reporting of intake
C. Memory recall bias
D. Tracking weekdays only
E. Parental tracking inaccuracies

109. An 8-year-old male with class I obesity is brought into the clinic by his mother for snoring and "holding his breath" in the middle of the night. Upon examination, significant tonsillar hypertrophy is present, however, the mother is resistant to surgery. A sleep study confirms obstructive sleep apnea, and a continuous positive airway pressure machine is prescribed, which the patient does not tolerate and refuses to wear. Which morning lab abnormalities may be seen in this patient?

A. Decreased bicarbonate
B. Elevated pH level
C. Polycythemia
D. Hyponatremia
E. Elevated liver enzymes

110. A 27-year-old male presents to a new primary care physician's office for evaluation of fatigue. He has not been seen by a physician "since high school," as he has felt well and has not been seriously ill. He denies alcohol or tobacco use and states that he tries to avoid fast food. Vital signs are within normal limits, besides a BMI of 28 kg/m². Physical examination reveals hyperpigmented skin in his axillary folds and the nape of his neck. Other physical exam findings are unremarkable. A cholesterol panel reveals total cholesterol to be 220 mg/dL (reference range < 200 mg/dL) and HbA1c of 6.0% (reference range: < 5.7%). What other physical examination finding is most likely present?

    A. Xanthoma
    B. Easy bruising
    C. Acrochordons
    D. Dry skin
    E. Corkscrew hairs

111. A mother brings her child to the pediatrician for his 18-month well-child exam. He has met all of his age-appropriate milestones, including starting to walk at 12 months old. She states that he has gained more "rolls" in the arms and legs and seems to be gaining weight faster than she recalls of her other children. Which would be the most accurate way to track this patient's weight parameters?

    A. Weight-for-height
    B. Body mass index
    C. Age-adjusted growth
    D. Weight-for-length
    E. CDC growth charts

112. A 46-year-old male with a BMI of 38 kg/m^2 presents for follow-up regarding his diabetes. He is being treated with metformin and empagliflozin; his last HbA1c was 6.8%. He has mild knee pain with prolonged exercise but otherwise feels well. According to the Edmonton Obesity Staging System, he would be classified as which of the following?

A. Stage 0
B. Stage 1
C. Stage 2
D. Stage 3
E. Stage 4

113. A 21-year-old male with a past medical history of depression and obesity presents to a dietician for a nutrition evaluation. He states that he has overeaten at night for as long as he can remember. He admits to craving sweets and even sometimes wakes up throughout the night to get a snack. Given his most likely underlying diagnosis, which of the following findings is likely to be seen in this patient?

A. Daytime fatigue
B. Excessive daily protein intake
C. Pica
D. Frequent daytime grazing
E. Morning anorexia

114. An electrophysiology study is being performed, which evaluates the resting metabolic rate of individual organs in an average person without excess body weight. A radiotracer is injected into a patient who is lying still, and a subsequent body scan is performed. The tissue with the highest metabolic rate displays the brightest on body scan imaging, with quantitative data extrapolated. Based on this scan, which tissue would most likely display the brightest on imaging?

A. Kidneys
B. Heart
C. Digestive system
D. Liver
E. Fat

115. A 33-year-old male presents to his family practice physician at his wife's request for "sleep-eating." He states that his wife has caught him multiple times in the middle of the night eating large amounts of food before returning to bed. He has no recollection of this in the morning but has noticed that he has consistently gained weight despite a relatively healthy diet and exercise. He does admit to working rotating shifts. Given this history, which medication is this patient most likely taking?

A. Diphenhydramine
B. Eszopiclone
C. Ramelteon
D. Trazodone
E. Ginkgo biloba

116. A 51-year-old female is undergoing a preoperative evaluation for a planned Roux-en-Y gastric bypass. She admits to often feeling tired during the day and occasionally falling asleep during conversations. Her spouse has told her that she snores very loudly, sometimes requiring him to sleep in another bedroom. Vital signs are within normal limits. BMI is 39 kg/m^2, and her neck circumference is 17 inches (43.2 cm). What is the next best step in evaluating for obstructive sleep apnea?

    A. Inquire if she has stopped breathing during sleep
    B. Place a referral for an overnight pulse-oximetry test
    C. Place a referral for polysomnography
    D. Perform a physical exam, focusing on the oral exam
    E. Order a daytime arterial blood gas

117. A 17-year-old female presents to her family medicine doctor for a sports physical. She has no prior medical history, although she feels more fatigued than usual. Vital signs reveal a heart rate of 60 BPM and a BMI of 22 kg/m^2. A physical exam reveals parotid gland enlargement and scrapes over the dorsum of her second metacarpal phalangeal joint. She is elusive when asked questions about her eating habits. Which medication is contraindicated given her underlying diagnosis?

    A. Trazodone
    B. Bupropion
    C. Topiramate
    D. Sertraline
    E. Buspirone

118. A 29-year-old male presents to an internist to establish care. His chief concern is related to his lack of upper body strength, in particular the muscle size. He states despite working out his arms for nearly 3 hours daily, his arms still appear smaller than he would like. He has difficulty focusing on his work as a car salesman, as he feels people notice his arms and admits to being very self-conscious. A physical exam reveals a healthy, muscular-appearing male in no distress. If inquired, the patient most likely would admit to experiencing which of the following?

A. Compulsive behaviors
B. Anxiety attacks
C. Severe calorie restriction
D. Nocturnal eating
E. Delayed sleep onset

119. A university is conducting a research study. The primary objective is to correlate quantitative sex hormone binding globulin (SHBG) levels with different patient characteristics. In particular, age, weight, and comorbid conditions such as polycystic ovarian syndrome (PCOS) are analyzed. Which of the following patients would have an increased SHBG level compared to their comparative matched cohort?

A. A patient with a BMI of 45 kg/m^2
B. A female with a diagnosis of PCOS
C. A younger individual
D. A male with decreased total testosterone
E. A patient six months status post gastric bypass

120. A pediatrician is evaluating a young patient in the office and determines that the growth charts utilized for most children in her practice is inadequate for this patient, and a specialized chart is utilized. Which of the following physical exam findings does the patient most likely have?

    A. Bicuspid aorta
    B. Macrocephaly
    C. Macroglossia
    D. Ovarian agenesis
    E. Upslanting palpebral fissures

121. A 41-year-old Caucasian male presents to his primary care physician for an annual health screen. His immunizations are up to date. A recent diabetes and hypertension screening completed through work was within normal limits. His height is 70 inches (178 cm), and his weight is 260 lbs (117 kg). By utilizing the chart below, his weight would best be described as being in which of the following categories?

BMI	28	29	30	31	32	33	34	35	36	37	38	39	40	41	42	43	44	45	46
5'4"	163	169	174	180	186	192	197	204	209	215	221	227	232	238	244	250	256	262	267
5'5"	168	174	180	186	192	198	204	210	216	222	228	234	240	246	252	258	264	270	276
5'6"	173	179	186	192	198	204	210	216	223	229	235	241	247	253	260	266	272	278	284
5'7"	178	185	191	198	204	211	217	223	230	236	242	249	255	261	268	274	280	287	293
5'8"	184	190	197	203	210	216	223	230	236	243	249	256	262	269	276	282	289	295	302
5'9"	189	196	203	209	216	223	230	236	243	250	257	263	270	277	284	291	297	304	311
5'10"	195	202	209	216	222	229	236	243	250	257	264	271	278	285	292	299	306	313	320
5'11"	200	208	215	222	229	236	243	250	257	265	272	279	286	293	301	308	315	322	329

(Note: Weight is in pounds)

    A. Normal weight
    B. Overweight
    C. Class I obesity
    D. Class II obesity
    E. Class III obesity

122. A 49-year-old female with a history of severe obesity is following-up with her pulmonologist regarding her pulmonary hypertension, confirmed with a right-heart catheterization. She has no prior tobacco or occupational exposures, and her polysomnography test was negative. Given this information, which of the following would most likely be seen in this patient?

A. Class 4 Mallampati score
B. Increased Epworth sleepiness scale
C. FVC/FEV$_1$ < 0.70
D. Increased respiratory disturbance index
E. Arterial blood gas PaCO$_2$ > 45 mmHg

123. A mother brings her previously healthy 10-year-old daughter to her family medicine physician for an annual examination. The patient has been spending more time on the computer and watching television, with decreased physical activity. Her weight has steadily increased. Her body mass index is in the 86th percentile for age and gender. The patient denies any symptoms or concerns. Which test should be ordered for evaluation purposes?

A. Fasting lipid profile
B. Aspartate aminotransferase
C. Fasting glucose
D. Creatinine
E. Thyroid-stimulating hormone

124. After injuring his finger, a 6-year-old male with class III obesity presents to the emergency department. The mother states that the child was trying to swing at a local park when his finger became stuck in the chain. The patient has full range of motion but increased swelling of his third digit. An x-ray is shown below. Which other finding is most likely?

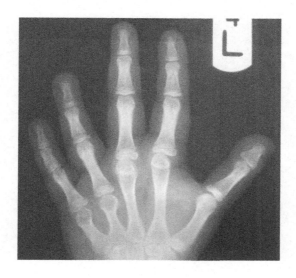

A. Pseudohypoparathyroidism
B. History of seizures
C. Almond-shaped eyes
D. Microorchidism

125. A 34-year-old female presents to her obstetrician for preconception counseling. She is wanting to become pregnant within the next year and wants to know how much weight gain would be appropriate during pregnancy. Her BMI is 31 kg/m². What is the most appropriate answer to her question?

A. Maintain current weight
B. 11-20 lbs
C. 15-25 lbs
D. 25-35 lbs
E. 28-40 lbs

III. Treatment

126. A 7-year-old female and her parents meet with the pediatrician to initiate discussions on treatment options for obesity. The family has tried numerous strategies at home without significant success and is now seeking guidance. Which of the following intensive behavioral lifestyle treatments is most likely to provide the most success?

A. Providing 30 hours of treatment over a 6-month time frame
B. Utilizing motivational interviewing focused on patient motivation
C. Encouraging an intense after-school basketball program
D. Initiate pharmacotherapy and follow up in 6 months

127. A 39-year-old male presents to the hospital with fatigue and decreased urine output. His past medical history includes obesity class II and prediabetes for which he is on metformin. His New Year's resolution was to lose 25 lbs (11.3 kg) prompting him to initiate high-intensity physical activity. In addition, his physician started him on an anti-obesity medication. During a recent workout, he twisted his ankle and has been taking multiple ibuprofen and naproxen to help with the pain. Recent labs display a creatinine of 2.1 mg/dL (reference range: 0.6–1.2 mg/dL) and a lactate level of 7.1 mmol/L (reference range: 0.5 to 2.2 mmol/L) with an increased anion gap. Which of the following medications was most likely initiated at his recent appointment?

A. Liraglutide
B. Bupropion
C. Orlistat
D. Topiramate
E. Semaglutide

128. A 44-year-old female presents to her primary care physician with dysuria and malodorous urine. She denies abdominal pain. She has type 2 diabetes and was recently started on dapagliflozin to help with weight loss and diabetes control. In addition, she initiated a new diet this week. Her urinalysis dipstick results are below. Given these findings, the diet she has started most likely encourages which of the following components?

Leukocyte	1+	Specific gravity	1.011
Nitrite	2+	Ketone	2+
Protein	Trace	Bilirubin	Not detected
Blood	1+	Glucose	3+

A. Significant carbohydrate restriction
B. Avoiding foods with a glycemic index > 70
C. Increasing omega-3 intake with extra virgin vegetable oil
D. Limiting fat intake to 20-25% of daily calories
E. Intake a minimum of 5 servings of fruit daily

129. A 14-year-old male presents for his annual checkup at his pediatrician's clinic. He has no prior medical history. His BMI is 31 kg/m^2. The pediatrician discusses healthy eating choices, exercise, and lifestyle changes to prevent weight-related complications. This discussion is an example of which of the following phases of prevention in chronic obesity?

A. Primary prevention
B. Secondary prevention
C. Tertiary prevention

130. A patient had a previous bariatric procedure performed ten years ago in which a band was placed around the top of the stomach, creating a small pouch. Although adjustable, the patient has had difficulty following up and thus is interested in a surgical revision. The patient has had three adjustments during the past decade, initially losing 32 lbs (14.5 kg), but has since regained this weight. Which is true of this bariatric procedure?

A. It is considered a malabsorptive procedure
B. The minimum BMI required for placement is 30 kg/m^2
C. The mortality rate is similar to other bariatric procedures
D. Adjustment requires conscious sedation
E. It is the most common weight loss procedure worldwide

131. A healthy 6-year-old female presents to her primary care physician with her father for an annual exam. She has no prior medical conditions and is up to date on immunizations. Her father has no concerns about her current health but is concerned about preventing weight gain, as her sibling has excess weight. The patient's BMI is in the 50th percentile, with consistent height and weight in the 55th and 60th percentile, respectively. Which of the following is the most appropriate recommendation for this child?

A. Consume 3 or more fruits and vegetables daily
B. Minimize screen time to < 3 hours daily
C. Allow the child to self-regulate meals
D. Encourage at least 8 hours of sleep nightly
E. Eat as a family at least 3 times weekly

132. A 53-year-old male is presenting for evaluation for weight loss. He has started the bridge-to-transplant program, which requires a BMI of 35 kg/m² or less in order to be listed on the kidney transplant list. His current BMI is 44 kg/m². Both medication and surgical options are discussed. He prefers to undergo bariatric and metabolic surgery. Which of the following surgical options is most preferred?

A. Single anastomosis duodeno-ileal bypass
B. Roux-en-Y gastric bypass
C. Vertical sleeve gastrectomy
D. Gastric balloon
E. Adjustable gastric band

133. A mother presents to her pediatrician with her breastfed 6-month-old daughter to discuss healthy habits to initiate over the next year. The mother is concerned given the family history of obesity that her child will gain excess weight. What recommendations should be given to the parents over the next year?

A. Limit television to less than 1 hour daily
B. Reward good behavior with healthy foods
C. Stop breastfeeding and transition to solid food now
D. Allow the child to feed themselves complementary foods
E. Ensure the child finishes food/milk during each feeding

134. A mother brings her 6-year-old daughter, who is in the 95th percentile for weight, to her pediatrician's office due to persistent constipation despite increased water intake. They have been using over-the-counter stool softeners without relief. The mother states that the child is not picky regarding food and eats "whatever is available." The physician recommends increasing whole grains. What effect will this indirectly have on the child?

A. Reduces HDL and triglyceride levels
B. Increases risk of irritable bowel syndrome
C. Increases nutrient-rich food intake
D. Increases saturated fat consumption
E. Cause diarrhea and potential fecal incontinence

135. A 57-year-old male presents to the emergency department two weeks after a Roux-en-Y gastric bypass for dehydration, nausea, and vomiting. His spouse has also noted some confusion recently. Vital signs reveal a heart rate of 110/min and a blood pressure of 89/58 mmHg. Physical exam reveals dry mucus membranes, nystagmus, and difficulty walking. He is alert but oriented to person only. Given his most likely nutritional deficiency, what other clinical sequelae may be seen if left untreated?

A. Macrocytic anemia
B. Dermatitis (pellagra)
C. Seizure disorder
D. Glossitis and cheilitis
E. Peripheral neuropathy

136. A 59-year-old male presents to his internist with the desire to start anti-obesity pharmacotherapy. The physician is interested in starting a particular combination medication but first inquires about a history of calcium phosphate stones, as this medication should be avoided in those with a history of renal nephrolithiasis. Given the most likely medication eluded to, what is a contraindication of this medicine?

    A.   Chronic malabsorption syndrome
    B.   Family history of medullary thyroid cancer
    C.   Concurrent history of glaucoma
    D.   History of epilepsy or risk of seizures
    E.   Uncontrolled hypertension

137. A 36-year-old female with diabetes mellitus type 2 presents to her primary care physician's clinic for a bariatric surgery evaluation. Her diabetes has been poorly controlled despite being on metformin, semaglutide, empagliflozin, and high-dose insulin. She exercises 250 minutes weekly and has been on a low glycemic index dietary plan for the past nine months. Despite this, her hemoglobin A1c is 8.9% (reference range: 4.2-5.7%). Her body mass index is 32 kg/m^2. Regarding her bariatric surgery eligibility question, would she be a good candidate?

    A.   No: Her body mass index is not in an appropriate range
    B.   No: She only has one obesity-related comorbidity
    C.   No: She should pursue an insulin pump instead
    D.   Yes: Her diabetes is difficult to control
    E.   Yes: She meets the criteria for Roux-en-Y gastric bypass only

138. A 52-year-old male presents to his primary care physician with concerns of decreased libido. He states he has no current sexual desire, and does not wake up with a morning erection. Physical exam reveals small testicles, gynecomastia, and a BMI of 52 kg/m². Morning testosterone levels are low on two occasions, while a prostate-specific antigen is within normal limits. What effect would starting testosterone likely have in this patient?

A. Increase HbA1c
B. Decrease fertility
C. Increase weight
D. Worsening lipid panel
E. Increasing blood pressure

139. A 47-year-old male with end-stage renal disease is presenting to his primary care physician's office with the desire to lose weight. To be considered for a renal transplant, he must lose an additional 22 lbs (10 kg). Although he has incorporated lifestyle modifications, he has failed to meet his weight loss goals. He is interested in bariatric medications. Which of the following would be the most appropriate medication to prescribe?

A. Phentermine/topiramate ER
B. Naltrexone/bupropion ER
C. Liraglutide
D. Phentermine monotherapy
E. Metformin

140. A patient presents to her internist with concerns about supplements she has been taking. She was started on L-carnitine and green tea extract at the recommendation of an herbalist. However, since starting, she has noticed increased anxiety, palpitations, and a slight tremor. Both of these supplements theoretically work by which mechanism?

A. Energy expenditure
B. Satiety
C. Carbohydrate metabolism
D. Blocking fat absorption
E. Increase fat oxidation

141. A 52-year-old female has presented for a follow-up visit to the obesity clinic. A rotating resident is interviewing the patient and is asking questions such as "What weight-loss techniques have worked for you in the past?" and "So, swimming was an exercise you could do long-term?" After further discussions, the resident expresses hope stating, "It sounds like you are ready to pursue and maintain weight loss." He summarizes the visit, and the patient leaves the office. Which skill did this resident utilize?

A. OARS
B. FRAMES
C. SMART goals
D. RULE

142. An obesity medicine specialist is working with an internal medicine resident and discusses ways to improve surgical outcomes in those undergoing metabolic and bariatric surgery, including decreased hospitalization and recovery times. Which of the following should routinely be performed to improve outcomes?

A. Preoperative carbohydrate loading
B. Intraoperative low-molecular-weight heparin
C. Nasogastric nutritional supplementation
D. Intraoperative high ventilator tidal volumes
E. Postoperative intravenous opioid administration

143. A surgeon consults an obesity medicine specialist after a 39-year-old female develops a provoked lower extremity deep venous thrombosis (DVT) extending to the femoral artery on post-operative day three from a Roux-en-Y gastric bypass. Post-op complications included persistent nausea and vomiting, which have now subsided. The surgeon requests assistance with anticoagulation therapy. What is the most appropriate recommendation to provide?

A. Initiate rivaroxaban and check anti-Xa levels in 3 days
B. Bridge anticoagulation with fondaparinux and warfarin
C. Start an unfractionated heparin drip and place an IVC filter
D. Consult vascular surgery for mechanical thrombectomy
E. Discharge patient with weight-based enoxaparin

144. A recently published study has shown weight-loss success and diabetes improvement with a subcutaneous injectable medication undergoing continued clinical testing. The medication contains GLP-1 and another hormone that is endogenously secreted by the pancreatic beta-islet cells. This dual medication has been shown to have more significant effects on weight than with a GLP-1 alone. The described medication combined with a GLP-1 is

    A. gastric inhibitory peptide
    B. oxyntomodulin
    C. glucagon
    D. amylin
    E. peptide YY

145. A 44-year-old female with a history of ovarian cancer recently completed chemotherapy. During cancer treatment, she lost substantial weight and currently has a BMI of 20 kg/m². She states she does not have a significant appetite and must force herself to remember to drink protein shakes, although she has no nausea. Her diabetes mellitus type 2 initially had improved with the unintended weight loss and she quit all of her medications during treatment. Her most recent hemoglobin A1c is 7.4% (reference range: ≤5.7%). Which is the most appropriate medication to initiate at this time?

    A. Semaglutide
    B. Sitagliptin
    C. Tirzepatide
    D. Insulin
    E. Dapagliflozin

146. A 26-year-old male is presenting for psychiatric evaluation as part of a multi-disciplinary team approach before bariatric surgery. He admits that he eats until he feels uncomfortably full, even eating large amounts when he doesn't feel hungry. This is something that has caused significant guilt and depression. He eats much more over a short period compared to his friends. He states it feels "like I lose control when food is around." Which of the following classes of medications is FDA-approved to treat his underlying condition?

A. Central nervous system stimulant
B. Anticonvulsant
C. Atypical antipsychotic
D. Selective serotonin neuromodulator
E. Glucagon-like peptide analog

147. A 14-year-old male presents for a sports physical for the upcoming football season. He has always been at the 95th-100th percentile of his weight compared to his peers. His weight today is 204 lbs (92.5 kg). He has unhealthy eating habits and consumes multiple sodas daily. The concern about his weight is discussed, including the health risks. He seems perplexed by this, as he feels he is at a good weight for football. After further discussion, he agrees to a focused follow-up visit regarding dietary modifications. Which of the following stages of change is this patient experiencing?

A. Pre-contemplation
B. Contemplation
C. Preparation
D. Action
E. Maintenance

148. A 57-year-old business executive returns to his primary care physician for follow-up regarding his exercise prescription. Although the prescription clearly states 300 minutes of exercise weekly in the form of brisk walking, he does not have that amount of time to devote to exercise and did not fulfill his prescription. His current BMI is 31 kg/m². What would be the most appropriate modification to his exercise prescription?

A. Change to water walking
B. Increase exercise intensity
C. Change to resistance training
D. Focus on dietary components instead
E. Confront him on his priorities

149. A general surgeon is discussing one potential bariatric surgical option with a patient in which 80% of the greater curvature of the stomach is resected laparoscopically, allowing for 2-3 ounces (60-90 mL) of volume intake. Which of the following is true regarding the described procedure?

A. Dumping syndrome is a common complaint
B. It is the second most common bariatric procedure
C. The procedure does not affect hunger hormones
D. Patients are prone to experience vitamin B₁₂ deficiency
E. This surgery is most effective for treating diabetes

150. A 39-year-old female with a history of type 2 diabetes and sleep apnea is presenting to her general surgeon after undergoing a Roux-en-Y gastric bypass six months ago. She has noted a weight loss of 47 lbs (21.3 kg) and is happy with the results. She regularly meets with her dietician. Her only complaint is that after she eats certain meals, she experiences facial flushing and lightheadedness. Given the most likely etiology of these symptoms, what other associated finding is she likely to encounter?

A. Intermittent constipation
B. Excessive belching
C. Wheezing
D. Reactive hypoglycemia
E. Bacterial overgrowth

151. A rapid response is called on a 33-year-old female 12 hours after undergoing a Roux-en-Y gastric bypass. She complains of progressively worsening mid-epigastric pain with radiation to her left chest and mild dyspnea. Vital signs reveal a heart rate of 120 BPM, respirations 24/min, and oxygen saturation of 99% on room air. A portable chest x-ray shows a new left-sided pleural effusion. A complete blood count reveals a white blood cell count of 13.4 x 10^3/mcL (reference range: 4.8-10.8 x 10^3/mcL). What is the next best step in management?

A. Start empiric ceftriaxone and azithromycin
B. Order a stat CTA of the chest
C. Administer 1 mg/kg low molecular weight heparin
D. Contact the attending surgeon
E. Order an electrocardiogram

152. A 39-year-old female presents to the clinic due to nausea, vomiting, and increased fatigue over the past three weeks. Past medical history includes class II obesity, migraines, and polycystic ovarian syndrome (PCOS). She is on oral combined birth control and phentermine/topiramate ER. She has lost 19 lbs (8.6 kg) over the past four months but has recently started to regain some weight over the past month. Which of the following could have prevented the underlying cause of her symptoms?

A. Adhering to the Risk Evaluation and Mitigation Strategy program
B. Referral to a dietician to discuss a low-carbohydrate diet
C. Prophylactic ondansetron to take before anti-obesity medication
D. Cognitive behavioral therapy to prevent anxiety from phentermine
E. Adding metformin to treat the current PCOS symptoms

153. A 39-year-old male presents to the obesity clinic for a 2-month follow-up appointment. He was started on semaglutide six months ago and has maintained exercise of 200 minutes weekly. He states he feels well and plans to continue his current treatment regimen. Vital signs are within normal limits. Over the past year, he has lost 34 lbs (15.4 kg), accounting for an 8% total body weight loss. He is now at his lowest weight since being seen at the clinic. If he maintains his current regimen, what can you predict about his weight loss in the future?

A. He will continue to lose weight but at a slower pace
B. Eventually he will plateau and regain weight
C. He will lose weight until he plateaus at his ideal body weight
D. Eventually he will relapse to his previous weight

154. A 44-year-old male is being evaluated in the intensive care unit after a biliopancreatic diversion with duodenal switch. The surgery was particularly time-consuming due to anatomic variation and significant scar tissue from prior abdominal surgeries. The nurse is concerned as his urine has darkened, and the urine output has decreased to < 40 mL per hour despite adequate fluid hydration. His abdomen is soft, with no bowel sounds appreciated. Which of the following tests will most likely be abnormal?

A. Urinalysis hemoglobin
B. Renal parenchymal ultrasound
C. Renal vasculature duplex
D. Urine eosinophil count
E. Urine microscopy

155. A 62-year-old female is presenting to her primary care physician's office to discuss semaglutide (Wegovy®) for weight loss. Her medical comorbidities include diabetes type II and hypertension. She is currently taking metformin, rosuvastatin, sitagliptin, and chlorthalidone. She drinks two alcoholic beverages nightly and quit tobacco products six years ago. Which of the following is the most appropriate action before starting semaglutide?

A. Obtain baseline lipase levels
B. Discontinue one of her current medications
C. Inquire about a family history of MEN 1 syndrome
D. Require alcohol cessation due to interactions
E. Obtain triglyceride levels

156. A 42-year-old female presents with chronic diarrhea, abdominal pain, and bloating for six months. She underwent a duodenal switch approximately eight years ago and has had minimal follow-up due to losing insurance. She admits to now feeling weak and lightheaded with exertion. Laboratory examination reveals macrocytic anemia with increased folate levels. Which of the following tests is most appropriate at this time?

A. Urea breath test
B. Carbohydrate breath test
C. Stool osmolality
D. Stool cultures
E. Endoscopic evaluation

157. A 37-year-old male with type 1 diabetes presents to his primary care practitioner to discuss anti-obesity medication. In particular, he would like to start semaglutide. His last HbA1c was 7.4% (reference range: < 5.7%) and he is on 18 units of glargine nightly and dosing the aspart based on carbohydrate counting. His current BMI is 31 kg/m^2, which has increased from 27 kg/m^2 since last year. Which of the following is the most accurate statement regarding his inquiry?

A. Semaglutide is contraindicated in patients with type 1 diabetes
B. I will discuss this with your endocrinologist
C. You do not meet the criteria for anti-obesity medications
D. Tirzepatide would be a safer alternative
E. I would like to discuss intermittent fasting or a ketogenic diet today

158. A 17-year-old female with a history of binge eating disorder meets with her primary care physician to discuss techniques to assist in weight loss. She has numerous allergies and is apprehensive about pharmacotherapy. In addition, she has a meniscus injury that limits her physical activity. The physician discusses meeting with a specialist to begin a structured approach that addresses maladaptive thoughts related to eating and physical activity through systematic tracking of daily habits, thoughts, and emotions. What intervention is being discussed?

A. Cognitive behavioral therapy
B. Mindfulness-based therapy
C. Motivational interviewing
D. Psychoanalytic therapy
E. Dialectical behavioral therapy

159. A geriatrician notices that many of his patients have lost muscle mass with debility or reduced physical activity but continue to gain excess fat mass. Although some of these patients have certain conditions predisposing them to muscle wasting, including malignancy, fractures, and neurodegenerative conditions, the majority experience frailty independent of any underlying diseases. Which of the following would be an important part of the multidisciplinary treatment plan in regard to preventing sarcopenia and subsequent frailty?

A. Prescribe megestrol acetate
B. Encourage resistance training
C. Target protein intake of 0.8 g/kg/day
D. Consider testosterone supplements (males)
E. Encourage water aerobics

160. A 26-year-old female presents to the emergency department with a laceration above her right eye from a fall. She underwent a single anastomosis duodeno-ileal bypass with sleeve gastrectomy (SADI-S) six months prior and has not followed up with any providers since the surgery. She states she felt light-headed when getting up to go to the restroom and "passed-out" in the bathroom. Her skin turgor is normal. Which of the following questions will assist in preventing future similar hospital admissions?

A. Have you been drinking sufficient fluids?
B. Are you taking your daily vitamins?
C. Have you discontinued your sitagliptin post-operatively?
D. Did you have any alcohol before the fall?
E. Are you still taking blood pressure medication?

161. A 26-year-old female was recently diagnosed with polycystic ovarian syndrome (PCOS) following a workup for abnormal menstrual cycles. She has noted worsening hirsutism which is bothersome. She is sexually active and uses barrier protection intermittently. A recent pregnancy test and oral glucose tolerance test were negative. She is interested in treatment for PCOS. Which treatment is most appropriate?

A. Oral contraception
B. Metformin
C. Spironolactone
D. Intrauterine device
E. Clomiphene

162. An 8-year-old male is presenting to his family medicine provider as a new patient after moving from another state. Past medical history includes depression, migraines, and asthma. His growth chart has consistently been in the overweight category based on body mass index percentile for the past two years. He denies excess hunger but does admit to being sedentary. Which is the most appropriate intervention at this time?

A. Recheck weight in three months
B. Evaluate for weight-promoting medications
C. Initiate pharmacotherapy
D. Screen for genetic etiologies of weight gain
E. Refer for metabolic and bariatric surgery

163. A clinician is going through additional training in order to initiate treatment options for her patients with overweight and obesity. She wants to address the physical, emotional, and behavioral aspects in a personalized way by utilizing follow-up visits, motivational interviewing, and individualized treatment options. Based on this, she is most likely going to offer

A. intensive health behavioral and lifestyle treatment
B. pharmacotherapy initiation
C. comprehensive obesity treatment
D. metabolic and bariatric surgical assessments

164. A patient presents to her nutritionist to discuss an article she read on the internet. It discussed making dietary changes by adding nutrients that have potentially favorable effects beyond basic nutrition. She most likely read an article on which of the following topics?

A. Supplements
B. Over-the-counter medications
C. Functional foods
D. Prescription medications
E. Herbal remedies

165. A 28-year-old healthy male presents to his primary care physician with frustration about his inability to lose a significant amount of weight. For the past six months, he has changed to a vegan diet and exercises 30 minutes daily. Although he has lost 8 lbs (3.6 kg), he feels he should have lost more. His current BMI is 31 kg/m². After reviewing the side effects of medications, he chooses one that he feels will be a safe option. After two months, he returns with no significant weight loss. Which of the following anti-obesity medications was he most likely prescribed?

A. Phentermine/topiramate ER
B. Orlistat
C. Naltrexone/bupropion ER
D. Liraglutide

166. A 24-year-old male is discussing his concerns about blood clots after his planned sleeve gastrectomy surgery next month. His father died from a pulmonary embolism (PE) one week after undergoing a total hip arthroplasty. The patient has no history of deep venous thrombosis, and besides his father, he knows of no other family history. He denies smoking. Which of the following would be the most appropriate statement regarding venous thromboembolism (VTE) in this patient?

A. Delay VTE prophylaxis until at least 48 hours after surgery
B. Low-molecular-weight heparin 40 mg twice daily is considered standard
C. Failure to wean from ventilator support may indicate VTE
D. He should be on extended chemoprophylaxis upon discharge
E. Given his family history, an IVC filter should be discussed

167. A psychiatrist is evaluating a patient in a psychiatric hospital for a recent episode of mania. The patient has a diagnosis of bipolar type I. The patient states that she has stopped her lithium due to excessive weight gain, leading to this current episode. The patient would like to discuss alternative options that would not cause this adverse effect. Which option should be discussed with the patient?

A. Valproate
B. Sertraline
C. Divalproex
D. Gabapentin
E. Lamotrigine

168. A 48-year-old male presents for follow-up with the dietician. He has been doing research and wants to discuss some dietary plans. He has obesity class I without other obesity-related comorbidities and is currently taking no medications besides a daily multivitamin. He asks for an opinion related to frequently used dietary plans. Which of the following recommendations is most accurate?

A. Intermittent fasting allows for a time of restricted eating followed by unregulated calorie consumption
B. The Dietary Approach to Stopping Hypertension (DASH) diet plan provides significant weight loss with cardiovascular benefits
C. Low carbohydrate diets are more effective long-term for weight loss compared to low-fat dietary plans
D. Eating low-density foods increases the sensation of fullness and thus promotes weight loss in comparison to high-density foods

169. A patient is meeting with a bariatric surgeon to discuss potential surgical options. Although she has done a lot of research, she still has not committed to one surgery. She asks about the estimated number of bariatric surgeries performed, including which are popular and which are becoming obsolete. Which of the following statements is accurate regarding bariatric surgery statistics over the past ten years?

A. The number of bariatric surgeries has declined in the past five years
B. Gastric banding has persistently made up 5% of bariatric surgeries
C. Roux-en-Y gastric bypass remains the most common surgery
D. Sleeve gastrectomy surgeries have nearly doubled in number
E. Intragastric balloons have been available since 2012

170. A 29-year-old female with a past medical history of migraine headaches and pre-diabetes is presenting to a local obesity medicine clinic frustrated about her lack of weight loss. She exercises 300 minutes/week, restricts her calories to 1200 kcal/day, and takes no medications. She has been working with a weight-loss coach for the past six months. She is interested in weight-loss surgery. Her BMI is 29 kg/m², and her vital signs and physical exam are otherwise unremarkable. Which of the following would be the most appropriate action to take now?

A. Further intensify lifestyle modifications
B. Begin weight-loss pharmacotherapy
C. Referral for bariatric surgery
D. Referral for dietician
E. Provide reassurance

171. You are discussing with a patient their interest in physical activity. After asking the patient to grade their motivation in readiness to initiate a workout plan, the patient states they are at a 6 out of 10. What is the most appropriate reply to their assessment?

A. Why did you not select a number higher than that?
B. Great- it seems like you are motivated
C. Why did you not select a 3?
D. What can I do to convince you to get it to a 10?
E. It doesn't seem like you are quite ready yet

172. A patient is six months post biliopancreatic diversion with duodenal switch and has been happy with her weight loss thus far. However, she has noticed that her hair has grown slower and started to fall out. This is very concerning to her. She admits to taking one prenatal vitamin daily and following all food restrictions. Recent thyroid levels and complete metabolic panel were normal. Given these findings, what micronutrient deficiency is the most likely explanation for her symptoms?

A. Selenium
B. Zinc
C. Copper
D. Vitamin K
E. Vitamin A

173. A family practice physician sees multiple patients during her dedicated bariatric clinic session. A number of them have approached her regarding evaluation for bariatric surgery. Which of the following patients would be the best current candidate for weight-loss surgery?

A. 29-year-old male (BMI 36 kg/m^2) who is a current tobacco user with a history of hypertension and obstructive sleep apnea
B. 34-year-old female (BMI 33 kg/m^2) with a history of cervical cancer status post hysterectomy with clean margins
C. 52-year-old female (BMI 55 kg/m^2) with a history of hypertension, refusing to undergo mammography and colonoscopy
D. 60-year-old male (BMI 34 kg/m^2) with a history of osteoarthritis, hyperlipidemia, diabetes type 2, and chronic kidney disease stage 2

174. A 48-year-old female with the disease of obesity presents for a follow-up appointment regarding increased liver enzymes. She recently completed a right upper quadrant ultrasound that revealed fatty liver infiltration. She denies any significant alcohol use. Which of the following diets should be recommended to her at this time?

A. Mediterranean-style
B. DASH diet
C. Low glycemic index
D. Low fat
E. High protein

175. A 42-year-old male presents to a dietary clinic for his initial consultation. He admits that his work schedule is hectic, requiring him to travel frequently, and thus, he feels his weight gain is most likely due to his fast-food intake. He is not interested in calorie counting. His weight loss goals include losing approximately 10% of his weight within the next year, based on mostly diet changes, as he already exercises every morning. His BMI is 37 kg/m^2 and he has no prior medical history. Given these preferences, which would be the best fit regarding weight-loss management?

A. Mediterranean diet
B. Paleo diet
C. Bariatric surgery
D. Meal replacement
E. Pharmacotherapy

176. A 52-year-old male presents for follow-up at the transplant center. He was diagnosed with cirrhosis secondary to long-standing metabolic-associated fatty liver disease. He has minimal ascites and his last hospitalization was three months ago for hepatic encephalopathy. His BMI is currently 38 kg/m^2, and he must lose 25 lbs (11.3 kg) before being placed on the liver transplant list. Which of the following anti-obesity medications is contraindicated in this patient?

A. Setmelanotide
B. Naltrexone/ bupropion ER
C. Semaglutide
D. Orlistat
E. Cellulose and citric acid hydrogel

177. A patient returns to the office extremely concerned because she recently found out her grandfather had medullary thyroid carcinoma (MTC). She started on semaglutide at her prior appointment to help with weight loss. Which of the following is the best advice to provide the patient?

A. "It is fine to continue the medication, as MTC is not associated with this class of medications."
B. "The associated risk of MTC has only been shown in animal studies, not in human trials."
C. "We must monitor calcitonin levels and order a RET oncogene test while on this medication."
D. "Unfortunately, your risk of developing MTC has increased significantly, given your family history."

178. A 37-year-old male presents to discuss bariatric surgical options. He had a friend who underwent a single anastomosis duodeno-ileostomy with sleeve gastrectomy (SADI-S) and has done well. He is wondering about the benefits and risks of this procedure compared to a Roux-en-Y gastric bypass (RYGB). What is the best advice to provide?

A. The SADI-S has more anastomotic sites than the RYGB
B. The SADI-S reduces ghrelin significantly more than RYGB
C. A RYGB requires more frequent monitoring of vitamin levels
D. The RYGB leads to increased remission rates of diabetes mellitus
E. The SADI-S is done through an open abdominal procedure

179. A recently graduated advanced practice nurse is prescribing pharmacologic therapy in the clinic. Although she has received her national provider identifier (NPI) number, she currently does not have her Drug Enforcement Agency (DEA) license. Because of this limitation, which of the following medications can she prescribe?

A. Diethylpropion
B. Phentermine/topiramate ER
C. Phendimetrazine
D. Naltrexone/bupropion ER

180. A 29-year-old female affected by obesity is presenting for help with losing and maintaining weight. During discussions, the importance of losing 5-10% of her baseline weight related to her health is reiterated, specifically related to improving current medical conditions and preventing future issues. This discussion falls into which of the following categories of the "5 A's of obesity management"?

A. Ask
B. Assess
C. Advise
D. Agree
E. Arrange/assist

181. A 67-year-old male presents for lifestyle modification education after recently having a cardiac stent placed for unstable angina. In particular, he is wondering about "good fats" that his wife has talked about. Which of the following is the most accurate statement?

A. Saturated fats are unlikely to be absorbed and thus preferred
B. Trans fats should only be consumed in moderation
C. Increasing polyunsaturated fats reduces cardiac risk factors
D. Coconut oil is preferred instead of vegetable oil
E. Tilapia is a cheaper alternative to salmon with similar benefits

182. A 52-year-old female presents to the emergency room by ambulance after a witnessed seizure. The patient is not on any current medications. She underwent a successful Roux-en-Y gastric bypass nearly two years ago, with hypertension currently in remission. Her husband states she has complained of lightheadedness and fatigue 1-2 hours after meals for the past few months. However, this is the first time she has had a seizure. Point of care glucose on arrival is 23 mg/dL (reference range: 74-106 mg/dL). Which of the following daily medications may have prevented her seizure?

A. Semaglutide
B. Metformin
C. Metoprolol
D. Acarbose
E. Sitagliptin

183. Vagal nerve blockade via laparoscopically implanted electrodes (vBloc®) is being discussed with a patient. Which of the following is accurate regarding this device?

A. It is approved for adolescents
B. It produces 8-10% weight loss
C. It increases ghrelin production
D. It is contraindicated in those on dialysis
E. It is approved for short-term use only

184. A 50-year-old male has initiated an aerobic training program in preparation for running a half marathon the following year. He would like help determining his target heart rate for high-intensity exercise. He has no prior cardiac history and is asymptomatic. Which recommended heart rate is most appropriate to target?

    A. 115-135 beats per minute
    B. 135-155 beats per minute
    C. 155-175 beats per minute
    D. 175-195 beats per minute

185. A 36-year-old male presents to urgent care with complaints of fatigue, weakness, and numbness in his lower extremities. He underwent a Roux-en-Y gastric bypass 9 years ago but has not had follow-up for the past 5 years. He is taking cyanocobalamin sublingual tabs and calcium. He has a positive Romberg test with diminished vibratory sensations and 4/5 muscle strength in all extremities. Lab work is shown below:

Test	Patient's Value	Reference Range
Hemoglobin	9.4 g/dL	13.5–17.5 g/dL
White blood cells	3100/mm^3	4500–11,000/mm^3
Platelet	200,000/mm^3	150,000–400,000/mm^3
MCV	116 μm^3	80–100 μm^3
LDH	175 U/L	100-280 U/L

Which of the following is the most likely deficiency leading to his findings?

    A. Iron
    B. Copper
    C. Folate
    D. Vitamin E
    E. Pyridoxine

186. An 8-year-old male with excess weight presents to his pediatrician, accompanied by his mother. The patient appears happy, has no other medical conditions, and takes no medications. The mother states the school year has been busy with music lessons and chess tournaments, which he prefers over sports. She says he is physically inactive but has eliminated soda from his diet. Given the mother's work schedule, they often pick up food from restaurants in the evening. Which of the following would be the most effective method to promote weight loss in this patient?

A. Initiate pharmacotherapy
B. Wake patient up early to exercise
C. Restrict dinner portion sizes
D. Sign the patient up for soccer
E. Involve the family in weight loss

187. A 31-year-old female with a body mass index of 36 kg/m^2 presents to her primary care physician after discussing weight loss medications with her friend. She is interested in starting a medication but is unsure of the best option. She denies any tobacco or alcohol abuse. Past medical history reveals a history of recurrent nephrolithiasis and epilepsy. Physical exam reveals truncal obesity with a small reducible umbilical hernia with minimal abdominal striae. Of the options below, which would be her best long-term option?

A. Phentermine/topiramate ER
B. Phentermine monotherapy
C. Liraglutide
D. Naltrexone/bupropion ER
E. Orlistat

188. A 59-year-old female presents to an obesity medicine specialist. She has tried numerous dietary plans and becomes frustrated with the associated restrictions and rules. Since the beginning of the COVID-19 pandemic, she has worked from home, exercises 200-300 minutes weekly, and does resistance training twice weekly. She is interested in anti-obesity medications but also wants to continue working on lifestyle modifications. Which of the following recommendations would be most useful for her?

A. Recommend increasing her weekly physical activity
B. Provide resources on mindful eating
C. Discuss phone-based applications to count calories and macronutrients
D. Initiate medications and put lifestyle changes on hold
E. Begin sertraline to help with depression and improve motivation

189. A 37-year-old female is following up with her bariatric surgeon after undergoing a successful Roux-en-Y gastric bypass procedure three weeks prior. Overall she is doing well, however, she points to her mid-epigastric region as having increased constant pain, which is not relieved with famotidine. Also, yesterday she noticed nausea, and today she has had two bouts of emesis. She does admit to starting smoking again, but only 4-5 cigarettes daily. Her last bowel movement was three days ago. Which of the following is the most likely diagnosis?

A. Internal hernia
B. Gastric outlet obstruction
C. Mesenteric ischemia
D. Anastomotic stricture
E. Marginal ulcer

190. A 31-year-old previously healthy male presents to his family care physician for evaluation of his chronic condition of obesity. He started seeing a dietician and is very happy with his progress regarding dietary changes and calorie counting. He has not begun to exercise but is interested. A history and physical is performed, with no limitations to exercise perceived. An exercise prescription is being written. Which of the following is directly part of this prescription?

A. Patient safety
B. Barriers to exercise
C. Motivational interviewing
D. Enjoyment of activity
E. Physical limitations

191. A 49-year-old female presents to her family practitioner with a complaint of weight gain. She was on fenfluramine in combination with phentermine in the distant past and would like to start on something similar, as it was very effective. She is started on phentermine 15 mg in the morning. What is the most common side effect this patient will likely experience?

A. Xerostomia
B. Nausea and vomiting
C. Diarrhea
D. Dysgeusia
E. Headaches

192. A 42-year-old female with a medical history of difficult-to-control diabetes mellitus type 2 and obesity class III presents for a bariatric seminar to learn more about surgical options. She is particularly interested in a more recently endorsed malabsorptive procedure. It is described as having a high diabetes remission rate and causing a significant reduction in hunger due to the removal of a portion of the stomach. Which surgical procedure is she referring to?

A. Single anastomosis duodeno-ileostomy with sleeve gastrectomy
B. Vertical sleeve gastrectomy
C. Roux-en-Y gastric bypass
D. Biliopancreatic diversion with a duodenal switch
E. One anastomosis gastric bypass

193. A 27-year-old female with a history of epilepsy is returning for a one month-follow up to her primary care physician's office. Three months ago, she was started on phentermine/topiramate ER after lifestyle changes failed to achieve her weight loss goals. Her current dose is 7.5/46 mg phentermine/topiramate ER daily. She is tolerating the medication well but is unsure of its effectiveness. During the past three months, her weight has decreased from 220 lbs (100 kg) to 216 lbs (98 kg). Which option would be the most appropriate to initiate at this time?

A. Monitor for weight loss for an additional month
B. Take an additional phentermine/topiramate ER 3.75/23 mg tab at night
C. Change the medication to naltrexone/bupropion ER
D. Titrate up to phentermine/topiramate ER 15/92 mg daily
E. Titrate off medication, then start liraglutide

194. A 31-year-old male presents for his initial 1-week post-bariatric surgery (sleeve gastrectomy) follow-up appointment with his dietician. He has continued a liquid diet and has been taking crushed vitamin supplementation. His current vitamin intake includes the following:

- Two adult multivitamins
- Elemental calcium of 1200 mg daily
- 1500 international units of vitamin D
- 65 mg of iron taken on an empty stomach

Which of the following recommendations should be made to this patient?

A. Take iron with calcium for increased absorption
B. Avoid concentrated carbohydrates to prevent dumping syndrome
C. Double the amount of vitamin D intake
D. Decrease the multivitamin to one tablet daily
E. Ensure the multivitamins contain vitamin selenium

195. A 31-year-old female status post Roux-en-Y gastric bypass is being seen 4 hours postoperatively on the general medical floor by the hospitalist. There were no immediate surgical complications. The patient has type 2 diabetes mellitus and was previously on empagliflozin, tirzepatide, and metformin. She has tolerated a small amount of oral liquid intake. Point-of-care glucose testing reveals a current glucose level of 150 mg/dL. What is the most appropriate management of this patient's diabetes?

A. Decrease empagliflozin by 50%
B. Continue to monitor glucose levels
C. Initiate semaglutide
D. Change metformin to extended-release
E. Start insulin drip to maintain glucose levels of 140-180 mg/dL

196. A 34-year-old male is presenting for a 2-week follow-up with his health coach. He had lost 3 lbs (1.4 kg) the first week but has regained that back. He states that work is busy, and he has difficulty avoiding eating fast food, which is convenient. The health coach agrees that losing weight does take effort and then states, "You are showing motivation to lose weight by coming to the office, but yet you continue to eat fast food frequently. How do those two go together?" What motivation interview principle did the coach display?

A. Empathy
B. Avoiding arguments
C. Developing discrepancy
D. Resolving ambivalence
E. Supporting self-efficacy

197. A 24-year-old female presents for smoking cessation counseling. She has mild depression symptoms and increased weight gain since starting the night shift. The clinician starts her on a single medication that can treat all of these components. Which of the following parameters may increase once starting this medication?

A. LDL
B. Triglycerides
C. Glucose levels
D. Blood pressure
E. Heart rate

198. A 35-year-old female is following up with her primary care physician two years after undergoing a Roux-en-Y gastric bypass. She has lost and maintained 65% of her excess body weight. Today, her vitamin D (OH-25) is 8 ng/mL (reference range > 30 ng/ml), her parathyroid hormone is slightly elevated, and her corrected calcium levels are normal. She undergoes a bone density scan, which is consistent with osteopenia. Which of the following is the most appropriate treatment at this time?

A. Calcitriol
B. Ergocalciferol
C. Calcium oxalate
D. Oral alendronate
E. Intravenous zoledronic acid

199. A 41-year-old male with a body mass index of 61 kg/m^2 presents for a surgery consultation regarding bariatric surgical options. Comorbidities include well-controlled obstructive sleep apnea, hypertension, and right knee osteoarthritis. Upon discussing goals, he states his primary goal is maximum weight loss. Given his prior medical history and weight loss goals, which of the following would be the most appropriate surgical option for him?

A. Laparoscopic adjustable gastric banding (LAGB)
B. Sleeve gastrectomy (SG)
C. Roux-en-Y gastric bypass (RYGB)
D. Biliopancreatic diversion with duodenal switch (BPD/DS)

200. A 43-year-old female presents to the office for increased weight since her last appointment. She was started on amlodipine for blood pressure and has noted a 2.2 lb (1 kg) weight gain despite no other changes to physical activity. What is the most likely explanation for this?

A. Increased interstitial edema
B. Increased appetite
C. Decreased energy expenditure
D. Activation of POMC/CART pathway
E. Placebo effect

201. A 52-year-old female presents to her primary care physician with intermittent post-prandial fullness, nausea, and occasional vomiting. She underwent a laparoscopic Roux-en-Y gastric bypass two years prior and has been very happy with her weight loss. A barium swallow and subsequent EGD fail to explain her findings. The following week she goes to the emergency department for biliary emesis. The most likely cause of her symptoms is a(n)

A. mesenteric defect
B. small intestinal bowel overgrowth
C. *H. pylori* infection
D. marginal ulcer
E. anastomotic stricture

202. A 41-year-old female presents to her primary care physician for concerns of diaphoresis, weakness, and tunnel vision approximately two hours after meals. She underwent a Roux-en-Y gastric bypass (RYGB) three years ago and subsequently lost 103 lbs (46.7 kg) with a current BMI of 26.1 kg/m². She denies ever having similar symptoms. She has decreased her carbohydrate intake, which helped minimally. Which of the following conditions most accurately describes her symptoms?

A. Dumping syndrome
B. Insulinoma
C. Postprandial hyperinsulinemic hypoglycemia
D. Nesidioblastosis
E. Noninsulinoma pancreatogenous hypoglycemia syndrome

203. A 39-year-old Caucasian female with a past medical history of obstructive sleep apnea adherent with CPAP and gout presents to her primary care office for follow-up regarding elevated blood pressures. Over the last three months, home and in-office blood pressures have ranged from 150-170/90-105 mmHg. Today, her blood pressure is 164/98 mmHg, and she has a BMI of 34 kg/m². Which of the following is the most appropriate medication to prescribe now?

A. Losartan
B. Naltrexone/bupropion ER
C. Chlorthalidone
D. Metoprolol

204. A patient reaches out to her family medicine physician for advice. She was told to discontinue semaglutide one week prior to an elective cholecystectomy. She has had significant weight loss with this medication and has concerns about weight regain. She has been on a stable dose for the past 6 months and has had no adverse effects. The patient was most likely instructed to discontinue this medication due to concerns for

A. postoperative nausea
B. perioperative hypoglycemia
C. reduced wound healing
D. gastric regurgitation
E. post-operative ileus

205. A pediatrician working in a rural community wants to provide the highest level of care for her patients. Upon researching the most updated guidelines, the evidence-based approach that will improve the health of her patients with overweight or obesity the most would include

A. discussing surgical options once patients complete puberty
B. evaluating all patients for lipid disorders and insulin resistance
C. starting patients in a staged management approach
D. familiarizing herself with community-based resources
E. require lab work evaluating for endocrinopathies

206. A 48-year-old female started tirzepatide for diabetes and has titrated up to the maximum dose. She has noticed clumps of hair falling out when washing her hair in the shower over the past 2 months and is concerned. She has lost 64 lbs (29 kg) after starting the medication and invoking aggressive lifestyle and behavioral changes. She takes a daily vitamin, and intakes 1400 kcal/day with 82 grams of protein. Which of the following best explains her presenting complaint?

A. Telogen effluvium
B. Micronutrient deficiency
C. Perimenopausal status
D. Tinea capitus
E. Protein malnourishment

207. A 7-year-old is presenting to his pediatrician for a well-child exam. He overall feels well and his exercise-induced asthma is controlled with an albuterol inhaler. The parents are present with him. Which of the following recommendations is most appropriate at this time?

A. Encourage 60 minutes of exercise daily
B. Limit bedroom television time to < 1 hour daily
C. Encourage a sleep duration of at least 8 hours nightly
D. Dessert should only be given when meal is completed
E. Limit eating at restaurants to once weekly

208. A 54-year-old male with a history of gout and class I obesity presents for a 2-week follow-up visit after initiating a ketogenic diet. Per urine ketone strips, he has been in ketosis for the past week. Which of the following lab findings are expected today compared to when he first initiated the diet?

A. Hyponatremia
B. Decreased uric acid levels
C. Increased serum pH levels
D. Hyperkalemia

209. A 51-year-old female is presenting to her primary care physician with plans to undergo a sleeve gastrectomy. She has a prior diagnosis of polycystic ovarian syndrome and hypertension, for which she is taking metformin and lisinopril. Overall she states she feels well. Her physical activity consists of briskly walking (5 metabolic equivalents) for 45 minutes daily. Physical examination is unrevealing. Her STOP-BANG score is 1. Which would be the most appropriate test to perform before surgery?

A. Pharmacologic stress test
B. Fasting lipid panel
C. Thyroid-stimulating hormone
D. Dexamethasone suppression test
E. Overnight polysomnography

210. A patient is researching different bariatric procedures and is considering a duodenal switch. In discussing this procedure with the patient, which of the following most accurately describes this procedure?

A. It is preferred in those with a BMI < 45 kg/m^2
B. The common channel is less than 20 cm in length
C. Digestive enzymes enter the digestive loop
D. A portion of the stomach is removed

211. A clinical trial is evaluating an oxyntomodulin analog, which is a potential investigational obesity therapy that has shown promising effects in animal studies. It is theorized that this medication will increase satiety, decrease food intake, and potentially have beneficial glucose effects in patients with type 2 diabetes mellitus. The beneficial effects of this intravenous peptide most likely occur as a result of which of the following mechanisms?

A. GLP-1 receptor agonist
B. Glucagon receptor antagonism
C. NPY/AgRP direct antagonist
D. Increase in central serotonin levels
E. Ghrelin binding and inactivation

212. A 29-year-old female presents to the clinic with concerns about an abnormal fasting lipid panel on screening blood work for life insurance.

Test	Value	Reference Range
Total cholesterol	287 mg/dL	< 200 mg/dL
LDL	188 mg/dL	< 130 mg/dL
HDL	31 mg/dL	> 40 mg/dL
Triglycerides (TG)	388 mg/dL	< 150 mg/dL

In discussing a carbohydrate versus fat-restricted diet, which of the following would be an accurate statement to provide to this patient?

A. A ketogenic diet is preferred to improve the LDL value
B. A diet consisting of < 30% fats will preferentially improve HDL
C. Genetic hypercholesterolemia responds to carbohydrate restriction
D. Low-fat diets do not affect insulin resistance or glucose levels
E. Carbohydrate-restricted diets would have a greater effect on TG

213. A 42-year-old female presents for her 3-month follow-up appointment with her diabetes specialist. The patient has noticed increased polyuria over the past month and admits to having some "slip-ups" following her carbohydrate-restricted diet. Medical history includes type 2 diabetes, heart failure with preserved ejection fraction, and mild diabetic nephropathy. Medications include metformin 2000 mg daily, lisinopril 10 mg daily, and hydrochlorothiazide 25 mg. Body mass index is 34 kg/m², whereas vital signs and physical examination are otherwise normal. Her most recent HbA1c is 8.6% (reference range: < 5.7%), an increase of 0.5% since her prior appointment. Which of the following is the most appropriate management change at this time?

A. Increase metformin
B. Initiate basal insulin
C. Start a DPP-4 inhibitor
D. Prescribe an SGLT-2 inhibitor
E. Lifestyle changes only

214. A 52-year-old male presents to a gastroenterologist for evaluation of esophageal dysphagia. He underwent an open Roux-en-Y gastric bypass 15 years prior. Although he has maintained significant weight loss, he has not been adherent to physical activity or taking vitamins. An image from the upper gastrointestinal series is shown below. Given this finding, which other feature is likely found on physical examination?

A. Koilonychia
B. Hepatomegaly
C. Dermatitis
D. External hemorrhoids
E. Actinic cheilitis

215. A patient presents to a bariatric seminar, as he is interested in undergoing surgery for weight loss. He has struggled with weight his entire life, and despite recommended dietary and physical activity changes, his body mass index is still > 60 kg/m². At the end of the seminar, he discusses with the surgeon an option that he has read about, but was not presented by the surgeon, which included placing a balloon into the stomach for weight loss. Which of the following is a true statement regarding this procedure for weight loss?

A. This device is not FDA-approved for use in the United States
B. Intragastric balloons account for 10% of bariatric procedures
C. Indications include a BMI between > 30-40 kg/m² with comorbidities
D. Intragastric balloons have been proven ineffective for weight loss
E. The balloons are placed for 12 months, then removed

216. A 26-year-old female with severe obesity presents for a metabolic and bariatric surgical consultation. Her prior medical history includes gastroesophageal reflux and obstructive sleep apnea. She takes prenatal vitamins and omeprazole and admits adherence regarding her continuous positive airway pressure machine. Physical examination reveals acanthosis nigricans on the back of her neck and narrow striae on her abdomen. A recent complete metabolic panel and thyroid-stimulating hormone level were normal. Which of the following must be completed before this patient undergoes bariatric surgery?

A. Preoperative *Helicobacter pylori* testing
B. Right upper quadrant ultrasound
C. Serum dehydroepiandrosterone-sulfate (DHEA-S)
D. Psychosocial-behavioral evaluation
E. 5% mandatory weight loss preoperatively

217. A 29-year-old female who is one month postpartum is being evaluated for weight management. She is currently breastfeeding, and her BMI is 36 kg/m^2. She states her BMI has never been below 30 kg/m^2 during her adult life. She would like to start treatment to help with returning to her pre-conception weight. Which option would be most appropriate to initiate at this time?

A. Semaglutide
B. Phentermine/topiramate ER
C. Naltrexone/bupropion ER
D. Cellulose and citric acid hydrogel
E. Metformin

218. A 39-year-old female is presenting to her general surgeon, who performed her gastric bypass four months prior. She is having vague episodes of sharp mid- to upper abdominal pain that lasts 2-3 hours and then resolves. During these episodes, she feels nauseated but denies emesis. These occur 2 hours after eating, but she is unsure of the correlation to certain foods. She does admit to taking naproxen occasionally for a headache but is on concurrent omeprazole. A right upper quadrant ultrasound reveals cholelithiasis without cholecystitis. In working up her abdominal pain, which of the following statements is true?

A. She should be given a trial of rifaximin
B. NSAIDs should never be used after bariatric surgery
C. Endoscopic evaluation is high-risk after bariatric surgery
D. Traditional ERCP is preferred for choledocholithiasis evaluation
E. Ursodeoxycholic acid may have prevented her symptoms

219. A 22-year-old female is presenting to the weight-loss clinic to discuss FDA-approved, long-term anti-obesity medications. She denies any prior eating disorders, including bulimia or anorexia nervosa, which are contraindications to the combination oral medication that you want to prescribe. In addition, this medication carries a black box warning for which of the following conditions?

A. Congenital defects
B. Suicidal ideation
C. Medullary thyroid carcinoma
D. Pancreatitis
E. Ventricular arrhythmia

220. A female patient meets with her dietician one final time before undergoing a Roux-en-Y gastric bypass. The dietician discusses starting a high-protein, liquid diet two weeks before the surgery. What is the reasoning behind this?

A. Develop good dietary habits for the postoperative period
B. To prevent surgical complications from organ injury
C. Reduce inflammation in the stomach and proximal intestines
D. Decrease colonic stool burden and risk of an intestinal leak
E. Increase the total percentage of post-operative weight loss

221. A 47-year-old female presents for a comprehensive metabolic and bariatric surgery consultation. Her BMI has consistently been over 50 kg/m^2 for the past ten years, which she attributes to pregnancies and genetics. She has a family history of endometrial cancer in her mother and prostate cancer in her father. Per the Centers for Disease Control and Prevention (CDC), aggressive weight loss will likely reduce the risk of malignancy affecting which of the following areas?

A. Thyroid
B. Lymph nodes
C. Lung
D. Skin
E. Oral

222. A 6-year-old male presents to a geneticist after he is found to have hyperphagia. Testing reveals that pro-insulin levels are increased. The child's BMI is 150% of the 95th percentile. Genetic testing returns positive for a variant of the proprotein convertase subtilisin/Kexin type 1 (PCSK1) gene. Which of the following should be administered to this child?

A. Amylin analogs
B. Metreleptin
C. Semaglutide
D. Setmelanotide
E. Gastric inhibitory polypeptide

223. A 33-year-old female presents for a pre-operative consultation with a desire to undergo a Roux-en-Y gastric bypass. She is concerned as she states that she has been on buprenorphine-naloxone for the past five years due to a history of intravenous heroin use. Since stopping heroin, she has had a steady increase in weight, and her current BMI is 41 kg/m². She has an accountability partner, has been sober for the past five years, and is now counseling others on the effects of substance use. Which of the following statements is accurate to present?

A. A history of substance use is a contraindication to surgery
B. Buprenorphine-naloxone must be stopped prior to surgery
C. The risk of alcohol use disorder is increased after surgery
D. An underlying eating disorder will improve after surgery
E. Weekly urine drug screens will ensure adherence after surgery

224. A 32-year-old female is being evaluated by psychiatry before bariatric surgery. During the interview, the patient understands the risks and benefits of the planned gastric sleeve but shows a lack of motivation to maintain the dietary and exercise changes. The patient is asked to write a list of potential pitfalls or concerns the patient has regarding maintaining weight postoperatively. What key process of motivational interviewing is being displayed?

A. Engagement
B. Focusing
C. Evoking
D. Planning

225. A multi-disciplinary weight management center has recently added the TransPyloric Shuttle (TPS)® to its list of options for weight loss. What is true regarding this device?

A. It is best for those with significant BMI levels as a bridge to surgery
B. It can only be kept in place for six months maximum
C. It is safe in pregnancy, although it must be removed before birth
D. Patients must be on chronic acid suppression while device is in place
E. Bowel obstruction is the most common adverse side effect

226. A 29-year-old female presents for a two-month follow-up appointment after her initial obesity medicine consultation. At the prior appointment, her medroxyprogesterone injection was discussed as being weight-positive. She was started on tirzepatide to assist in weight loss. She has since changed to an oral estrogen-progesterone contraceptive pill and is tolerating the tirzepatide well. Which lab finding may occur within the next year if her current medications are not addressed?

A. Increased renin levels
B. Hypokalemia
C. Increased urine anion gap
D. Hypoglycemia
E. Positive urine HCG

227. A 21-year-old female is having frequent migraines leading to missed days of work. Most headaches last up to two days and she has approximately eight debilitating headaches per month. She has tried NSAIDs and sumatriptan for abortive therapy and topiramate and propranolol for prevention. None of these have been effective. Recent head imaging was normal. She does not want to start on medications that will cause weight gain. Which is the best pharmacologic treatment for this patient?

A. Atenolol
B. Amitriptyline
C. Acetazolamide
D. Erenumab
E. Valproic acid

228. A 34-year-old male with a past medical history of anxiety and diabetes presents to his primary care physician two years after undergoing a sleeve gastrectomy. He initially lost 60 lbs (27.2 kg) within the first year, but then over this past year, he has slowly regained approximately 30 lbs (13.6 kg). Medications include metformin, detemir, and fluoxetine. He does admit to nonadherence with his recommended daily vitamins but continues to exercise three times weekly. Given these findings, which of the following most likely explains his postoperative weight regain?

A. Dilated gastric pouch
B. Excess insulin administration
C. Dietary indiscretion
D. Psychologic issues
E. Vitamin deficiencies

229. A 49-year-old female who was recently widowed after her husband had complications from obesity presents to her family medicine physician for weight loss counseling. Her BMI is 42 kg/m^2, and she has a past medical history of hypertension, diabetes, and asthma. Comprehensive lifestyle changes are discussed. What is a reasonable weight loss goal, in terms of total body loss, for this patient within the next six months, according to the "2013 ACC/AHA/TOS Guidelines for the Management of Overweight and Obesity in Adults"?

A. 0-5%
B. 5-10%
C. 10-15%
D. 15-20%

230. A 33-year-old female with a past medical history of class III obesity, diabetes type 2, tobacco abuse, and polycystic ovarian syndrome presents for a bariatric evaluation. She is interested in a "gastric bypass." Her medications include metformin, oral contraceptive birth control, and a prenatal vitamin. After a thorough history and physical examination, you discuss preoperative recommendations, including a physical activity plan and healthy dietary patterns. What other perioperative education would be necessary for this patient?

A. Avoid becoming pregnant for at least 6 months after surgery
B. Birth control must be discontinued 1 week before surgery
C. Her hemoglobin A1c should be less than 9% preoperatively
D. Metformin is contraindicated after Roux-en-Y gastric bypass
E. Tobacco products must be stopped 6 weeks before surgery

231. A 24-year-old female presents to her primary care physician's office for an evaluation regarding weight gain. She states she has been exercising five times weekly for approximately 30 minutes during her sessions. She has decreased her calories to 1200 kcal daily, focusing on a low-fat diet, but she still has noticed a 10 lb (4.5 kg) weight gain in the past year. Medical history includes bipolar disease, which is well-controlled on aripiprazole. Previous laboratory work was within normal limits, including HbA1c, thyroid stimulating hormone, and complete metabolic panel. Which would be the most effective in treating her weight gain?

A. Prescribe metformin
B. Prescribe orlistat
C. Intensify calorie restrictions
D. Change aripiprazole to olanzapine
E. Intensify exercise regimen

232. A 12-year-old female who has struggled with obesity for the past five years is presenting to a bariatric center for a vertical sleeve gastrectomy evaluation. She has hypertension and severe obstructive sleep apnea that did not respond to tonsillectomy. She is sexually active and developmentally is at a Tanner stage 3. Her BMI is currently 37 kg/m². Psychiatry evaluation reveals mild depression and a lack of understanding of the risks regarding the surgical procedure. Which of the following is a contraindication for this adolescent to undergo bariatric surgery?

A. Tanner stage
B. Body mass index
C. Sexual activity
D. Depression
E. Risk appreciation

233. A 28-year-old female is presenting to her primary care physician's office six months after undergoing laparoscopic adjustable gastric banding (LAGB). She states two weeks ago, she had eaten too quickly, with subsequent nausea and vomiting. Since then, she has been unable to keep solids down and will regurgitate undigested food after small meals. In addition, her acid reflux has significantly worsened during this time. Which of the following is the next best step in management?

A. CT of the abdomen
B. Remove fluid from the band
C. Surgical revision
D. Dietary changes
E. Start omeprazole

234. A 35-year-old female presents for follow-up three years after undergoing a sleeve gastrectomy. She states she had significant weight loss within the first year post-operatively but has since plateaued in her weight, approximately 30 lbs (13.6 kg) short of her goal. She has followed all recommendations but admits to an increased appetite. She would like to discuss anti-obesity medications to assist in helping with reaching her goals. Which of the following is the most appropriate recommendation to provide?

A. Weight-loss medications are contraindicated after bariatric surgery
B. Cellulose and citric acid hydrogel is preferred post-operatively
C. Revision surgery is most appropriate to reach your target weight
D. Body contouring surgery will likely allow you to reach your goal
E. Starting semaglutide and phentermine will reduce weight

235. A 13-year-old female presents to her pediatrician for continued weight gain. Her BMI is 140% of the 95th percentile range, remaining consistent over the past year despite lifestyle changes. Recent lab work displayed an ALT level of 48 U/L (reference range: 8–20 U/L) and an HbA1c of 6.9% (reference range: <5.7%). She continues to snore at night despite a tonsillectomy last year. Which of the following would be the most appropriate action to provide the best long-term health benefits for this patient?

A. Offer referral for metabolic and bariatric surgery now
B. Start the patient on metformin
C. Initiate a six-month trial of dietary modifications
D. Prescribe pioglitazone for metabolic liver disease
E. Initiate a staged approach to treating obesity

236. A mother brings her 12-year-old daughter to her primary health care provider for evaluation of anti-obesity medications. Despite seeing a dietician and trainer, monitoring caloric intake, and undergoing intensive health behavior and lifestyle treatment she has not improved her growth chart curve. Genetic testing was negative and she has no other medical conditions. She is interested in pharmacotherapy. Which of the following is the most appropriate FDA-approved medication for this indication?

A. Tirzepatide
B. Metformin
C. Phentermine
D. Semaglutide
E. Setmelanotide

237. A 41-year-old female with class III obesity and depression is diagnosed with severe obstructive sleep apnea after completing a polysomnography. Since diagnosis, she has been adherent to her continuous positive airway pressure. She retakes the STOPBANG score and compares it to her score before she initiated treatment and notices that it has decreased by 1 point. Which STOPBANG component most likely improved?

A. Body mass index
B. Daytime somnolence
C. Blood pressure
D. Depression
E. Neck circumference

238. A 29-year-old female presents to a gastroenterologist to learn more about endoscopic sleeve gastroplasty, as she admits to a strong phobia of abdominal surgeries. In terms of hormone changes after surgery, this procedure is most similar to which of the following?

A. Sleeve gastrectomy
B. Laparoscopic adjustable gastric banding
C. Roux-en-Y gastric bypass
D. Single anastomosis duodenal-ileal bypass with sleeve gastrectomy

239. A patient meets with a personal trainer to discuss exercise options. Her father recently passed away unexpectedly in the setting of heart disease, so she wants to be proactive and begin exercising. She enjoys numerous activities but would prefer outdoor activities. An exercise prescription is written to include performing resistance training two days per week. In addition, the prescription includes performing an outdoor activity of moderate intensity for 30 minutes, five days weekly. Which of the following activities would qualify for this exercise prescription?

A. Walking at 2 miles per hour
B. Playing singles tennis
C. Bicycling at 8 miles per hour
D. Jogging at 5 miles per hour
E. Swimming laps

240. A 59-year-old male is interested in initiating the exchange diet into his daily routine. He plans to eliminate one of his snacks daily and substitute two servings of vegetables for two starches.

American Diabetes Association Exchange Servings				
1 Serving	Protein	Carbohydrate	Fat	Calories
Starches	3 g	15 g	<1 g	80 kcal
Vegetables	2 g	5 g	0 g	25 kcal
Fat	0 g	0 g	0 g	45 kcal
Fruit	0 g	15 g	0 g	60 kcal
Dairy	8 g	15 g	0-8 g	90-150 kcal
Protein	7 g	0 g	2-5 g	55-75 kcal
Snacks	3 g	15 g	0-1 g	80 kcal

How many daily calories will he reduce by making these changes?

A. 80 kcal/day
B. 130 kcal/day
C. 190 kcal/day
D. 240 kcal/day
E. 270 kcal/day

241. A 19-year-old female presents to her obstetrician to discuss options for birth control. She wants to maintain a healthy weight, given her family history of diabetes and early-onset coronary artery disease. She is sexually active and does not want to become pregnant. Which of the following is associated with the most weight gain?

A. Intrauterine device
B. Barrier method
C. Progesterone-only pill
D. Etonogestrel implant
E. Progesterone depo injections

242. A 32-year-old male presents to his primary care physician for yellowing of his eyes and noticing increased fatigue. He takes no prescribed medication but does admit to taking a combination herbal supplement for weight loss. Although it is recommended to take twice daily, he has been taking approximately ten daily, and has noticed a 14 lb (6.4 kg) weight loss. AST, ALT, bilirubin, and INR are markedly elevated. Which of the following ingredients in his supplement is most likely contributing to his current condition?

A. Chitosan
B. Ephedra
C. Glucosinolates
D. Green tea extract
E. Raspberry ketone

243. A 29-year-old male presents to his dietician after starting a very low-calorie diet. He has done some research and determined that he would like to maintain less than 800 kcal/day and eliminate all fat from his diet. Currently, he is consuming 1300 kcal/day without significant weight loss. The dietician discusses the importance of close monitoring and recommends adding some fat to his diet instead of eliminating it altogether. Without this recommendation, what possible complications could arise?

A. Electrolyte imbalance
B. Gout flares
C. Cholelithiasis
D. Electrolyte derangements
E. Cold intolerance

244. A 26-year-old female underwent a one-anastomosis gastric bypass and has since had a persistent burning sensation in her mid-epigastric region. She states that proton pump inhibitors have not helped and sucralfate provided no relief. She denies any other symptoms, including fever, nausea, or vomiting. Endoscopic evaluation reveals no strictures or anastomotic ulcers, and a histologic sample shows mild stomach inflammation. A CT of the abdomen is unremarkable. Which of the following is the most likely cause of her symptoms?

A. Cardiac ischemia
B. Bile acid gastritis
C. *H. pylori* infection
D. Recalcitrant acid reflux
E. Esophageal spasm

245. A 44-year-old male presents to his primary care clinician for a three-month follow-up appointment. He has a history of obesity class II, hypertension, obstructive sleep apnea, and hyperlipidemia. He started an off-label medication for weight loss at his prior appointment and is tolerating it well. His lab work before and after initiating the anti-obesity medication, is shown below. Which of the following medications was likely started?

Test	Initial	Today	Reference Range
Sodium	138 mEq/L	136 mEq/L	136–145 mEq/L
Potassium	3.8 mEq/L	4.1 mEq/L	3.5-5.0 mEq/L
Chloride	99 mEq/L	107 mEq/L	95-105 mEq/L
Bicarbonate	24 mEq/L	18 mEq/L	22–28 mEq/L
BUN	16 mg/dL	18 mg/dL	6-20 mg/dL
Creatinine	0.8 mg/dL	0.9 mg/dL	0.6–1.2 mg/dL
Glucose	88 mg/dL	83 mg/dL	70–110 mg/dL

A. Phentermine
B. Metformin
C. Bupropion
D. Topiramate
E. Tirzepatide

246. A 31-year-old female presents to her primary care physician's office with complaints of significant anxiety. She has tried counseling and has noted slight improvements, but the anxiety still interferes with her life. She denies depression. She is concerned that initiating pharmacotherapy for anxiety could cause her to gain weight. Vital signs are normal. BMI is 32 kg/m^2. If pharmacotherapy is started, which would be the most appropriate?

A. Bupropion
B. Fluoxetine
C. Venlafaxine
D. Aripiprazole
E. Propranolol

247. A 38-year-old male with a history of obesity presents to his internist's office for an annual exam. The patient denies any new symptoms since his last appointment but has noticed some weight gain, especially around his waist. His current weight is 241 lbs (109.3 kg), an increase of 14 lbs (6.4 kg) since last year, placing his BMI at 39 kg/m^2. His lipid panel is within normal limits, however, his HbA1c is currently 5.9% (reference range: < 5.7%), and his fasting glucose level is 119 mg/dL (reference range: < 100 mg/dL). Which of the following would be the most appropriate recommendation at this time?

A. Initiate metformin therapy
B. Obtain C-peptide levels
C. Recheck HbA1c levels in 3 months
D. Recommend resistance training
E. Initiate an SGLT-2 inhibitor

248. A 52-year-old male presents for a follow-up for weight loss. He was started on phentermine 15 mg in the morning and states it works well, but he notices the effects wear off by midafternoon. He wants to avoid increasing the morning dose of phentermine due to some tremors he noticed on the higher dose. He has a history of nephrolithiasis and cannot afford GLP-1 receptor agonists due to a lack of insurance coverage. Which of the following would be a potential treatment option?

A. Initiate tirzepatide
B. Add diethylpropion in the afternoon
C. Add topiramate
D. Continue current regimen
E. Add metformin

249. A previously healthy 28-year-old female with a current BMI of 28 kg/m^2 presents for a follow-up appointment with her primary care. Over the past six months, she has intensified her exercise regimen to 200 minutes/week, restricted her diet to 1300 kcal/day, and eliminated fast food and soda. However, she is frustrated that she has not met her weight loss goals and is interested in pharmacotherapy. If prescribed, which would most likely help her accomplish her 10% weight loss goal if titrated to maximum recommended strength?

A. Phentermine/topiramate ER
B. Phentermine monotherapy
C. Liraglutide
D. Naltrexone/bupropion ER

250. A 17-year-old female who has struggled with the disease of obesity since childhood is meeting with a dietician to discuss weight loss goals. Her estimated total energy expenditure (TEE) is 1900 kcal/day. In conjunction with maintaining a food diary, the patient utilizes a smartphone application to monitor her caloric intake. She should be counseled to reduce her calories below TEE by a minimum of what amount to promote weight loss?

A. 300 kcal/d
B. 600 kcal/d
C. 900 kcal/d
D. 1200 kcal/d

251. A 67-year-old male presents with concerns of uncontrolled diabetes and increased weight gain. He is petrified of needles and refuses medications that require administration through needles, including insulin. Medications include metformin ER and dapagliflozin. He exercises 30 minutes daily and follows recommendations from his dietician. Which of the following is the next best step in management?

A. Initiate oral semaglutide
B. Discuss tirzepatide
C. Start pioglitazone
D. Intensify exercise routine
E. Prescribe continuous glucose monitoring

252. A 59-year-old female presents to her bariatric surgeon's office one week before undergoing a Roux-en-Y gastric bypass. Her current comorbidities include hyperlipidemia, hypothyroidism, obstructive sleep apnea, osteoarthritis, hypertension, and type 2 diabetes. She is hopeful of decreasing or discontinuing some of her medications after surgery. Despite improvements in many obesity-related comorbidities, which of the following conditions may likely need to have medications increased after her bariatric surgery?

A. Hyperlipidemia
B. Diabetes
C. Hypertension
D. Hypothyroidism
E. Osteoarthritis

253. A medical student is rotating with a surgeon who is about to perform a Roux-en-Y gastric bypass. He describes the procedure as one in which he will create a gastric pouch, then connect this new pouch to the jejunum, bypassing the duodenum. He describes a potentially severe complication, an anastomotic leak, which may follow the procedure, associated with high morbidity and prolonged hospital stays. What is true of this potential complication?

A. Barium studies are the preferred imaging
B. Failure to extubate may be the presenting sign
C. Procalcitonin has no role in evaluation
D. It is more frequently seen in a sleeve gastrectomy

254. A patient with type 1 diabetes and obesity class I presents to the clinic to discuss an FDA-indicated adjuvant medication to help reduce appetite and insulin intake. A subcutaneous medication is initiated after a thorough discussion, including hypoglycemia symptoms. Which mechanism or class of medication is associated with the initiated medication?

    A. Amylin analog
    B. Biguanide
    C. GLP-1 receptor agonist
    D. GLP-1 and GIP agonist
    E. Sympathetic amine

255. A 37-year-old male with a past medical history of chronic migraines and well-controlled hypertension is presenting to his primary care physician for evaluation of obesity management. He has lost 9 lbs (4 kg) with lifestyle modifications but has plateaued and wants to start pharmacotherapy. His current BMI is 32 kg/m². Insurance does not cover combination anti-obesity medication. Which of the following off-label medications would be the most appropriate medication to start now?

    A. Topiramate
    B. Phentermine
    C. Bupropion
    D. Naltrexone
    E. Metformin

256. A 29-year-old female, two months post-partum who is currently breastfeeding, presents to her family practitioner to jump-start weight loss. She states her goals are to lose weight healthily and not disrupt milk production. She is up multiple times nightly with her infant and always feels tired. She walks for 15 minutes daily and drinks 1-2 sodas daily. Her pre-pregnancy weight was 178 lbs (80.7 kg). Currently, she is at 212 lbs (96.2 kg). Which of the following would be an example of a SMART goal to set for this patient while utilizing shared-decision making?

A. Decrease calories to < 1000 kcal/day
B. Increase exercise as much as tolerated
C. Lose 5 lbs (2.3 kg) weekly until at pre-pregnancy weight
D. Decrease soda intake by 3 cans weekly until discontinued
E. Start and titrate liraglutide to a goal of 3 mg daily

257. A neurologist calls to discuss a mutual patient who needs treatments for partial seizures. The neurologist offers a few options listed below but would like your feedback based on the patient's comorbidities. The patient has diabetes mellitus type II with retinopathy, obesity class I, and hypertension. Which of the following options is most appropriate to recommend?

A. Carbamazepine
B. Gabapentin
C. Valproate
D. Zonisamide
E. Pregabalin

258. A 45-year-old male with a past medical history of acid reflux, class III obesity, hypertension, and osteoarthritis presents for a bariatric surgery evaluation. He takes a proton pump inhibitor twice daily but admits that he still has gastroesophageal symptoms regularly. A barium swallow evaluation is performed, as shown below. If bariatric surgery is pursued, which of the following should be recommended?

A. Sleeve gastrectomy
B. Biliopancreatic diversion with a duodenal switch
C. Adjustable gastric banding
D. Intra-gastric balloon
E. Roux-en-Y gastric bypass

259. A 58-year-old male presents to clinic after undergoing an MRI spectroscopy scan displaying significant visceral adiposity. He inquires about the most effective manner to reduce this specific fat storage and positively impact his life. Which of the following should be recommended?

A. Intermittent fasting
B. Moderate weight loss
C. Liposuction
D. Orlistat
E. Vigorous exercise

260. A 61-year-old male presents to his primary care office with a desire to start a newer medication to treat his diabetes and help with weight loss. The medication discussed has two mechanisms of action. Which of the following is a contraindication to this medication?

A. History of prior alcohol-induced pancreatitis
B. End-stage renal disease
C. Suicidal ideation
D. Family history of medullary thyroid carcinoma
E. History of nephrolithiasis

IV. Practice Management

261. A 45-year-old male reluctantly presents to a bariatric seminar. He has wanted to attend for the past few years, but always cancels due to concerns of what others may think. In particular, his coworkers have already verbalized that he is less valuable compared to more active and fit employees. Thus, if he takes 2-3 weeks off from work for surgery, he feels this may exacerbate their views. What is the term that describes this labeling of decreased value that his coworkers have imparted on him?

A. Bias
B. Self-efficacy
C. Implicit bias
D. Prejudice
E. Stigma

262. A primary care physician is treating a patient who is interested in bariatric surgery. The patient wants to understand the potential mortality, morbidity, and predicted amount of weight loss she could experience, given her comorbidities. More specifically, she wants to compare and contrast these parameters between a sleeve gastrectomy and a Roux-en-Y gastric bypass to help her decide the best option for her. In addition to referring her to a bariatric surgeon, what resource will likely be able to assist in providing her with the information she is looking for?

A. American College of Sports Medicine
B. Metabolic and Bariatric Surgery Accreditation Quality Improvement
C. Obesity Medicine Association
D. The Obesity Society
E. United States Preventive Services Task Force

263. A cardiologist is teaming up with a bariatric clinic to provide multidisciplinary expertise regarding exercise safety. They have created an algorithm to screen asymptomatic individuals who would benefit from performing an exercise electrocardiogram stress test before engaging in a robust exercise program. Which patient would most likely fall into a moderate-risk category for suffering a cardiac event during exercise and, therefore, should be recommended for an exercise stress test before beginning aerobic exercise?

A. 52-year-old male starting moderate-intensity exercise
B. 49-year-old female initiating vigorous-intensity exercise
C. 61-year-old male starting water-walking
D. 41-year-old male beginning vigorous-intensity workouts

264. A mother of a 12-year-old son with cognitive delays and class III obesity has brought a formal complaint to the medical board regarding the denial of a metabolic bariatric surgery evaluation. The surgeon states that although the patient meets criteria for surgery based on body mass index and comorbidities, he is concerned that the cognitive disability would make post-operative follow-up more difficult. Thus, he denied the adolescent entrance into the comprehensive bariatric program. This physician may be found in violation of which of the following principles?

A. Respect for autonomy
B. Beneficence
C. Nonmaleficence
D. Justice
E. American disability act

265. A Master of Public Health candidate is interviewing clinicians for her dissertation focused on the biased treatment of those living with obesity. In particular, she wants to understand the clinician-patient relationship, including support staff, regarding the perception of those with obesity in the medical setting. Which of the following is the most accurate statement regarding this topic?

A. Patients with obesity seek out medical care as a safe haven for bias
B. The FDA treats medications for obesity similarly to other medications
C. Clinicians with a normal BMI are more comfortable discussing weight
D. Physicians self-report that obesity is a disease similar to diabetes
E. Patients with obesity tend to receive longer office visits

266. An employer of a mid-level business is evaluating ways to improve productivity while decreasing costs. He would like to implement a physical activity initiative in which his employees would reap the cost-savings of an overall healthier workforce. Which of the following has the highest cost for an employer of workers affected by obesity compared to workers with a healthy weight?

A. Absenteeism
B. Health insurance premiums
C. Presenteeism
D. Retirement plans
E. Accidental death insurance

267. A 19-year-old female presents to her primary care physician. She has a diagnosis of systemic lupus erythematosus with nephritis, and she has gained nearly 50 lbs (22.7 kg) since starting treatment. Her current BMI is 33 kg/m². Which of the following is the best primary diagnosis code used for billing in this patient?

A. E66.01: Severe obesity due to excess calories
B. E66.1: Drug-induced obesity
C. E66.9: Obesity, unspecified
D. Z68.33: Body mass index (BMI) 33.0-33.9, adult
E. Z68.53: BMI pediatric, 85% to less than 95th percentile for age

268. A primary care physician will start seeing bariatric patients in his clinic as part of a multi-disciplinary approach to treating patients planning to undergo bariatric surgery. He plans to perform a preoperative screening, education, and postoperative follow-up visits. In preparing his office for this influx of patients with obesity, what would be recommended to make the patients feel more comfortable when presenting to his office?

A. Ensure his scales can weigh up to 300 lbs (136 kg)
B. Ensure standard chairs have handrails on either side
C. Order additional medium and large blood pressure cuffs
D. Ensure reading material in the waiting room is obesity-sensitive
E. Provide additional obesity-culture training only to the nursing staff

269. A physician is meeting with a United States senator regarding reimbursement for obesity therapy, including pharmacotherapy. The senator discusses the cost burden associated with obesity and his concerns that additional finances for coverage of extra office visits, bariatric surgery, and pharmacotherapy would ultimately not be worth the extra cost. Which of the following statements is true regarding the value of obesity therapy?

A. A patient with a BMI of 35 kg/m^2 infers an additional annual average medical cost of $500 compared to someone with a BMI of 25 kg/m^2
B. Nationally, the burden of obesity accounts for $50 billion in additional healthcare costs
C. Anti-obesity interventions cumulatively could generate $20 billion in savings for Medicare within ten years
D. Although bariatric surgery provides decreased morbidity, no studies have confirmed improved mortality rates
E. Physicians should only use FDA-approved anti-obesity medications despite the cost, as off-label medications have little evidence.

270. A school counselor is evaluating a 9-year-old male. The child states that two other boys in his class relentlessly tease him about his weight during recess. This has caused the student to withdraw from friends and academically decline. He is very conscious of what he eats now and states, "I wish they would just leave me alone!" The counselor calls the parents to discuss the situation. Which of the following would be the most constructive advice to provide to the parents?

A. Encourage them to seek medical care for the child's weight
B. Reassure the parents this will likely resolve with disciplinary action against the students initiating the bullying
C. Recommend scheduled counseling for the child
D. Encourage parents to teach the child to stand up for himself
E. Inform the parents that ignoring bullying is an effective technique

271. A 14-year-old male with Down syndrome and class II obesity with obstructive sleep apnea, hyperlipidemia, and prediabetes presents for follow-up at a bariatric center. The patient has been evaluated for bariatric surgery and was started on lifestyle modifications. His mother states he eats what he is given and rarely snacks. The patient and his family have been walking together every night for 1 hour. However, he has not lost any weight despite these measures. When discussing the procedure, the patient does not show an understanding of the procedure but states, "I want to be skinny." What is the most appropriate surgical management?

A. Obtain surgical consent from the parents
B. Continue to educate the patient and only perform the surgery when he can understand and provide consent
C. Two physicians that agree that surgery is appropriate, along with the parent's consent, is sufficient for pre-operative consent
D. Do not perform surgery due to a lack of understanding
E. Intensify lifestyle modifications

272. An obesity clinic is trying to determine the best way to reach different ethnicities by utilizing cultural-specific resources effectively. Given the clinic's central location, its patient population consists of many minority groups. Generally speaking, which strategy would be the most effective therapeutic addition for a culturally tailored approach to weight loss?

A. Provide a heart disease class for American Indians
B. Have Caucasians teach weight-loss strategies to Chinese Americans
C. Discuss alcohol avoidance within the Muslim population
D. Utilize a faith-based setting for African Americans

273. A 27-year-old male with a body mass index of 34 kg/m^2 presents to his primary care physician for follow-up from an emergency department visit for intractable nausea that has since resolved. He is very disappointed with his experience, as he requested hospital records and found in the emergency room notes that the physician used wording that he felt was hurtful and counterproductive. Which of the following statements would be an appropriate opening identifying statement regarding his weight?

A. A 27-year-old morbidly obese male
B. A 27-year-old individual affected by obesity
C. A 27-year-old obese patient
D. A class 1 obese 27-year-old male

Answer Explanations

1. (Content: I-B-7) A 41-year-old male is seen in the hospital on postoperative day one status post Roux-en-Y gastric bypass. Home medications include glargine 30 units nightly and aspart sliding scale with meals. Since surgery, he has not required any insulin to maintain normal glucose levels and has plans to be discharged on a low dose of immediate-release metformin. The increased endogenous hormone responsible for this diabetic medication adjustment

    A. is only secreted in the small intestine
    B. is secreted in response to fat and protein ingestion
    C. reduces hepatic gluconeogenesis
    D. has the same quantitative effects as seen after sleeve gastrectomy
    E. causes gallbladder contraction

(C) Glucagon-like peptide 1 is secreted in the distal small bowel and colon. This hormone has an incretin effect in response to carbohydrate ingestion, including glucose-dependent insulin secretion, **reduction of hepatic gluconeogenesis via glucagon suppression**, and delays in gastric emptying leading to increased satiety and reduced appetite. This hormone is responsible for the weight-independent, immediate improvements in diabetes after gastric bypass, as levels significantly increase after bypassing the proximal intestines.

Anorexigenic (Meal-Terminating) Intestinal Hormones		
Hormone	**Secretion Site**	**Action**
Cholecystokinin (CCK)[1]	Duodenum and jejunum (I-cells)	Stimulates gallbladder contraction, slows gastric emptying, and reduces appetite
Gastric inhibitory peptide[3] (i.e., glucose-dependent insulinotropic peptide) (GIP)	Duodenum and jejunum (K-cells)	Insulin incretin effect and slows gastric emptying
Glucagon-like peptide 1 (GLP-1)[2]	Distal small bowel and colon (L-cells)	**See paragraph above**
Oxyntomodulin (OXM)[3]	Distal small bowel and colon (L-cells)	Decrease appetite and increase energy expenditure
Peptide YY (PYY)[3]	Distal small bowel, colon, and rectum (L-cells)	Appetite suppression and delays gastric and intestinal emptying

[1]Secreted in response to fat/protein ingestion and gastric distention
[2]Secreted in response to carbohydrate ingestion. Reduced in obesity and type II diabetes
[3]Secreted in response to feeding

Reference: Miller GD. Appetite Regulation: Hormones, Peptides, and Neurotransmitters and Their Role in Obesity. Am J Lifestyle Med. 2017;13(6):586-601. Published 2017 Jun 23. doi:10.1177/1559827617716376

2. (Content: I-A-3) A 24-year-old female presents for genetic counseling regarding obesity. She is frustrated by the lack of ability to lose weight and being classified as "overweight" at a very young age despite her tall stature. She admits to wanting to give up regarding weight loss since obesity "is a family curse." She has diabetes and is on metformin. Previous testing indicated that she had significantly elevated circulating insulin levels. Which of the following genetic abnormalities is most likely present?

A. **MC4R**
B. POMC
C. FTO
D. PCSK1
E. LEPR

(A) Many of the above genes are involved in early-onset and often severe levels of obesity. **Melanocortin 4 receptor deficiency (MC4R)** is the most common monogenic defect predisposing to obesity, shared within families. It is characterized by tall stature, increased bone mineral density ("big boned"), and high insulin levels with insulin resistance.

MC4R mediates most of the anorectic effects of leptin; therefore, a deficiency leads to early-onset obesity via leptin resistance. Interestingly, leptin is also independently involved in linear bone growth, with increased levels causing tall stature, as seen in MC4R deficiency.

Other genetic abnormalities leading to early-onset obesity are listed below.

- **POMC:** Proopiomelanocortin gene mutations lead to an adrenal crisis in neonates due to ACTH deficiency, which is produced from POMC (hypothalamus) as well as alpha-melanocyte-stimulating hormone, which is involved in reducing food intake.
- **LEPR:** Leptin receptor gene deficiency leads to difficulty suppressing their appetites and insulin resistance, but they do not have tall stature.
- **Congenital leptin deficiency:** Similar to those with LEPR deficiency clinically, but with undetectable or severely suppressed leptin levels.

Importantly, diagnosis allows for treatment options. Setmelanotide is approved for POMC and LEPR deficiency and Bardet-Biedl syndrome; leptin replacement (metreleptin) is approved for congenital leptin deficiency with lipodystrophy.

Reference: Up To Date: "Genetic contribution and pathophysiology of obesity"

3. (Content: I-D-4) A 51-year-old female presents to the health clinic with questions about a diet she heard about through a health magazine. Although she cannot remember the name of the diet, it promoted a higher intake of omega fat than other diets she has researched. Benefits included lowering cardiovascular disease and preventing type 2 diabetes, both of which run in her family. In addition, she will still be able to consume seafood, an important component given her fishing hobby. What is the most likely diet that this patient is referencing?

A. Vegan
B. Pescatarian
C. Lacto-ovo
D. Mediterranean
E. Low carbohydrate

(D) **A Mediterranean diet** (meal pattern) differs from other dietary plans as it allows moderate fats (35-40% macronutrient consumption), with extra virgin olive oil being the primary source of omega-3 fat. Fruits, vegetables, nuts, legumes, avocados, and whole grains are staples of the diet, which also allows moderate alcohol intake. Although limited amounts of poultry, dairy, and red meat are allowed, fish and seafood can be consumed in moderation.

Several studies have shown improvements in <u>primary</u> cardiovascular disease prevention and associated risk factors with a Mediterranean diet. Also, the Lyon Heart Study displayed <u>secondary</u> cardiovascular disease benefits.

Note: Although the Primary Prevention of Cardiovascular Disease with a Mediterranean Diet (PRIDIMED) has been retracted due to randomization errors, recalculation still displays a cardiac benefit from this diet.

Reference: Lyon Diet Heart Study: Benefits of a Mediterranean-Style, National Cholesterol Education Program/American Heart Association Step I Dietary Pattern on Cardiovascular Disease. Penny Kris-Etherton , Robert H. Eckel , Barbara V. Howard , Sachiko St. Jeor , Terry L. Bazzarre

4. (Content: I-B-5) A 31-year-old female wants to know her total energy expenditure. She estimates her non-exercise activity thermogenesis to be 300 kcal/day, her thermic effect of meals to be 10% of her total expenditure, and her calories from exercise to be 400 kcal/day. What other testing is necessary to determine her total energy expenditure accurately?

A. **Indirect calorimeter**
B. Skinfold calipers
C. Duke's treadmill score
D. Bioelectric impedance analyses
E. Basal body temperature

(A) **Indirect calorimetry** can determine the resting metabolic rate, as it is used as a proxy for resting energy expenditure, the last component needed in this patient to determine her total energy expenditure.

Indirect calorimetry estimates energy expenditure by measuring carbon dioxide production and oxygen consumption. Patients must wear a sealed mask, with gas exchange monitored through an electronic device. Testing can be done in the office. It is inexpensive, non-invasive, and reimbursable (CPT code: 94690).

Direct calorimetry: In contrast to indirect, direct calorimetry measures the heat generated by an organism via an enclosed chamber. Water circulates the chamber, and the incoming and outgoing water temperature differences are measured, which can then be used to calculate total energy expenditure.

The formula below calculates total energy expenditure (TEE) and approximate percentages of each component.

REE: Resting energy expenditure (basal metabolic rate)
TEM: Thermic effect of meals
EEPA: Energy expenditure from physical activity (exercise and non-exercise activity thermogenesis)

Note: Resting energy expenditure can also be estimated by the Mifflin St. Jeor (preferred in those with obesity) and Harris-Benedict equations.

Reference: Obesity Medicine Association: Obesity Algorithm (2023)

5. (Content: I-A-5) A research team is developing a thesis regarding intrauterine predisposition to factors, such as how maternal obesity affects the developing fetus through adulthood. So far, the longitudinal study has shown that a mother's body mass index correlates with comorbidities of cognitive deficits and autism spectrum disorders. This type of research is best associated with which of the following?

A. Neurohormonal physiology
B. **Epigenetics and environment**
C. Behavioral determinants
D. Mutations of genetic DNA
E. Socioeconomic and culture

(B) The term **epigenetics** refers to the modification of genetic expression (not genetic mutations), often in the setting of inheritable changes. It is essential to understand that these effects do not modify the DNA sequence, only their expression via DNA methylation.

The consequences of maternal obesity and the intrauterine environment affect the brain of the developing fetus. Studies have shown that increased maternal inflammatory markers, glucose, and lipids affect postnatal neurodevelopment and metabolism.

In addition to metabolism, the following increased risks were appreciated when maternal BMI was > 30 kg/m^2.

- Attention deficit disorders
- Autism spectrum disorders
- Cognitive deficits
- Impaired stress response

Note: Another important epigenetic point is that higher birth weight is directly related to a higher risk of obesity later in life.

In addition to the above, adverse childhood events (ACEs) have been associated with an increased risk of obesity in children, adolescents, and even adults. Abuse, violence, incarceration or death of parents, divorce, etc., are all considered ACEs and cumulatively increase the risk of obesity later in life.

Reference: Assessing the fetal effects of maternal obesity via transcriptomic analysis of cord blood: a prospective case–control study. AG Edlow L Hui HC Wick I Fried DW Bianchi. First published: 29 December 2015

6. (Content: I-B-4) A longitudinal study was completed looking at the effects of sleep on weight. Both weight and the time of quality sleep, measured through a smartwatch device, were documented over 10 years. At the end of the study, what hormones or receptor levels would be expected to be increased in those who received 5 hours of sleep compared to those who received 8 hours?

    A. Leptin and neuropeptide Y
    B. α-MSH and peptide YY
    C. POMC receptors and ghrelin
    D. Cortisol and leptin
    E. Ghrelin and orexin A

(E) Long-term studies have been completed that have shown a progressive decrease in the duration of sleep for most Americans. There was a correlation between those who received fewer hours of sleep with increased weight compared to those who slept for longer periods of time, indicating sleep deprivation and subsequently increased hunger hormones lead to increased weight. These patients with decreased amounts of sleep would likely have **increased ghrelin from the stomach and increased release of orexin from the NPY/AgRP pathway,** with subsequent decreased leptin, leading to increased appetite and decreased energy expenditure.

Short amounts of sleep (approximately 5-6 hours) were correlated with a 60% increased rate of obesity and 20% with overweight. Shockingly, there was a 200% increased prevalence of obesity among those who slept <5 hours nightly.

Overall, the trend of sleep patterns indicates more people are receiving < 6 hours of sleep and a decrease in those that received ideal sleep (7-8 hours) in the United States from 1977 → 2009 when this study was conducted.

Not only does sleep length play a role, but also interruptions of sleep that may occur from restless leg syndrome, obstructive sleep apnea, bed partner movements (including pets), circadian misalignment, and sleep-maintenance insomnia.

Reference: Jean-Louis G, Williams NJ, Sarpong D, Pandey A, Youngstedt S, Zizi F, Ogedegbe G. Associations between inadequate sleep and obesity in the US adult population: analysis of the national health interview survey (1977-2009). BMC Public Health. 2014 Mar 29;14:290. doi: 10.1186/1471-2458-14-290. PMID: 24678583; PMCID: PMC3999886.

7. (Content: I-B-2) A 65-year-old male is following up with his dietician after starting a low-fat diet six weeks ago. He has increased his exercise to 250 minutes/week and has noticed a 1% total body weight loss since initiating these lifestyle changes. He comments that he has always had to work hard to maintain or lose weight, and it seems that if he stops dieting for a few weeks, he regains weight rapidly. In contrast, he states that his wife can eat whatever she likes, has always remained thin, and seldomly exercises. Compared to his wife, this patient most likely has which of the following?

A. Decreased energy harvest from food
B. Higher fasting-induced adipose factor expression
C. **Increased levels of Firmicutes in his gut**
D. Higher AMPK

(C) The gut microbiome has been studied as it relates to obesity and the effects of dieting. The two most common gut bacteria are Firmicutes and Bacteroides, comprising 92% of gut flora. In general, those who are leaner, such as his wife, have higher levels of Bacteroides and decreased levels of Firmicutes compared to someone affected by obesity. Interestingly, with weight loss, gut bacteria will alter (Firmicutes will decrease, while Bacteroides increases). These levels will also eventually resemble lean individuals in those who undergo gastric bypass. Compared to his lean wife, this patient likely **has higher Firmicutes levels.**

Note: In rat studies, increased calories were found in stool samples of lean rats, indicating that rats with obesity had increased calorie absorption (i.e., energy harvesting and complex carbohydrate absorption) compared to lean rats.

Gut bacteria outnumber the number of human cells; therefore, the gut microbiome is an intriguing research area related to obesity. Ongoing studies include the effects of fecal transplants, probiotics (active, good bacteria), and prebiotics (sugars that serve as food for good bacteria).

Memory aid: Firmicutes is proportionally increased in those with excess fat.

Reference: Clarke SF, Murphy EF, Nilaweera K, et al. The gut microbiota and its relationship to diet and obesity: new insights. Gut Microbes. 2012;3(3):186-202. doi:10.4161/gmic.20168

8. (Content: I-B-8) A research study is underway in which patients fast for 8 hours, followed by consuming a meal of 500 kcal. Several hormones are monitored every 2 hours during the fasting and postprandial period for 12 hours. Six hours into the fast, ghrelin hormone levels are at their peak. What other finding would most likely be present during this time?

A. Y1 and Y5 receptor stimulation
B. Leptin hormone elevation
C. Suppressed agouti-related peptide hormone levels
D. Activation of the POMC/CART pathway
E. Orexin A and B hormone suppression

(A) In periods of fasting, ghrelin levels increase, which activates the orexigenic pathway, with subsequent **Y1 and Y5 receptor stimulation** on the orexin/melanin-concentrating hormone second-order neuron. These second-order neurons signal other brain regions, leading to decreased energy expenditure and increased hunger.

Note: AgRP inhibits melanocortin (MC4) receptors
POMC: Proopiomelanocortin; **CART:** Cocaine and amphetamine-regulated transcript; **α-MSH:** α melanocyte-stimulating hormone; **MC3R/MC4R:** Melanocortin 3 and 4 receptors; **NPY:** Neuropeptide Y; **AgRP:** Agouti-related peptide; **MCH:** Melanin-concentrating hormone

Reference: Varela L, Horvath TL. Leptin and insulin pathways in POMC and AgRP neurons that modulate energy balance and glucose homeostasis. EMBO Rep. 2012;13(12):1079-1086. doi:10.1038/embor.2012.174

9. (Content: I-A-4) A 31-year-old female presents to her primary care physician for follow-up regarding weight-gain. Over the past three months, she has noticed a weight gain of approximately 10 pounds (4.5 kg), which is discouraging because she has been trying to get healthy and lose weight before her wedding in 2 months. She quit smoking with the help of bupropion and has been walking daily. She had a copper intrauterine device inserted four months ago. Although she goes to bed later due to wedding planning, she states she still sleeps 8 hours nightly. Which of the following is most likely playing a role in her weight gain?

A. Bupropion
B. Intrauterine device
C. **Decreased tobacco**
D. Sleep habits

(C) **Tobacco cessation** is a common cause for patients to gain weight. It is likely related to decreased metabolic rate, increased caloric intake, change in food preference, and increased lipoprotein lipase activity. In addition, nicotine has an appetite suppression component. The average weight gain is 4-5 kg, although nearly 10% gain over 13 kg after cessation. These effects are more common in women, nonwhites, and heavier smokers.

Note: Bupropion is an anti-depressant that is also used in smoking cessation. It has weight-negative properties.

Patients should be counseled on the possibility of weight gain while quitting tobacco and develop habits to mitigate this effect, including utilizing chewing gum. Compared to the often minimal weight gain, the long-term benefits of smoking cessation are more significant. Patients should be reminded of this and encouraged not to use weight gain as an excuse to delay smoking cessation.

Reference: Smoking cessation and weight gain. Filozof C, Fernández Pinilla MC, Fernández-Cruz A. Obes Rev. 2004;5(2):95
Reference: Smoking cessation, lung function, and weight gain: a follow-up study. Chinn S, Jarvis D, Melotti R, Luczynska C, Ackermann-Liebrich U, AntóJM, Cerveri I, de Marco R, Gislason T, Heinrich J, Janson C, Künzli N, Leynaert B, Neukirch F, Schouten J, Sunyer J, Svanes C, Vermeire P, Wjst M, Burney P Lancet. 2005;365(9471):1629.

10. (Content: I-C-2) Several medical students are trying to create a project to determine the best way to impact childhood obesity rates, as this rate has nearly tripled in the past 30 years. They begin to review epidemiologic data on a national level to see who is most affected by obesity prevalence, focusing on children 2-19 years old. They compare age, race, gender, and financial status. During their research, what are they most likely to find?

A. The highest prevalence of obesity is in Hispanic female children
B. Class 3 obesity in children has declined over the past decade
C. Asian adolescents had higher obesity rates than Hispanics
D. The highest income class had the lowest obesity rates
E. The prevalence of obesity was nearly 40% in all children

(D) Obesity affects nearly 20% of all children 2-19 years old. The prevalence is highest in those in the lowest (18.9%) and middle (19.9%) income levels, likely explained by the increased cost of healthy food and the lack of grocery stores in lower-income neighborhoods. In contrast, the **highest-income households had the lowest obesity rates (10.9%).**

The obesity epidemic disproportionately affects ethnic minorities, with African American girls and Hispanic boys having the highest prevalence. Class 3 obesity (140% of the 95th percentile BMI range) is growing most rapidly. Besides socioeconomic status and race, other risk factors are:

- Sedentary lifestyle and increased screen time
- Poorly balanced diet (sugary drinks, processed foods, etc.)
- Family history

The consequences of obesity are significant, ranging from psychiatric (depression, eating disorders), obstructive sleep apnea, gallstones, acid reflux, kidney stones, slipped capital femoral epiphysis, pseudotumor cerebri, hypertension, dyslipidemia, diabetes/insulin resistance, polycystic ovarian syndrome, metabolic syndrome, and intertrigo and/or candida skin infections to name a few.

Reference: CDC: https://www.cdc.gov/obesity/data/childhood.html#Prevalence (Accessed 12/11/2023)

11. (Content: I-B-4) A 19-year-old female presents to her family practice practitioner to request a referral to a lymphedema clinic. She states that since she was 15 years old, she has gained excessive weight, predominantly in her lower extremities. She says her grandmother had similar findings on her upper extremities after undergoing a mastectomy, and she was treated at a lymphedema clinic with good results. She has a normal waist circumference and a BMI of 26 kg/m². Her lower extremities have a sensation of round peas when the fatty tissue is palpated. What other findings would be expected in this patient?

    A. Decreased lymphatic flow
    B. Positive cuff sign
    C. Marked pitting edema
    D. Eventual progression to arms
    E. Positive Stemmer's sign

(B) This patient's presentation is classic for lipedema, which is abnormal subcutaneous fat deposition affecting the lower extremities; this is in contrast to lymphedema, which is a pathology of the lymphatic system (fluid), as seen in her grandmother. One differentiating physical exam finding is a **"cuff sign,"** **which occurs due to fat tissue overhanging the minimally involved feet.**

Lipedema treatment includes decongestive lymphatic therapy, exercise (aqua therapy), pain control, and potentially even surgery (liposuction).

Lymphedema versus Lipedema		
Condition	**Lymphedema**	**Lipedema**
Pathophysiology	Lymphatic pathology	Lipodystrophy
Demographics	Men and women, affecting any age	Women, between the ages of 15-30
Family history	Not common	Common
Physical findings	-Firm, with marked pitting edema -Stemmer's sign[1] -Foot involvement	Soft and minimally pitting, with a "round pea" sensation[2] -Cuff sign (foot spared)

[1]Negative Stemmer's sign occurs when you can grasp thin skin by pinching the upper surface of the second toe (lipedema). A positive test is when you can only grasp a lump of tissue (lymphedema), not the thin skin.
[2]Not to be confused with Dercum's disease with is painful lipomas affecting those with obesity

Reference: Okhovat JP, Alavi A. Lipedema: A Review of the Literature. Int J Low Extrem Wounds. 2015;14(3):262-267. doi:10.1177/153473461455428A

12. (Content: I-B-1) A 33-year-old female recently underwent a sleeve gastrectomy and is losing weight appropriately. She is most impressed by her decreased appetite, irrespective of meals, which has helped maintain a significant calorie deficit. The hormone most likely responsible for her decreased appetite initially acts on what area of the brain?

A. Dorsal vagal complex
B. Amygdala
C. Nucleus of the tractus solitarius
D. **Arcuate nucleus**
E. Lateral hypothalamus

(D) Sleeve gastrectomy, with the removal of up to 80% of the fundus of the stomach, reduces ghrelin levels, thereby significantly decreasing appetite via decreased activation of the NPY/AgRP orexigenic pathway. All peripheral hormones from the intestines and adipose tissue, as well as nutrients, act on first-order central neurons in the **arcuate nucleus of the hypothalamus.** These peripheral hormones either activate the weight-gaining (NPY/AgRP) or the weight-losing (POMC/CART) neuron systems.

The arcuate nucleus is the location of the first-order appetite neurons, which relay signals to second-order neurons deeper within the hypothalamus, ultimately activating or inhibiting certain regions of the brain to manage hunger and satiety.

Many peripheral hormones are affected after bariatric surgery. The predominant hormone impacting weight and appetite for the two most common bariatric surgeries are discussed below:

- **Gastric bypass:** Significant increase in GLP-1 (both basal levels and post-prandial), activating the POMC/CART anorexigenic pathway
- **Sleeve gastrectomy:** Significant decrease in ghrelin and increase in peptide YY (PYY), which <u>decreases</u> the activation of the NPY/AgRP orexigenic pathway

Reference: Ochner CN, Gibson C, Shanik M, Goel V, Geliebter A. Changes in neurohormonal gut peptides following bariatric surgery. Int J Obes (Lond). 2011;35(2):153-166. doi:10.1038/ijo.2010.132

13. (Content: I-D-1) A dietician is reviewing terminology with one of her students. She discusses a term that describes the value of the amount of a nutrient estimated to meet the requirement of half of all healthy individuals in a population. What term is she defining?

   A. **Estimated average requirement**
   B. Adequate intake
   C. Recommended daily allowance
   D. Tolerable upper intake level
   E. Daily value

(A) The definition of **estimated average requirements (EAR)** refers to the amount of a nutrient estimated to meet the requirement of half of all healthy individuals in the population.

Nutrient requirements and safety thresholds are commonly reported in terminology that must be understood. Some of these are discussed below:

- **Tolerable upper intake level (UL):** This is the highest intake of a nutrient that is likely to pose no risk of toxicity for almost all individuals.
- **Recommended dietary allowance (RDA):** This is the average daily dietary intake of a nutrient sufficient to meet the requirements of nearly all healthy persons within a particular population (age, gender, pregnancy, elderly, etc.).
- **Adequate intake (AI):** This definition is only used if an RDA cannot be determined. It is the recommended intake value based on observed or experimentally determined approximates for a group of healthy persons.
- **Daily value (DV):** A recommended amount an individual should consume for a specific nutrient (i.e., fat, calcium, etc.).

Reference: National Agricultural Library: U.S. Department of Agriculture

14. (Content: I-B-7) A human research study is ongoing and is recruiting patients with a body mass index > 30 kg/m^2 who have not previously been diagnosed with thyroid disease and do not have symptoms of overt hypothyroidism. Inclusion criteria requires a thyroid-stimulating hormone (TSH) level > 5 mcU/mL (reference range 0.4-4.2 mcU/mL). At the end of the study, 130 patients met the above criteria. The patients were then provided resources to assist in losing 5% of their total body weight. Which lab finding would be expected after they achieved their weight-loss goal?

    A. Increased thyroid-releasing hormone
    B. Increased T$_4$ (thyroxine) levels
    C. Decreased T$_3$ (triiodothyronine) levels
    D. Unchanged thyroid levels

(C) Leptin, produced by adipose tissue, is thought to play a role in thyroid hormone production and levels. It is theorized that leptin stimulates thyroid-releasing hormone, thereby stimulating thyroid-stimulating hormone and subsequent T$_4$ and T$_3$, acting similar to mild secondary hyperthyroidism- not subclinical hypothyroidism as previously thought. Therefore, with weight loss (decreased adipose tissue), the decreased leptin would reduce thyroid stimulation and **thus decrease thyroid hormone, including T$_3$ (triiodothyronine) levels.**

A study appears to confirm this theory. Participants lost 10% of their body weight, with a proportional decrease in T$_3$ levels. At their decreased weight, leptin was then exogenously administered, with a subsequent increase in T$_3$ levels, correlating to the notion that leptin (whether endogenous or exogenous) contributes to increased thyroid levels.

Note: Anorexic patients tend to have the lowest TSH and T$_3$ levels.

Reference: Rosenbaum M, Goldsmith R, Bloomfield D, et al. Low-dose leptin reverses skeletal muscle, autonomic, and neuroendocrine adaptations to maintenance of reduced weight. J Clin Invest. 2005;115(12):3579-3586. doi:10.1172/JCI25977
Reference: Blüher S, Mantzoros CS. Leptin in humans: lessons from translational research. Am J Clin Nutr. 2009;89(3):991S-997S. doi:10.3945/ajcn.2008.26788E

15. (Content: I-B-4) A 49-year-old male presents to the office to discuss weight-related complications. He states he was recently promoted to chief operating officer of a Fortune 500 company and the fear of messing up and losing the associated lifestyle, prestige, and salary is "driving me mad." Per chart review, it is noted that since starting this new position, he has gained nearly 45 lbs (20.4 kg). Compared to before the promotion and now, which hormonal change is most likely?

   A. Insulin sensitivity increase with glucagon suppression
   B. Activation of α-MSH and increased levels of leptin
   C. Poor quality of sleeping activating the POMC/CART pathway
   D. NPY activation related to excess cortisol section
   E. Suppressed ghrelin levels due to vagal nerve suppression

(D) Even in the absence of confirmed Cushing's disease, a pathologic hypercortisolism disease, patients with chronic stress have many similar pro-obesity hormonal changes. An elevated baseline stress level causes increased cortisol release and hyper-responsiveness to the hypothalamic-pituitary axis. This chronic state has been shown to increase the risk of both metabolic syndrome and heart disease.

Note: Acute stress (e.g. witnessing a trauma) activates the sympathetic system leading to a short-term decreased appetite in most patients.

Increased cortisol levels associated with the stressed state affect neuroendocrine hormones, including increasing insulin and leptin resistance. In addition, cortisol has a direct and indirect effect on the orexigenic pathway in the central nervous system, **leading to activation of the NPY/AgRP pathway.**

Not only does stress increase factors that play a role in promoting obesity, but obesity is a cause of stress for many patients. This cycle can feed into itself, synergistically having an impact on weight.

Treatment in this situation is focused on stress reduction. This could include reducing stressors, increasing wellness activities, therapy, and pursuing stress-relieving hobbies. If these are unlikely to improve symptoms long-term, career changes and more drastic measures may provide the best long-term medical benefits for the patient.

Reference: van der Valk, E.S., Savas, M. & van Rossum, E.F.C. Stress and Obesity: Are There More Susceptible Individuals?. Curr Obes Rep 7, 193–203 (2018). https://doi.org/10.1007/s13679-018-0306-y

16. (Content: I-C-1) A researcher is looking to evaluate different climates' effects on obesity rates. He believes warmer temperatures should allow more outdoor activity, thus lowering obesity rates. He wants to begin his research in the state with the lowest obesity rates. Which state should he start his research?

A. **Colorado**
B. Mississippi
C. Oklahoma
D. Florida
E. West Virginia

(A) Climate does not seem to play as strong of a role in decreasing obesity, although the landscape and outdoor activities may, to some extent. **Colorado** has consistently been one of the states with the lowest rate of obesity, while states in the Southeast tend to have the highest rate.

Obesity is the most common chronic disease in the U.S. with 42.4% of adults having obesity (BMI ≥ 30 kg/m²) and nearly 73.6% meeting the criteria for overweight or obesity (BMI ≥ 25 kg/m²).

The image below shows the percent of self-reported obesity data for the United States from the 2022 BRFSS data (most up-to-date information as of 12/2023).

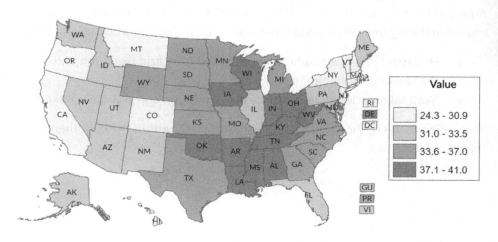

Note: The NHANES survey does in-person weighing (smaller cohort) and is considered more accurate compared to the BRFSS survey, which is self-reported over the phone, and tends to under-report weight.

Reference: https://www.cdc.gov/obesity/data/prevalence-maps.html (Accessed 12/11/2023)

17. (Content: I-B-6) An endocrinologist is discussing with a medical student the vast number of hormones that play a role in obesity and satiety. In particular, one hormone is an insulin sensitizer, in which levels are inversely related to body fat mass. In addition, the endogenous levels of this hormone decrease in the setting of type 2 diabetes. The hormone described above most likely originates from which of the following structures?

A. **Adipose tissue**
B. Gastric fundus
C. Duodenum
D. Beta cells of the pancreas
E. Alpha cells of the pancreas

(A) Adiponectin is exclusively produced in the **white adipose tissue;** it is the most abundantly produced and secreted hormone from this tissue. Its levels increase in the setting of lower weight and decrease in the context of high body fat composition. Also, adiponectin levels are strongly inversely related to systemic inflammation and insulin resistance.

Note: Amylin is secreted by the beta islet cells of the pancreas and is co-secreted with insulin. In type 2 diabetes, insulin and amylin levels are increased, although they are less effective (i.e., resistance).

Adiponectin has many different effects on different organs, with the most important being related to insulin management, as discussed below:

- **Hepatic:** Enhances insulin sensitivity and fatty acid oxidation and decreases gluconeogenesis
- **Skeletal muscle:** Increases fatty acid oxidation and glucose uptake

Also, adiponectin reduces inflammation, particularly within the endothelium of the vasculature.

Reference: Erin E. Kershaw, Jeffrey S. Flier, Adipose Tissue as an Endocrine Organ, The Journal of Clinical Endocrinology & Metabolism, Volume 89, Issue 6, 1 June 2004, Pages 2548–2556, https://doi.org/10.1210/jc.2004-0395

18. (Content: I-A- 2) A grandmother brings her 9-year-old granddaughter for a wellness visit. The grandmother gained full custody when the child's parents were incarcerated for child neglect and physical abuse. The child is reserved and demonstrates poor eye contact. The child's growth chart is in the 87th percentile for weight based on age and gender. Which of the following is the most appropriate advice to provide to the grandmother?

    A. Now that the homelife is stabilized, her weight should improve
    B. The child should be monitored for anorexia given life stressors
    C. The child is at risk for developing obesity given her parent's actions
    D. Enrollment in social sports like basketball will be beneficial
    E. Trazodone may help with depression symptoms and improve sleep

(C) This patient has experienced multiple adverse child events (ACEs) that **increase the risk of health problems including obesity** both now, and for many years to come. Treatment should be focused on promoting safe and nurturing family relationships by teaching resilience. In addition, recovery from these events will likely require therapy to promote healing from the trauma.

The presence of ≥ 2 early ACEs correlated with an increased risk of obesity later in childhood and adolescence. The excess stress related to ACEs may contribute to maladaptive coping (e.g., binge eating, eating for comfort) and poor sleep hygiene. In addition, weight gain may be a protective measure used by abuse victims in order to prevent further abuse.

In particular, the following ACEs have a higher correlation with causing obesity:

- Death of a parent
- Family economic hardship
- Sexual abuse
- Witnessing domestic violence
- Physical abuse

Other ACEs include emotional abuse, neglect (both emotional and physical), and household dysfunction including incarcerated parents, substance abuse, untreated mental illness in the family, and parental divorce.

Reference: Schroeder K, Schuler BR, Kobulsky JM, Sarwer DB. The association between adverse childhood experiences and childhood obesity: A systematic review. Obes Rev. 2021 Jul;22(7):e13204. doi: 10.1111/obr.13204. Epub 2021 Jan 27. PMID: 33506595; PMCID: PMC8192341.
Reference: Obesity Medicine Association: Pediatric Obesity Algorithm (2023-2024)

19. (Content: I-A-3) A pediatric patient presents for genetic testing regarding an abnormal appetite. The patient is described as having a small head size with narrow hands and feet. The patient's mouth is open and eyebrows are thickened. Which of the following is the most likely etiology of his findings?

    A. Prader-Willi syndrome
    B. Borjeson-Forssman-Lehmann syndrome
    C. MC4R deficiency
    D. Trisomy of chromosome 21
    E. Cohen syndrome

(E) **Cohen syndrome** is caused by an 8q22 mutation leading to a small head size, narrow hands and feet, joint hypermobility, "open mouth" expression, low white blood cell count (neutropenia), retinal dystrophy, and thick hair and eyebrows.

Patients with Cohen syndrome often have central adiposity with thinner arms and legs. Other characteristics include a cheerful and easygoing disposition, hearing deficiencies, and possible seizures.

Note: Children with developmental delays may have an increased risk of obesity attributed to dysregulated appetites, being placed on weight-promoting medications, food sensitivity/selectivity issues, physical activity limitations, and are more prone to receiving food as rewards.

The table below displays a memory aid of the characteristic findings of Cohen syndrome.

Cohen Syndrome (Memory Aid)	
C	**C**ognition (intellectual disability with microcephaly) and facial **C**ountenance (facial findings showing a prominent nasal bridge, thick hair and eyebrows, widely-spaced central incisors, small jaw, high palate, and narrow sloping forehead), **C**heerful
O	**O**pen-mouth expression
H	**H**ypotonia and joint **H**ypermobility, **H**ands narrowed, **H**earing deficiencies
E	**E**ye abnormalities: myopia, retinal dystrophy, and strabismus
N	**N**eutropenia (low white book cell count)

Reference: Wang H, Falk MJ, Wensel C, et al. Cohen Syndrome. 2006 Aug 29 [Updated 2016 Jul 21]. In: Adam MP, Mirzaa GM, Pagon RA, et al., editors. GeneReviews® [Internet]. Seattle (WA): University of Washington, Seattle; 1993-2023. Available from: https://www.ncbi.nlm.nih.gov/books/NBK1482/

20. (Content: I-B-4) A 44-year-old male with a past medical history of insomnia presents for an annual wellness exam. He denies any current complaints, but does admit to right knee pain that is worsened with prolonged walking. He has a moderate score on the Epworth sleepiness scale. His body mass index is 31 kg/m², his waist circumference is 81.3 cm (32 inches), and his body fat composition is 24%. Laboratory work, including a hemoglobin A1c, complete metabolic panel, and lipid panel, is unremarkable. An x-ray of his right knee shows moderate osteophytes and joint space narrowing. Which of the following best describes his condition?

A. Sick fat disease
B. Obesity class II
C. Obesity based on % body fat
D. **Fat mass disease**
E. Abdominal obesity

(D) This patient's knee osteoarthritis and moderate probability of obstructive sleep apnea are direct effects of his excess body weight, causing increased mechanical forces. This is consistent with **fat mass disease**.

Both fat mass disease and sick fat disease (adiposopathy) are pathogenic components of obesity. Fat mass refers to the mechanical forces acting on the body, whereas sick fat disease refers to the inflammatory/hormonal effects.

Other components that may be seen in fat mass disease are listed below:

- Heart failure with a preserved ejection fraction
- Obesity hypoventilation syndrome (external restrictive lung disease)
- Thrombotic events due to tissue compression of the pelvic floor and lower extremities which directly impairs venous return
- Hypertension due to perivascular adipose tissue restricting vessel wall expansion

Often, comorbidities of obesity have a component of both sick fat disease and fat mass, which are not mutually exclusive.

Reference: De Lorenzo A, Soldati L, Sarlo F, Calvani M, Di Lorenzo N, Di Renzo L. New obesity classification criteria as a tool for bariatric surgery indication. World J Gastroenterol. 2016;22(2):681-703. doi:10.3748/wjg.v22.i2.681

21. (Content: I-A-3) A 6-year-old male is being seen by a pediatric endocrinologist for severe obesity. The mother states that the patient had a normal birth weight and even required nutrient supplementation due to failure to thrive early on. However, since age three, he has had extreme hunger, which has led to progressive weight gain. The child currently weighs 178 lbs (80.7 kg). A genetic mutation is discovered, and subsequent treatment with hormone replacement is initiated with impressive results. Which of the following neuromodulators was most likely activated with the hormone replacement?

A. Orexin A and B
B. **Alpha melanocyte-stimulating hormone**
C. Agouti-related peptide
D. Melanin-concentrating hormone

(B) This patient's findings are most consistent with leptin deficiency, an infrequent genetic cause of secondary obesity due to a mutation of the LEP gene. Treatment with exogenous leptin causes drastic weight loss by activating the anorexigenic pathway, which stimulates different **neurotransmitters and neuromodulators, including α-MSH,** thus leading to satiety.

Neurotransmitters Associated with Hunger/Satiety	
Orexigenic	**Anorexigenic**
-Neuropeptide Y (NPY)[1] -Agouti-related peptide (AgRP)[1] -Orexin A and B[2] -Melanin-concentrating hormone[2]	-Proopiomelanocortin (POMC)[3] -Cocaine and amphetamine regulated transcript (CART)[3] -α-Melanocyte-stimulating hormone -Serotonin

[1]Inhibited by insulin, leptin, PYY, and serotonin
[2]Inhibited by leptin, stimulated by NPY/AgRP
[3]Inhibited by NPY and GABA, stimulated by serotonin, leptin, and insulin

Reference: Varela L, Horvath TL. Leptin and insulin pathways in POMC and AgRP neurons that modulate energy balance and glucose homeostasis. EMBO Rep. 2012;13(12):1079-1086. doi:10.1038/embor.2012.174
Reference: Up to Date: "Physiology of leptin"

22. (Content: I-B-1) Researchers are looking at potential intravenous medications to assist with weight loss. One treatment that has shown promise is a synthetic form of a gastrointestinal hormone produced in both the large and small intestines and rectum and is found to be elevated within 1 hour after meals. Its contributions to weight loss are due to its potent appetite suppressant effect and ability to delay gastric emptying and intestinal transit time. The hormone level increases irrespective of macronutrient intake. What is the hormone most likely being studied?

A. Ghrelin
B. Cholecystokinin
C. Glucagon-like peptide 1
D. Oxyntomodulin
E. Peptide YY

(E) In clinical research, **peptide YY (PYY)** is being studied as a pharmacologic therapy for obesity. Daily intravenous infusions show decreased appetite and short-term weight loss. This endogenous hormone is usually produced and secreted from the distal small bowel, colon, and rectum, acting as a natural potent appetite suppressant. In addition, it delays gastric and intestinal motility.

Note: Thus far, intranasal and oral formulations of synthetic PYY have been unsuccessful in leading to prolonged weight loss.

Most anorexigenic hormones have been or are currently being studied for pharmaceutical-targeting therapy. Oxyntomodulin is still under investigation, while cholecystokinin has been ineffective long-term due to tachyphylaxis.

Glucagon-like peptide 1 (GLP-1) has been one of the most successful pharmacologic anorexigenic hormones causing weight loss thus far. While all formulations are used for diabetes management, two GLP-1 receptor agonist monotherapies are explicitly FDA-approved for weight loss: liraglutide (Saxenda®) and semaglutide (Wegovy®). More recently, a GLP-1/GIP dual incretin injectable medication (Zepbound®) was approved for obesity management in 2023, having only been FDA-approved for diabetes mellitus type 2 (Mounjaro®) the year prior.

Reference: Daily, intermittent intravenous infusion of peptide YY(3-36) reduces daily food intake and adiposity in rats. Prasanth K. Chelikani, Alvin C. Haver, Joseph R. Reeve Jr., David A. Keire, and Roger D. Reidelberger 01 Feb 2006; https://doi.org/10.1152/ajpregu.00674.2005

23. (Content: I-A-4) A previously healthy 9-year-old female presents to her pediatrician for a well-child check. Her growth chart is shown below. Her percentile BMI has steadily increased over the last four visits despite lifestyle changes incorporated within her family. She has breast bud development. Which of the following conditions may be contributing to these findings?

A. Excessive caloric intake
B. Precocious puberty
C. Bulimia
D. Achondroplasia
E. Hypothyroidism

(E) This patient presents with increased weight despite decreased linear bone growth or linear bone growth arrest, which is concerning for an endocrinopathy such as **hypothyroidism.**

In contrast to children with excess weight due to increased caloric intake, those with endocrinopathies such as hypercortisolism (i.e., Cushing syndrome) or thyroid disorders will significantly increase weight compared to height. This mismatch should prompt further evaluation with consideration of the following labs:

- TSH and free T_4
- Dexamethasone suppression test and 24-hour urine cortisol

In contrast, excessive caloric intake and precocious puberty tend to cause accelerated linear bone growth proportionate to weight gain. Although syndromic obesity could cause decreased bone growth, excessive weight gain usually occurs earlier and is often accompanied by developmental delay. Also, remember that MC4R deficiency (monogenic obesity) causes tall stature.

Reference: Obesity Medicine Association: Pediatric Obesity Algorithm (2023-2024)

24. (Content: I-A-1) A 7-year-old female presents with her mother for a dietician evaluation and education session. The family drinks a lot of sweetened tea in the home and inquires about changing from sugar to nonnutritive sweeteners (NNS). The best response to her inquiry would be that NNS

    A. are a preferred alternative to sucrose
    B. increase the risk of ADHD in children
    C. may help with weight loss, as they are calorie-neutral
    D. can cause a dysregulation in appetite
    E. are regarded as "not safe for children" by the FDA

(D) Although nonnutritive sweeteners (NNS) seem like a good alternative on the surface level as a caloric-neutral option, they should be used cautiously, as some are up to 20,000 times sweeter than natural sugar (i.e., sucrose). This can lead **to a dysregulation in appetite**, especially in children, leading to craving and preferring sweeter tasting foods.

Although deemed safe by the Food and Drug Administration (FDA), NNS tend to promote dietary preferences for sweet foods, often leading to calorie-dense foods that promote weight gain. Therefore, NNS are generally not considered effective for weight loss.

Contrary to initial concerns, NNS are not associated with children developing ADHD, psychiatric conditions, congenital disabilities, malignancies, or autoimmune conditions when exposed as a child or in utero.

Note: In 2023, the World Health Organization (WHO) released a guideline advising not to use NNS for weight control, except for those with diabetes. The WHO noted high intake of NSS were associated with higher risks of strokes, hypertension, and cancer (particularly saccharin increasing the risk of bladder cancer).

Reference: Use of non-sugar sweeteners: WHO guideline. Geneva: World Health Organization; 2023. Licence: CC BY-NC-SA 3.0 IGO
Reference: Obesity Medicine Association: Pediatric Obesity Algorithm (2023-2024)

25. (Content: I-A-3) A 5-year-old male with the disease of obesity is seen in the pediatric clinic for follow-up after meeting with a childhood obesity specialist. The patient has had many difficulties, including significant intellectual disability, retinal dystrophy, and polydactyly. Renal malformations have led to polyuria and polydipsia, requiring a percutaneous endoscopic gastrostomy tube to be placed to keep up with fluid replenishment. Given these findings, the patient most likely carries which of the following diagnoses?

    A. Prader-Willi syndrome
    B. Cohen syndrome
    C. Borjeson-Forssman-Lehmann syndrome
    D. Albright hereditary osteodystrophy
    E. Bardet-Biedl syndrome

(E) All of the above syndromes are associated with genetic mutations that lead to obesity and intellectual disability. However, autosomal recessive **Bardet-Biedl syndrome (BBS)** is also characterized by microorchidism (men), retinal dystrophy, polydactyly, renal malformations, polyuria, and polydipsia. It is the second most common cause of syndromic obesity. Ciliary dysfunction with impaired signaling leads to many of the characteristic findings of BBS.

The other obesity-related genetic syndromic causes associated with concurrent intellectual disability are as follows:

- **Prader-Willi:** Not inherited; loss of function on chromosome 15. Hypotonia with poor suck in neonatal period. Hyperphagia, short stature, "almond-shaped" eyes. It is the most common syndromal cause of genetic obesity followed by BBS.
- **Albright Hereditary Osteodystrophy:** Short stature, round face, pseudohypoparathyroidism, shortened fourth metacarpals
- **Cohen syndrome:** Autosomal recessive. Small head size, narrow hands and feet, joint hypermobility, "open mouth" expression, low white blood cell count, retinal dystrophy, thick hair and eyebrows
- **Borgeson-Forssman-Lehmann Syndrome:** X-linked (males), seizures, large earlobes, short toes, gynecomastia, and small genitals

Note: Be familiar with the genetic patterns (i.e., autosomal dominant, autosomal recessive, X-linked, etc.) of obesity. These will show up on test day!

Reference: Up To Date: "Genetic contribution and pathophysiology of obesity"

26. (Content: I-B-7) A research lab is performing studies on hormonally active tissue. In the study, tissue is obtained from pathological specimens upon autopsy. One tissue biopsy displays resistin, interleukin 6, and estrogen. Which of the following tissues did this biopsy most likely come from?

    A. Ovaries
    B. Lymph nodes
    C. Adrenal glands
    D. Adipose
    E. Intestines

(D) **Adipose tissue** is very hormonally active, with over 600 adipokines identified, with some summarized below:

- Adiponectin: Promotes insulin sensitivity and has anti-inflammatory effects. This is the most abundant adipose-derived hormone.
- Leptin: Regulates hunger and satiety
- Resistin: Involved in insulin resistance and inflammation
- Interleukins, prostaglandins, and cytokines: Pro-inflammatory
- Estrogen: Sex hormone that increases malignancy risk (specifically breast and endometrial), and also affects fertility/ menstrual cycles.
- Angiotensinogen: Increases blood pressure
- PAI-1: Inhibitor of fibrinolysis, thereby increasing risk of blood clots

Image citation: Modified from VectorStock (image license purchased)
Reference: Richard AJ, White U, Elks CM, et al. Adipose Tissue: Physiology to Metabolic Dysfunction. [Updated 2020 Apr 4]. In: Feingold KR, Anawalt B, Blackman MR, et al., editors. Endotext [Internet]. South Dartmouth (MA): MDText.com, Inc.; 2000-. Available from: https://www.ncbi.nlm.nih.gov/books/NBK555602/

27. (Content: I-B-3) A 26-year-old patient is frustrated that they have been diagnosed with obesity based on a body mass index (BMI) of 31 kg/m^2. She is an active bodybuilder and has competed in several national championships. Which of the following is the best response to her concerns?

A. You meet the diagnostic criteria for obesity
B. I want to order a CT scan to see if you meet criteria for obesity
C. **The BMI is a useful screening test for most patients**
D. Body mass index has been determined to be an inaccurate tool
E. Would it be alright if I discussed some ways to improve your health?

(C) BMI is a screening tool for obesity, but cannot determine body composition including the percentage of body fat. In this muscular patient, BMI, which accounts for only weight and height, does not take into account lean body mass. The American Medical Association (AMA) recently adopted a new policy recognizing the limitations of BMI and encouraging it to be used in conjunction with other measures such as waist circumference (although limited data in pediatrics available), visceral fat, body composition, and genetic or metabolic factors.

In addition, BMI may over/under-represent adiposity in certain ethnic and racial groups, as cut-off values are based on primarily Caucasian individuals. Regardless, even with its limitations, **in the general population BMI correlates with the amount of fat mass**, but it should not be used as the sole criterion to determine obesity in all individuals. BMI should also not be solely used as the cut-off to deny appropriate therapy to individuals.

The AMA supports alternative measures for diagnosing obesity where available and promotes further research in this area, especially as it relates to pediatrics. BMI is unlikely to be replaced anytime soon given its ease of reproducibility, lack of cost to obtain, and insurance and guideline-based therapy directly related to BMI values. However, an understanding of its limitations, and seeking out alternative measures in appropriate individuals is vital to avoid misrepresentation of patients' risk factors.

Reference: AMA: Use of BMI alone is an imperfect clinical measure by Sara Berg, MS. https://www.ama-assn.org/delivering-care/public-health/ama-use-bmi-alone-imperfect-clinical-measure
Reference: AMA adopts new policy clarifying role of BMI as a measure in medicine. https://www.ama-assn.org/press-center/press-releases/ama-adopts-new-policy-clarifying-role-bmi-measure-medicine

28. (Content: I-B-5) A previously healthy 29-year-old male with a diagnosis of obesity presents to the clinic for a physical examination. He is an accountant and thus is relatively inactive during the day. Vital signs are within normal limits. His BMI is 35 kg/m². He is frustrated that despite exercising and eating similarly to his identical twin brother, he is nearly 40 lbs (18.1 kg) heavier than his brother, who is a mail carrier. Which of the following best explains the weight difference between him and his twin brother?

    A. Basal metabolic rate
    B. Non-exercise activity thermogenesis
    C. Intentional exercise
    D. Resting energy expenditure
    E. Dietary thermogenesis

(B) **Non-exercise activity thermogenesis (NEAT)** is the energy expended for everything that does not include sleeping, eating, or dedicated physical exercise. For this patient, given other similar variables, his sedentary work (accountant) compared to his brother's occupation (mail carrier) most likely explains the difference in energy expenditure and weight differences.

NEAT includes many daily activities, ranging from yard work to fidgeting. These cumulative events increase metabolic rate substantially, impacting an individual's non-resting energy needs (150-500 kcal/day), and may explain the difference in weight amongst individuals. NEAT can vary significantly between individuals (several-fold), whereas the thermic effect of meals displays minimal variability.

In order to increase NEAT in individuals, a pedometer can be used to monitor and encourage increased daily steps.

- < 5000 steps daily is considered sedentary (average for a US adult)
- 5000-7500 steps daily is low active
- 7500-1000 steps daily is somewhat active
- > 10,000 steps daily is considered active

In addition to helping with weight, increased NEAT also reduces the risk of cardiovascular disease compared to those with a more sedentary lifestyle.

References: Non-exercise activity thermogenesis (NEAT). Author: Levine, James. MD, PhD. Best Practice and Research Clinical Endocrinology and Metabolism. 2002 Dec; 16 (4):679-702.

29. (Content: I-D-1) On a medical mission trip, a 7-year-old patient is being seen in the clinic. He appears very malnourished, but he seems unphased by his lack of nutrition. His abdomen is distended, and anasarca is present. He is supplemented with low doses of protein in incremental amounts to prevent refeeding syndrome. Which of the following must be consumed in his diet, as his body cannot produce it?

A. Alanine
B. Aspartate
C. Glycine
D. Leucine
E. Proline

(D) This patient is presenting with Kwashiorkor, a severe <u>protein</u> malnourishment (not <u>total calorie</u> deficiency). The question essentially asks which of the above is an essential amino acid. Of the options, only **leucine** is considered an essential amino acid.

Severe malnutrition can be differentiated into the following:

- **Marasmus:** Total calorie deficit. Emaciated, irritable, thin sparse hair, low weight, no edema.
- **Kwashiorkor:** Protein deficiency, weight variable, anasarca with ascites, typically apathetic, stripes in the hair (flag sign).

The table summarizes the amino acids.

Amino Acids			
Essential Amino Acids[1]		**Non-essential Amino Acids**	
-Histidine	-Phenylalanine	-Alanine	-Glutamine
-Isoleucine	-Threonine	-Arginine	-Glycine
-Leucine	-Tryptophan	-Asparagine	-Ornithine
-Lysine[2]	**-Valine**	-Aspartate	-Proline
-Methionine		-Cysteine	-Serine
		-Glutamate	-Tyrosine

[1]Must be consumed (the human body cannot make them)
[2]Lysine deficiency is relatively common in vegans.
Bolded amino acids are branch-chain amino acids.

Memory aid of Essential Amino Acids: PVT TIM HaLL (Private Tim Hall)

Reference: Up to Date: "Malnutrition in children in resource-limited countries: Clinical assessment"

174

30. (Content: I-A-5) A researcher is trying to create a calculator that will take into account epigenetic factors contributing to childhood obesity rates to predict which children are most prone to obesity. He plans to have a smartphone application that contains a checklist of risk factors for childhood obesity, thus providing a percent risk of obesity based on current risk factors. Practitioners would then be able to discuss with the parents how reducing certain risk factors could improve the odds of a healthy weight in their children. Which of the following should be taken into account for his predictive calculator?

    A.   Kids have similar obesity rates whether one/both parents have obesity
    B.   A cesarean delivery increases the child's risk of obesity
    C.   Maternal smoking leads to decreased childhood obesity rates
    D.   Breastfed infants have fewer infections but increased obesity rates
    E.   Insufficient gestational weight gain is protective against obesity

(B) Epigenetics is the study of changes caused by gene expression rather than the genetic code (i.e., how the environment affects people). Many correlations have been discovered between childhood obesity and maternal and early infancy environment. Of the above, **newborns delivered via cesarean section are linked with a future increased childhood obesity rate.**

Other significant correlations that increase childhood obesity rates are:

- Maternal insulin resistance and increased preconception BMI
- Both extremes of gestational weight
- Tobacco abuse during pregnancy
- Premature infants
- Bottle-fed (compared to breast-fed) due to lack of self-regulation
- Parents: 1 with obesity (3x risk), both with obesity (10x risk)

Note: After the age of 6, an individual's personal weight becomes a stronger predictor of their adult weight. Conversely, prior to the age of 6, parental weight serves as a more indicative factor for the potential development of obesity.

In addition, many studies on the neonatal intestinal microbiome are underway, including the association of C-sections with infants having higher maternal skin microbes in the gut versus vaginal delivery.

Reference: Obesity Medicine Association: Pediatric Obesity Algorithm (2023-2024)

31. (Content: I-D-2) A 36-year-old female status post sleeve gastrectomy six years prior presents to her primary care physician complaining of numbness in her lower extremities. She has lost 120 lbs (54.4 kg) postoperatively. She is currently taking prenatal vitamins. Physical examination reveals diminished vibratory sense bilaterally in her lower extremities and a positive Romberg test. What is the most likely underlying cause of this patient's clinical presentation?

A. **Decreased intrinsic factor production**
B. Anti-parietal antibodies
C. Tissue transglutaminase antibodies
D. Impaired terminal ileum absorption
E. Decreased dietary intake

(A) This patient is presenting with subacute combined degeneration consistent with the diagnosis of vitamin B_{12} deficiency. The most likely cause is related to her sleeve gastrectomy. Vitamin B_{12} is absorbed in the terminal ileum, with assistance from the co-factor intrinsic factor, which is produced by parietal cells in the stomach. After a sleeve gastrectomy (80% stomach resection), a majority of these parietal cells are also resected, thus **decreasing intrinsic factor production.**

B_{12} deficiency is relatively uncommon in those with normal dietary intake. Some common causes of cyanocobalamin deficiency (B_{12}) are listed below:

- **Pernicious anemia:** Autoimmune condition that leads to antibodies directed at parietal cells, leading to decreased intrinsic factor.
- **Medications:** Metformin (long-term use) interferes with B_{12} absorption in the ileum, and proton pump inhibitors decrease acid secretion.
- **Vegans:** Insufficient supplementation, as B_{12} is usually found in animal protein. This takes years to develop.
- **Malabsorption:** Inflammation that affects the terminal ileum, such as celiac disease (tissue transglutaminase antibodies) or Crohn's disease, can prevent the absorption of B_{12}.

Reference: Up to Date: "Causes and pathophysiology of vitamin B_{12} and folate deficiencies"

32. (Content: I-A-4) A 29-year-old professional bull rider sustained a significant head injury during one of his performances. He is intubated and undergoes imaging showing a right frontal head injury with cerebral edema. After a prolonged recovery period he is finally discharged from an inpatient rehab facility. His wife notices that he no longer enjoys her cooking, but rather wishes to discuss gourmet dishes and their intricacies from different television shows he now watches. Which of the following conditions is most consistent with his presentation?

    A. Gilbert's syndrome
    B. Gourmand syndrome
    C. Gorlin syndrome
    D. Gardner syndrome
    E. Gilles de la Tourette syndrome

(B) **Gourmand syndrome** is a unique and rare condition that arises due to an injury affecting the right frontal lobe. Patients with this particular injury become obsessed with fine foods, often fixating on them in writing, reading, and discussions.

This syndrome is considered benign and affects those with lesions affecting the right anterior cerebral hemisphere, which is associated with impulse control. It often occurs months after an injury, and is similar, but more specific in its manifestations, to an addictive or obsessive-compulsive disorder. It was first recognized and studied in 1997, with only 36 people officially being diagnosed with this syndrome.

Reference: Regard M, Landis T. "Gourmand syndrome": eating passion associated with right anterior lesions. Neurology. 1997 May;48(5):1185-90. doi: 10.1212/wnl.48.5.1185. PMID: 9153440.

33. (Content: I-B-5) A patient is enrolled in a research study determining which variables have the strongest alterations on resting energy expenditure. Indirect calorimetry is performed weekly, with different variables changed prior to undergoing the study. The initial baseline calorimetry reading the week prior at rest, supine, and in a dark room showed a resting energy expenditure of 1750 kcal/day. Today, it showed 2300 kcal/day. Which of the following performed prior to testing caused this discrepancy?

    A. Fasting for 48 hours
    B. Taking sodium bicarbonate tablets
    C. Exercise
    D. Ice bath

(C) Numerous variables can affect the measurement of resting energy expenditure (REE), which is determined by indirect calorimetry. Of the options, all would decrease REE except for **exercising** prior to testing.

REE is determined by the abbreviated Weir Equation

- Resting Energy Expenditure = VO_2 + VCO_2

Therefore, any increase in oxygen consumption (VO_2) or carbon dioxide production (VCO_2) would increase REE.

Resting Energy Expenditure (REE) Variables	
Increases REE	**Decreases REE**
Elevated VCO_2 and RQ	**Decreased VCO_2 and RQ**
• Metabolic acidosis	• Metabolic alkalosis
• Hyperventilation	• Hypoventilation
• Excessive carbohydrate intake	• Starvation/ketosis
• Hypermetabolism	• Hypometabolism
Elevate VO_2	**Decreased VO_2**
• Hyperthermia	• Hypothermia
• Shivering & excess movement	• Hypothyroidism
• Overfeeding	• Fasting/starvation
• Exercise	• Paralysis

VO_2 = oxygen uptake/consumption; VCO_2 = Carbon dioxide production/elimination

Reference: Mtaweh H, Tuira L, Floh AA, Parshuram CS. Indirect Calorimetry: History, Technology, and Application. Front Pediatr. 2018 Sep 19;6:257. doi: 10.3389/fped.2018.00257. PMID: 30283765; PMCID: PMC6157446.

34. (Content: I-E-1) A patient presents to an exercise physiologist to discuss different workout routines. The physiologist discusses different exercise options and their effect on excess post-exercise oxygen consumption (EPOC). Which of the following would have the highest levels of EPOC?

    A. Bicep curls
    B. Aerobic exercise
    C. Muscle strengthening
    D. High-intensity interval training
    E. Yoga

(D) EPOC is a term that reflects the oxygen consumption after a workout is completed. In other words, it is the post-exercise energy required to bring your body back into a baseline resting metabolic rate and includes muscle repair, lactate removal, energy storage replenishment, and removal of waste products. At the conclusion of a workout, although breathing and heart rate slow down, they will not reach a nadir until the body has recovered.

EPOC, also referred to as "afterburn", is highest among anaerobic activity, of which the most lactate in the muscle is produced. The highest levels therefore are seen in those engaging in **high-intensity interval training (HIIT)**, especially if more muscle groups are utilized.

Caloric expenditure of up to 15% of the HIIT workout is expended on EPOC. Thus, if 300 kcal are burned during a workout, up to 45 additional kcal will be consumed during EPOC.

Reference: Jung WS, Hwang H, Kim J, Park HY, Lim K. Effect of interval exercise versus continuous exercise on excess post-exercise oxygen consumption during energy-homogenized exercise on a cycle ergometer. J Exerc Nutrition Biochem. 2019 Jun 30;23(2):45-50. doi: 10.20463/jenb.2019.0016. PMID: 31337205; PMCID: PMC6651650.
Reference: Arney, Blaine E. M.S., ACSM-EP; Foster, Carl Ph.D., FACSM, MAACVPR; Porcari, John Ph.D., FACSM, MAACVPR, ACSM-RCEP. EPOC: IS IT REAL? DOES IT MATTER?. ACSM's Health & Fitness Journal 23(4):p 9-13, 7/8 2019. DOI: 10.1249/FIT.0000000000000487

35. (Content: I-A-3) A 15-year-old male presents for an annual physical exam. The patient has hearing loss requiring a cochlear implant and visual impairment. In addition, the patient has type 2 diabetes mellitus. A recent echocardiogram displayed worsening dilated cardiomyopathy. His younger brother has similar findings. The patient's growth chart reveals severe obesity. The condition is most likely due to which of the following genetic abnormalities?

A. **ALMS 1 mutation**
B. Chromosome 11p15.5 dysregulation
C. X-linked inheritance
D. Genetic imprinting
E. MC4R mutation

(A) This patient with intellectual disability, dilated cardiomyopathy, insulin resistance, and hearing impairment with an endocrinopathy most likely has Alstrom syndrome, an autosomal recessive condition caused by an **ALMS 1 mutation.**

Alstrom syndrome is a rare condition that often leads to early-onset obesity. Similar to other syndromic causes of obesity, phenotype variability is commonly present.

The other choices and their associated condition are listed below:

- Chromosome 11p15.5 dysregulation: Beckwith-Wiedemann syndrome
- X-linked: Fragile X syndrome and Wilson-Turner syndrome
- Genetic imprinting: Prader-Willi syndrome
- MC4R mutation: MC4R deficiency

The table below contains the most common associations noted with Alstrom syndrome in a mnemonic format:

Alstrom Syndrome Memory Aid (ALMS 1)	
A	Autosomal recessive with an **A**LMS 1 mutation, **A**nosmia
L	**L**oss of vision with retinal dystrophy
M	Cardio**M**yopathy (dilated) leading to heart failure
S	**S**ensorineural hearing loss, **S**hort stature
1	**1**ntelectual disability with cognitive impairment

Reference: Marshall JD, Maffei P, Collin GB, Naggert JK. Alström syndrome: genetics and clinical overview. Curr Genomics. 2011 May;12(3):225-35. doi: 10.2174/138920211795677912. PMID: 22043170; PMCID: PMC3137007.

36. (Content: I-B-1) A 31-year-old female presents to her dietician's office five months after undergoing a sleeve gastrectomy. During this period, she has lost 43 lbs (19.5 kg) and is encouraged and motivated to continue working toward weight loss. She has followed all dietary recommendations and vitamin replacement. What is the most accurate statement regarding the hormone most affected by this surgery, contributing to her weight loss?

    A. Patients with Prader-Willi syndrome have normal levels
    B. Those with a vagotomy would have similar qualitative levels
    C. Glucose suppresses the hormone for extended periods
    D. Sleep deprivation reduces this hormone, while stress increases it
    E. Leptin levels are directly proportionate to this hormone

(B) Ghrelin is the only gastrointestinal orexigenic hormone. It is made in the gastric fundus and body, as well as the proximal small intestines. A large portion of the cells that secrete this hormone during a sleeve gastrectomy are removed, leading to decreased ghrelin levels. This **decrease is also seen in those who have undergone a vagotomy,** which inhibits ghrelin production.

Ghrelin increases hunger by stimulating the orexigenic pathway through NPY/AgRP receptors in the central nervous system and, to some extent, through the vagal nerve. Important characteristics of Ghrelin are discussed below.

Characteristics of Ghrelin	
Factors that ↑ levels	An empty stomach, fasting, weight loss, stress, sleep deprivation, Prader-Willi syndrome
Factors that ↓ levels	Stretched stomach, post meals, status post vagotomy or sleeve gastrectomy, weight gain, leptin, carbohydrates (fast rebound), protein (prolonged suppression)
Ghrelin level mechanism	Increases gut motility and food intake (through hunger), leading to increased weight gain. Decreases energy expenditure and decreases insulin secretion.

Reference: Miller GD. Appetite Regulation: Hormones, Peptides, and Neurotransmitters and Their Role in Obesity. Am J Lifestyle Med. 2017;13(6):586-601. Published 2017 Jun 23. doi:10.1177/1559827617716376

37. (Content: I-B-7) A pathophysiologist is lecturing medical students on the hormones that regulate appetite. In particular, one of these hormones plays a role in energy balance and is directly proportionate to the amount of adipose tissue in the body. As adiposity increases, this hormone increases, signaling satiety and increasing the rate of energy expenditure. Which of the following is most likely being discussed?

A. Pancreatic polypeptide
B. Cholecystokinin
C. Leptin
D. Glucagon-like peptide 1
E. Ghrelin

(C) **Leptin** is one of the long-acting adiposity signaling hormones in contrast to the short-acting meal-terminating hormones secreted by the intestines. It has a role in central signaling regarding energy sufficiency. As adipose tissue increases, leptin increases, thus signaling satiety and increasing energy expenditure. Its levels are proportionate to body fat mass, and thus with weight loss, levels will decrease, leading to increased appetite. It also:

- Stimulates the anorexigenic neuron system (POMC/CART)
- Inhibits the orexigenic neuron system (NPY/AgRP)

Interestingly men have lower levels of leptin compared to women at similar body mass index values, which may indicate more leptin resistance in females.

In individuals without insulin resistance, insulin may also contribute to satiety by acting on the hypothalamus. However, in conditions like diabetes and polycystic ovarian syndrome (PCOS) where insulin resistance is a prominent feature, the effectiveness of insulin in promoting satiety may be diminished. Similarly, in those with obesity with adiposopathy, relative leptin resistance can occur having a less pronounced central satiety effect.

Note: Pancreatic polypeptide hormone is secreted by the F cells of the endocrine pancreas in response to food intake (calories). This hormone reduces gastric emptying and hunger (centrally) and is associated with low levels in obesity and Prader-Willi syndrome.

Reference: Picó C, Palou M, Pomar CA, Rodríguez AM, Palou A. Leptin as a key regulator of the adipose organ. Rev Endocr Metab Disord. 2022 Feb;23(1):13-30. doi: 10.1007/s11154-021-09687-5. Epub 2021 Sep 14. PMID: 34523036; PMCID: PMC8873071.

38. (Content: I-D-3) A 39-year-old female presents to the emergency department for dyspnea on exertion and chest pain. She states she flew in from Europe to go skiing with friends in Colorado. She had a duodenal jejunal bypass liner placed 9 months prior and has lost 43 lbs (19.5 kg) and wanted to celebrate with her friends. A CT scan is negative for pulmonary embolism and shows no pulmonary edema. Lab work is shown below:

Lab	Patient's Value	Reference Range
Hemoglobin	8.4 g/dL	12.0–16.0 g/dL
MCV	78 μm^3	80–100 μm^3
Platelets	490,000/mm^3	150,000–400,000/mm^3

Which of the following deficiencies is most likely contributing to her presentation?

    A. Folic acid
    B. B_{12}
    C. Pyridoxine
    D. Iron
    E. Thiamine

(D) This patient is presenting with symptomatic anemia, which likely became more apparent with higher altitudes and exertion. **Iron,** which is primarily absorbed in the duodenum, may become deficient with an endoluminal sleeve which blocks absorption of the proximal small intestine. Iron deficiency most commonly presents with microcytic anemia and can cause thrombocytosis. In contrast, vitamin B_{12} and folic acid deficiency cause macrocytic anemia, often with pancytopenia as these nutrients are involved in DNA synthesis and would be deficient across all cell lines.

Note: Knowledge of this device is not needed to correctly answer this question. Endoluminal sleeves (EndoBarrier®) are not currently FDA-approved for use in the United States but are undergoing clinical trials (STEP-1), and are available in some European countries. This endoscopically-placed 60 cm sleeve which looks like a plastic liner, is placed into the first part of the intestine (duodenum/ jejunum) for a maximum of 12 months. Food enters the plastic liner, whereas digestive enzymes pass around the liner, meeting at the end of sleeve, thus mimicking a bypass by delaying digestion and subsequent absorption of food.

Reference: Obesity Medicine Association: Obesity Algorithm (2023)
Reference: American Diabetes Association; Diabetes Care 1 April 2023. https://doi.org/10.2337/dc22-1952

39. (Content: I-A-3) A 7-year-old patient presents to his family medicine physician with his father for ongoing obesity management. Physical examination reveals a broad forehead with large earlobes and strabismus. Upon record review, a loss of function mutation to the FMR1 gene (Xq27.3) is noted. Which of the following other findings is most likely present in this patient?

    A. Polydactyly
    B. Decreased testicular size
    C. Organomegaly
    D. Hypertonia
    E. Elongated face

(E) This patient presents with an X-linked genetic condition (Xq27.3) with a broad forehead, large earlobes, and strabismus consistent with Fragile X syndrome. Obesity is associated with 60% of patients with this condition, with a relatively common prevalence (1 in 2,500 births). This condition is also associated with an **elongated face.**

Fragile X syndrome is one of the most frequent etiologies of inherited intellectual disability. It affects males twice as frequently as females, and often has stronger phenotypical characteristics (full mutation) associated with it.

Characteristic findings of this condition include:

- Large ears
- Testicular enlargement with normal testicular function
- Elongated and narrow face with a broad, prominent forehead
- Prominent jaw
- Strabismus
- Hypotonia
- Joint hyperlaxity
- Developmental and cognitive delays including autism spectrum disorder
- Arched palate
- Behavioral changes (anxiety, attention deficit, hyperactivity)

Approximately 50% of females with a full mutation have normal intellect, with the remaining 50% having more mild phenotypes than males.

Reference: Up to Date "Fragile X syndrome: Clinical features and diagnosis in children and adolescents"

40. (Content: I-B-7) A 9-year-old male presents to a geneticist as the patient has had a speech delay and learning difficulties including dyslexia. On review of his growth chart, he has remained persistently in the 97th percentile for weight. On examination, a scar is noted on the hand which his mother states is related to the removal of a "sixth digit" as a neonate. Which of the following cellular structures is likely involved in this patient's underlying syndromic condition?

A. Endoplasmic reticulum
B. Lysosomes
C. Golgi apparatus
D. Cilia
E. Cell wall

(D) This patient is presenting with learning difficulties, a history of polydactyly (i.e., 6th digit), speech delay, and early-onset obesity most consistent with Bardet-Biedl syndrome (BBS), the second most common cause of syndromic obesity.

Cilia, which are hair-like structures on the surface of cells, are particularly important in sensory and signaling functions. **Ciliary dysfunction** in BBS is associated with impaired signaling pathways critical for the development and maintenance of various organs, whereas impaired sensory function leads to retinal photoreceptor cell dysfunction, as an example. Ciliopathy is the underlying mechanism contributing to the diverse BBS clinical manifestations.

Diagnostic Criteria for Bardet-Biedl Syndrome	
Primary Features	**Secondary Features**
-Rod-cone dystrophy (93%)	-Speech delay (54-81%)
-Central obesity (72-92%)	-Developmental delay (50-91%)
-Postaxial polydactyly (63-81%)	-Diabetes mellitus (6-48%)
-Genital anomalies (59-98%)	-Dental anomalies (51%)
-Renal anomalies (53%)	-Congenital heart disease (7%)
-Learning difficulties (61%)	-Brachydactyly (46-100%) or syndactyly (8-95%)
	-Ataxia/poor coordination (40-86%)
	-Anosmia/hyposmia (60%)
Diagnostic criteria: Four primary features or three primary features + two secondary features	

Reference: Forsythe E, Beales PL. Bardet-Biedl syndrome. Eur J Hum Genet. 2013 Jan;21(1):8-13. doi: 10.1038/ejhg.2012.115. Epub 2012 Jun 20. PMID: 22713813; PMCID: PMC3522196.

41. (Content: I-D-1) A 26-year-old female presents to the emergency department via ambulance in cardiac arrest with the following rhythm strip:

Per her husband, she was planning to lose a significant amount of weight before a friend's wedding next month and started over-the-counter supplements and a new diet. She has congenital long QT syndrome and class III obesity (BMI 54 kg/m^2). Which of the following dietary plans most likely contributed to this patient's presentation?

A. **Ketogenic diet**
B. Intermittent fasting
C. Very low-calorie diet
D. Mediterranean diet
E. Meal-replacement plan

(A) This patient presents with torsades de pointes (rhythm strip) which is most likely caused by a severely prolonged QTc. Severe obesity, as seen in this patient, is itself a risk for a prolonged QT interval. In addition, a **ketogenic diet** has been associated with a prolonged QTc and can induce torsades in those with concurrent risk factors. In addition, ketogenic diets may predispose to selenium deficiency which also increases the risk of arrythmias.

Note: Historical "high-protein liquid diets" resembled more of a fad diet to be used on a short-term basis, with minimal to no carbohydrates that pushed patients into ketosis. They were associated with a high risk of arrhythmias including torsades. Current-day meal replacements provide sufficient carbohydrates, protein, and multivitamins to be safely used longer-term.

Reference: Watanabe M, Tuccinardi D, Ernesti I, Basciani S, Mariani S, Genco A, Manfrini S, Lubrano C, Gnessi L. Scientific evidence underlying contraindications to the ketogenic diet: An update. Obes Rev. 2020 Oct;21(10):e13053. doi: 10.1111/obr.13053. Epub 2020 Jul 10. PMID: 32648647; PMCID: PMC7539910.
Reference: D'Imperio S, Monasky MM, Micaglio E, Negro G, Pappone C. Impact of Dietary Factors on Brugada Syndrome and Long QT Syndrome. Nutrients. 2021 Jul 21;13(8):2482. doi: 10.3390/nu13082482. PMID: 34444641; PMCID: PMC8401538.
Reference: Sudhakaran S, Yazdani L, Wheelan KR, Rao PK. The ketogenic diet and the QT interval. Proc (Bayl Univ Med Cent). 2019 Oct 11;33(1):77-79. doi: 10.1080/08998280.2019.1664220. PMID: 32063779; PMCID: PMC6988628.

42. (Content: I-B-1 and I-A-1) A 33-year-old female presents to her primary care physician for follow-up regarding her polysomnography results. Her results reveal her apnea-hypopnea index was > 30, indicating severe obstructive sleep apnea; the test was split with continuous positive airway pressure (CPAP) titration. She has a prescription for a CPAP machine but has not picked it up yet. Given these findings, which neurohumoral hormone would be expected to be decreased?

A. Ghrelin
B. Orexin
C. Leptin
D. Neuropeptide Y

(C) This patient with severe obstructive sleep apnea has a decreased duration of quality sleep, which has been shown to have adverse health outcomes directly related to obesity. Sleep deprivation and/or reduced sleep quality is associated with decreased **leptin** levels, leading to increased appetite and reduced energy expenditure.

In a study completed in 2004, those who consistently slept 5 hours, compared to those receiving 8 hours of quality sleep, had the following findings:

- BMI increase of 3.6%
- Leptin decrease of 15.5%
- Ghrelin increase of 14.9%

Note: Ghrelin is produced by the stomach in fasting states and stimulates hunger (i.e., appetite), whereas leptin is one of the many inhibitors of ghrelin.

Sleep apnea is the most common sleep-related breathing disorder, with obesity being the strongest risk factor. Untreated, this condition can lead to increased blood pressure, cardiovascular disease, pulmonary hypertension, and ultimately increased morbidity and mortality. It decreases sleep quality. Studies have shown that treating obstructive sleep apnea does not cause a significant reduction in weight. However, exercise, despite weight loss, may improve OSA.

Reference: Mignot, Emmanuel, et al. Stanford.edu/med-sleep-1208.html, Dec 2004

43. (Content: I-C-1) A physician is discussing with a medical student the ethnic disparities within obesity. Of the following ethnicity and gender combinations in adults, which would likely have the most significant disparity of increased obesity (based on percentage)?

A. Asian males
B. Hispanic males
C. White females
D. Black females

(D) Race/ethnic disparities seen in obesity are significant, of which Black and Hispanic populations have higher obesity rates compared to Caucasian and Asians. This is seen in both adults and children. When gender is considered, **Black females** have significantly higher percentages of obesity than Black males.

Interestingly, gender differences in obesity were seen when household income and education level were taken into consideration:

- Women: Increased obesity was seen in those with <u>more</u> poverty and <u>less</u> education.
- Men: More obesity is seen in those with <u>middle</u>-class incomes and those with <u>moderate</u> education (completed some college).

Note: In adults, the highest rate of obesity tends to occur in middle-age from 40-59 years old. In children, prevalence is highest between 12-19 years of age.

The table summarizes obesity rates (percentage) in different groups.

Obesity: Race/Ethnic Categorization (Percentages)			
Race/Ethnicity	Men (Boys)	Women (Girls)	Both: Adult (Child)
White	44.7 (17.4)	39.8 (14.8)	42.2 (16.1)
Black	41.1 (19.4)	56.9 (29.1)	49.6 (24.2)
Asian	17.5 (12.4)	17.2 (10.1[1])	17.4 (8.7)
Hispanic	45.7 (28.1)	43.7 (23.0)	44.8 (25.6)

[1]This sub category is based on 2016 data as 2017-2018 did not meet reliability standards.

Reference: Ogden CL, Fakhouri TH, Carroll MD, et al. Prevalence of Obesity Among Adults, by Household Income and Education — United States, 2011–2014. MMWR Morb Mortal Wkly Rep 2017;66:1369–1373. DOI:
Reference: NCHS, National Health and Nutrition Examination Survey, NCHS Fact sheet, July 2020.
https://www.cdc.gov/nchs/data/factsheets/factsheet_nhanes.htm (Accessed 12/14/2023)

44. (Content: I-B-3) A patient is presenting to discuss weight loss options. He has tried several dietary plans without success and has trouble maintaining a persistent exercise schedule. Which of the following statements would be most accurate?

A.   Caloric absorption is similar amongst individuals with identical intake
B.   For every 3500 kcal you decrease in your diet, you will lose 1 lb
C.   Losing weight is all about willpower and motivation
D.   It is easier to maintain weight loss, rather than lose it
E.   **Both subcutaneous and visceral fat can negatively affect health**

(E) Myths related to obesity are rampant not only among our patients but also among physicians. All of the above are incorrect myths except that **both subcutaneous and visceral fat negatively affect health.** The weight from adipose (visceral or subcutaneous) causes numerous health problems, often referred to as fat-mass disease, including osteoarthritis, obstructive sleep apnea, heart failure with preserved ejection fraction, and even hypertension. Subcutaneous fat also can secrete pro-inflammatory hormones, similar to visceral fat, although its effects are less robust as it does not directly affect surrounding organs.

Obesity is a complex disease process, incorporating neurohormonal, behavioral, and genetics into both central and peripheral signal processing. Findings seen in calorimeters (3500 kcal = 1 lb) do not correlate well in a living being. Although motivation and willpower are helpful in losing weight, these are by no means the answer to weight loss, nor the reason patients fail to lose weight.

In addition, 'calories in= calories out' has also been debunked as one patient may take in the same caloric intake as a patient with excess weight, but energy expenditure, caloric harvesting, and adipose storage can vary vastly. Other common myths that are inaccurate include:

- If you miss breakfast, your body goes into starvation mode and holds onto calories, leading to weight gain
- Lean individuals have less weight only due to a higher metabolism
- 1 lb of added muscle causes 50 kcal/day of energy expenditure (again, our bodies are not calorimeters)
- Slower weight loss leads to more sustained results

Reference: Obesity Medicine Association: Obesity Algorithm (2023)

45. (Content: I-D-2) A 46-year-old female presents for an annual follow-up with her obesity medicine specialist. She underwent a successful biliopancreatic diversion and duodenal switch seven years ago. She has been adherent with all nutritional visits and supplemental vitamin intake. She had lost 162 lbs (73.5 kg), but has regained 10 lbs (4.5 kg) in the past year. She denies any new symptoms. Laboratory work reveals a microcytic anemia with a decreased ferritin level. Which gastrointestinal area is most likely responsible for this patient's laboratory abnormalities?

A. Stomach
B. Duodenum
C. Jejunum
D. Ileum
E. Colon

(B) A biliopancreatic diversion with duodenal switch bypasses both the duodenum and a portion of the jejunum, leading to decreased mineral absorption. This patient has a microcytic anemia with decreased ferritin, most consistent with iron deficiency anemia. Iron is **primarily absorbed in the duodenum** (and some in the proximal jejunum).

Areas of vitamin and mineral absorption within the gastrointestinal tract are discussed below:

- **Duodenum:** Iron (majority) and calcium
- **Jejunum:** Folate, carbohydrates, amino acids, and potassium. The proximal portion can absorb iron as well. Fat-soluble vitamins (also from ileum)
- **Ileum:** B_{12}, potassium, minerals, bile salts, fats, and fat-soluble vitamins
- **Colon:** Vitamin K, biotin, water, sodium, and chloride

Iron supplementation can be attempted orally. Hemoglobin should improve within two weeks; however, iron stores (i.e., ferritin) can take up to 6 months. If no improvements are seen, consider parenteral replacement.

Reference: Up to Date: "Bariatric surgery: Postoperative nutritional management"
Reference: Ciobârcă D, Cătoi AF, Copăescu C, Miere D, Crișan G. Bariatric Surgery in Obesity: Effects on Gut Microbiota and Micronutrient Status. Nutrients. 2020 Jan 16;12(1):235. doi: 10.3390/nu12010235. PMID: 31963247; PMCID: PMC7019602.

The image below shows where nutrients are primarily absorbed. The line outlying the stomach shows the area affected by the sleeve gastrectomy, whereas the dark line indicates the area affected by a Roux-en-Y gastric bypass.

Note: Sources may slightly vary on primary areas of absorption. Knowing the general areas of absorption and how the different metabolic and bariatric surgeries affect absorption is sufficient for boards.

Nutrient Absorption in Gastrointestinal Tract

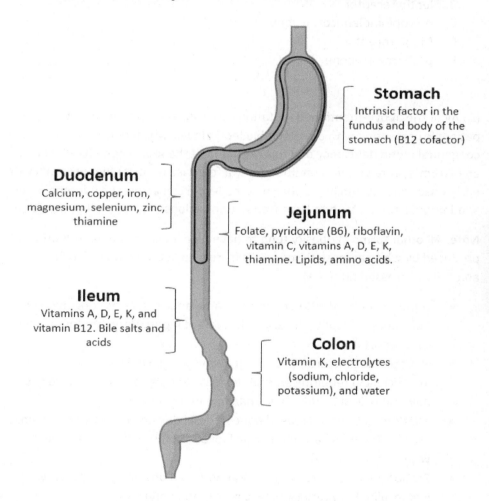

Stomach
Intrinsic factor in the fundus and body of the stomach (B12 cofactor)

Duodenum
Calcium, copper, iron, magnesium, selenium, zinc, thiamine

Jejunum
Folate, pyridoxine (B6), riboflavin, vitamin C, vitamins A, D, E, K, thiamine. Lipids, amino acids.

Ileum
Vitamins A, D, E, K, and vitamin B12. Bile salts and acids

Colon
Vitamin K, electrolytes (sodium, chloride, potassium), and water

Image citation: Image created by Charu G. Copyright owned by Kevin Smith, DO
Reference: Up to Date: "Bariatric surgery: Postoperative nutritional management"
Reference: Ciobârcă D, Cătoi AF, Copăescu C, Miere D, Crișan G. Bariatric Surgery in Obesity: Effects on Gut Microbiota and Micronutrient Status. Nutrients. 2020 Jan 16;12(1):235. doi: 10.3390/nu12010235. PMID: 31963247; PMCID: PMC7019602.

46. (Content: I-A-3) A 6-year-old male presents to an obesity management center for evaluation and treatment of severe obesity. His parents state that he has always had unquenchable hunger and they feel guilty for restricting food. Laboratory work reviews normal cortisol levels, undetectable leptin, and a hemoglobin A1c of 5.8% (reference range < 5.7%). He has normal mentation and flesh-colored striae on the abdomen. The most likely cause of this patient's findings is a mutation in the

A. **leptin gene**
B. leptin receptor
C. pro-opiomelanocortin gene
D. MC4R receptor
E. prohormone gene

(A) All of the above-mentioned mutations are causes of monogenic obesity. This patient is presenting with undetectable leptin levels which only occurs in congenital leptin deficiency due to a mutation of the **leptin gene (LEP).** This is an extremely rare genetic condition (only a few case reports) that presents with early-onset obesity and hyperphagia, as no leptin can active the hypothalamus. In addition, patients tend to have frequent infections due to T-cell dysfunction.

Note: All other forms of obesity tend to have high levels of leptin, as leptin is produced by white adipose tissue and is increased in the setting of high adiposity (increased fat mass).

- Leptin receptor (LEPR) deficiency: Same appearance as congenital leptin deficiency, except with very high levels of leptin. Very rare (only a few case reports).
- Pro-opiomelanocortin (POMC) gene mutation: Low cortisol (adrenal insufficiency) requiring steroid replacement. Patients often have red hair and pale skin. Rare (less than one in one million).
- MC4R mutations: Increased bone mineral density and accelerated linear growth. Patients have high insulin levels. Common (2-6% of patients with severe obesity).
- Prohormone convertase (PCSK1 gene): High pro-hormone levels with low insulin. Very rare (several case reports only).

Reference: Up to Date: "Obesity: Genetic contribution and pathophysiology"
Reference: Obesity Medicine Association: Pediatric Obesity Algorithm (2023-2024)

47. (Content: I-A-4) A PhD candidate is working with a pediatric infectious disease physician to determine if there is an association between a prior upper respiratory infection and the development of obesity. She looks for serum antibodies and finds a correlation between a positive viral assay and an increased body mass index and waist circumference. Which of the following viruses most likely correlated with her findings?

A. Parvo B19
B. HPV-16
C. Covid-23
D. Pneumonia serotype 15B
E. **Adenovirus-36**

(E) **Human adenovirus-36 (Adv-36)** has been found in multiple studies to have a correlation with obesity. In children, a prior infection had a statistically significant correlation with higher body mass index values and waist circumference.

Adv-36 is one of 52 serotypes of adenovirus and has been shown to cause adipogenesis in animals and humans. The virus has been determined to increase genetic expression affecting the regulation of fatty acid synthase, ultimately leading to enhanced fat accumulation. Adv-36 adipogenic effects have been studied in animals, with newly infected animals (chickens, monkeys, and rats) gaining 15-30% body weight post-infection.

Prevalence of this virus has been shown to range from 30-65% in those with obesity. One study of 500 patients determined the prevalence of Adv-36 to be 30% in those with obesity and only 11% in those with normal weight, with those infected approximately 25 kg heavier.

Interestingly, serum cholesterol and triglycerides are noted to decrease after infection, which was attributed to increased storage, and thus less circulating levels of these components. Insulin sensitivity also improved after infection.

Reference: Ponterio E, Gnessi L. Adenovirus 36 and Obesity: An Overview. Viruses. 2015 Jul 8;7(7):3719-40. doi: 10.3390/v7072787. PMID: 26184280; PMCID: PMC4517116.
Reference: Salehian B, Forman SJ, Kandeel FR, Bruner DE, He J, Atkinson RL. Adenovirus 36 DNA in adipose tissue of patient with unusual visceral obesity. Emerg Infect Dis. 2010 May;16(5):850-2. doi: 10.3201/eid1605.091271. PMID: 20409382; PMCID: PMC2953992.
Reference: Atkinson RL, Lee I, Shin HJ, He J. Human adenovirus-36 antibody status is associated with obesity in children. Int J Pediatr Obes. 2010 Apr;5(2):157-60. doi: 10.3109/17477160903111789. PMID: 19593728.

48. (Content: I-B-5) A nutritionist is discussing how energy relates to food intake and nutrition labels. How much energy would it take to raise 1 kilogram of water by 1 °C?

A. **1 Calorie**
B. 10 kilocalories
C. 100 Calories
D. 1,000 Calories
E. 10,000 calories

(A) Calories are a measure of energy. In particular, one calorie is the amount of heat required to raise the temperature of 1 gram of water by 1 °C. Therefore, to raise 1,000 grams (1 kilogram) of water 1 °C, it would take 1000 calories, which is equivalent to **1 Calorie** (notice the capitalization).

Note: 1,000 calories = 1 Calorie = 1 kilocalorie

When referencing food (i.e., food labels) or exercise, often the term Calorie is used, which refers to 1 kilocalorie (kcal). As this is a unit of energy, it should be noted that one kcal = 4.184 kilojoules of energy.

Reference: Obesity Medicine Association: Obesity Algorithm (2023)

49. (Content: I-D-3) A 23-year-old male presents to his family practice physician after he read an article on high-dose calcium intake related to weight loss. He is currently taking twice the recommended daily allowance, but hasn't noticed a significant weight loss at this point. He asks if this is an effective obesity treatment. His current BMI is 27 kg/m^2. His only complaint is constipation. Given his current status, which of the following is most likely increased in this patient?

    A. Parathyroid hormone activity
    B. Vitamin D levels
    C. Lipogenesis
    D. Lipolysis
    E. Fat storage levels

(D) Patients with high calcium intake tend to have **increased lipolysis** (fat breakdown) and decreased lipogenesis (fat production) and fat storage. In fact, epidemiologic data suggest a lower prevalence of overweight, obesity, and insulin resistance in people with high calcium intake.

Note: This study does not recommend taking above the recommended daily allowance for calcium, but instead taking adequate calcium intake. Also, this plays a small role when compared to exercise and diet.

The two mechanisms proposed to explain calcium intake on body weight is that increased dietary calcium suppresses PTH and vitamin D, thereby decreasing intracellular calcium in adipocytes, which inhibits lipogenesis and stimulates lipolysis (the opposite is true with low calcium intake).

The other mechanism is that dietary calcium intake binds and inhibits fatty acid absorption in the gastrointestinal tract.

Important: The prevalence of vitamin D (a fat-soluble vitamin) deficiency in obesity is > 30% due to body dilution, as skin surface area is not proportionate to patient volume. This deficiency does not increase weight.

Findings	Low Calcium Intake	High Calcium Intake
PTH, Vit D, Intracellular Ca^{2+}	↑	↓
Lipogenesis	↑	↓
Lipolysis	↓	↑

Reference: Dietary Calcium Intake and Obesity; Sarina Schrager. The Journal of the American Board of Family Practice May 2005, 18 (3) 205-210; DOI: https://doi.org/10.3122/jabfm.18.3.205
Reference: Obesity Medicine Association Board Review 2023

50. (Content: I-B-3) A group of physicians are developing a program to address patients with coronary artery disease who are at the highest risk of mortality within the next five years. To simplify the program, they only evaluate the body mass index and waist circumference. Those with the highest mortality risk will be entered into an intensive physical, dietary, and behavioral modification program. Which of the following parameters of patients should receive priority entrance into this class?

A. BMI 22 kg/m²; Waist circumference 85 cm
B. BMI 22 kg/m²; Waist circumference 101 cm
C. BMI 26 kg/m²; Waist circumference 85 cm
D. BMI 30 kg/m²; Waist circumference 85 cm
E. BMI 30 kg/m²; Waist circumference 101 cm

(B) A large study (> 15,000 participants) of patients with coronary artery disease were evaluated to see which group had the highest mortality rate. They discovered that patients with increased waist circumference had higher associated 5-year mortality throughout all BMI ranges. Interestingly, **patients with a normal BMI but increased waist circumference had the highest 5-year mortality risk.** This displayed the importance of visceral fat as it relates to adiposopathy.

The table below compares the risk of mortality in a subject that had a normal BMI (22 kg/m²) and increased waist circumference (101 cm) compared to other subjects (all statistically significant with $P < 0.0001$):

Subjects	BMI	WC	Comparison Subject: BMI 22 kg/m² WC 101 cm Hazard Ratio
Subject 1	22 kg/m²	85 cm	1.10
Subject 2	26 kg/m²	85 cm	1.20
Subject 3	30 kg/m²	85 cm	1.61
Subject 4	30 kg/m²	101 cm	1.27

Reference: Combining Body Mass Index With Measures of Central Obesity in the Assessment of Mortality in Subjects With Coronary Disease; Thais Coutinho, Kashish Goel, Daniel Corrêa de Sá, Rickey E. Carter, David O. Hodge, Charlotte Kragelund, Alka M. Kanaya, Marianne Zeller, Jong Seon Park, Lars Kober, Christian Torp-Pedersen, Yves Cottin, Luc Lorgis, Sang-Hee Lee, Young-Jo Kim, Randal Thomas, Véronique L. Roger, Virend K. Somers, Francisco Lopez-Jimenez; J Am Coll Cardiol. 2013 Feb, 61 (5) 553-560.

51. (Content: I-B-8) A 49-year-old female is discussing a recent incident with her health coach. She states that she recently dropped off her only child at college. A week later, she walked by a bakery and the smell brought back memories of her and her child baking bread on the weekends. Despite recently finishing up lunch and not being hungry, she indulged in two large pieces of bread. Which area of activation played the largest role in this incident?

A. Amygdala
B. Hippocampus
C. Pre-frontal cortex
D. Hypothalamus
E. Occipital lobe

(B) This patient's desire to eat bread was triggered by memories, not internal hunger stimuli. The **hippocampus** is activated with memories and in the setting of food, can override physiologic satiety. Obesity is very complex, with several areas affecting energy expenditure and food intake. Two primary paths are discussed below:

- **Homeostatic:** This consists of the complex POMC/CART and NPY/AgRP pathways located in the hypothalamus, which responds to peripheral neurohormonal inputs. This is the body's primary regulatory center.
- **Hedonic:** These pathways can override the homeostatic pathway. In other words, activation of the centers below can activate hunger, promoting food intake even if not initially hungry.
  - *Limbic system:* This is primarily driven by dopamine and mediates cravings, rewards, compulsions, and food addiction.
  - *Emotion/Memories:*
    - Amygdala: This area activates in response to food cues (advertisements, visuals, etc.).
    - Hippocampus: Memories or prior experiences activate this area (i.e., the smell of a dessert reminds you of a family celebration).
  - *Pre-frontal cortex:* This area is involved in impulse control, spontaneity, planning, and decision-making.

Reference: Farr OM, Li CR, Mantzoros CS. Central nervous system regulation of eating: Insights from human brain imaging. Metabolism. 2016 May;65(5):699-713. doi: 10.1016/j.metabol.2016.02.002. Epub 2016 Feb 6. PMID: 27085777; PMCID: PMC4834455.

52. (Content: I-A-3) A 4-year-old male with weight and height consistently in the 95th percentile presents to his pediatrician for follow-up regarding tumor surveillance. He recently underwent an abdominal ultrasound showing hepatosplenomegaly without concerning findings for malignancy. What genetic characteristic is most likely associated with this condition?

A. Autosomal recessive inheritance
B. Chromosome 15q deletion
C. Chromosome 8q22 mutation
D. **Chromosome 11p15.5 dysregulation**
E. ALMS 1 mutation

(D) This patient presents with excess weight at a young age, hepatosplenomegaly, and requires tumor surveillance. These findings are associated with Beckwith-Wiedemann syndrome, which is due to **genetic dysregulation of chromosome 11p15.5.**

Beckwith-Wiedemann syndrome is a fetal overgrowth syndrome that commonly presents with enlarged organs (hepatomegaly, splenomegaly, nephromegaly, and macroglossia) and predisposes the patient to tumor growth. Therefore, frequent surveillance with abdominal ultrasounds and tumor markers are necessary, as Wilms tumors and hepatoblastoma are possible.

Genetic Patterns of Early-Onset Childhood Obesity	
Autosomal recessive	-Bardet-Biedl syndrome -POMC deficiency -Congenital leptin deficiency -Cohen syndrome (8q22 mutation) -Alstrom syndrome -MC4R deficiency[1]
X-linked syndromes	-Fragile X -Wilson-Turner -Borjeson-Forssman-Lehmann
Paternal chromosome 15q deletion[2]	Prader-Willi syndrome
Maternal chromosome 15q deletion[2] (Ubiquitin protein ligase E3A)	Angelman syndrome
ALMS 1 mutation	Alstrom syndrome
Chromosome 11p15.5 dysregulation	Beckwith-Wiedemann syndrome

[1]Can be inherited via an autosomal recessive or dominant pattern; [2]Imprinting error

Reference: Up to Date: "Beckwith-Wiedemann Syndrome"
Reference: Obesity Medicine Association: Pediatric Obesity Algorithm (2023-2024)

53. (Content: I-A-5) A 24-year-old pregnant female is considering breastfeeding her child. However, she works a full-time job and is concerned about the logistics of pumping while at work. Which of the following statements is most accurate as it relates to breastfeeding?

A. Breastfed infants will initially gain weight more rapidly
B. The risk of childhood obesity is increased with breastfeeding
C. Guidelines recommend exclusive breastfeeding for 12 months
D. Non-breastfed infants are placed at an undue risk of obesity
E. Complimentary food should be introduced at 4 months of age

(A) **Breastfed infants will gain weight faster compared to formula-fed infants** in the first 3 months, and then a slowing of the velocity of weight gain. However, long term, there are lower rates of obesity in breastfed infants, as infants are better at self-regulating their caloric intake.

Mothers should never be made to feel guilty for their decision not to breastfeed, or the potential inability to breastfeed. However, education on the benefits of breastfeeding is appropriate. The first 1000 days of life have a significant impact on the development of the child. Monitoring for trends of weight gain and providing education on healthy habits during this time is crucial.

Note: Caregivers should also be reminded that the presence of excess weight in children does not indicate poor parenting.

The American Academy of Pediatrics recommends:

- Exclusive breastfeeding for the first 6 months
- Continued breastfeeding while complimentary foods are introduced
- Continued breastfeeding for 1 year or longer as mutually desired by infant and mother

Reference: Joan Younger Meek, Lawrence Noble, Section on Breastfeeding; Policy Statement: Breastfeeding and the Use of Human Milk. Pediatrics July 2022; 150 (1): e2022057988. 10.1542/peds.2022-057988
Reference: Obesity Medicine Association: Pediatric Obesity Algorithm (2023-2024)

54. (Content: I-B-6) A 37-year-old female presents to her surgeon for a 12-month follow-up after a successful sleeve gastrectomy. She has followed all diet and exercise regimens as prescribed by her dietician and electrophysiologist. However, she has noticed that even though she has increased her exercise time to 220 minutes weekly, she has not seen a significant decrease in weight as expected. She has lost 95 lbs (43 kg) postoperatively but has plateaued. Which of the following most likely explains this plateau effect?

    A. Increased total energy expenditure
    B. Increased muscle efficiency
    C. Adaptive thermogenesis
    D. Modified set-point
    E. Increased leptin levels

(B) This patient who fails to lose additional weight despite increased exercise, is experiencing **increased muscle efficiency,** in which her muscles burn fewer cumulative calories, although exercising for longer durations of time. This occurs because of muscle hypertrophy (efficiency) and less body weight to move. Another way to think of this is a 300-pound patient will burn more calories than a 200-pound patient (more mass, thereby increasing the required energy to move). Although she is likely experiencing adaptive thermogenesis, this does not explain her lack of weight loss with additional exercise.

There are many reasons why patients plateau or experience weight gain, as discussed below:

- **Neurohormonal:** Leptin, cholecystokinin, peptide YY all decrease, thus removing inhibitory actions on ghrelin, increasing appetite
- **Energy:** Decrease in resting energy expenditure due to weight loss
- **Adaptive thermogenesis:** Reduction in resting metabolic rate
- **Set-point fallacy:** Incorrect belief that once you achieve a lower weight, your body will maintain this decreased weight naturally
- **Commitment amnesia:** Lack of maintaining behavior, dietary, and physical activity levels that were required to lose the initial weight

Reference: Obesity Medicine Association: Obesity Algorithm (2023)

55. (Content: I-E-1) A 29-year-old male plans to run a marathon in the next four months. He has been training daily and can run nearly 18 miles without stopping. What is true of the muscle fibers he predominantly utilizes to prepare for this marathon?

A. Energy is from glycolysis
B. Creates forceful contractions
C. Fatigue susceptible
D. **Increased mitochondria are present**

(D) A person training for longevity is working on strengthening their slow-twitch or type 1 muscle fibers. These fibers produce their energy by utilizing adenosine triphosphate (ATP) made within the **mitochondria, which are abundant** in these slow-twitch muscle fibers.

Skeletal muscles are made up of bundles of individual muscle fibers called myocytes. These myocytes each contain many myofibrils, which are strands of actin and myosin proteins (making up the contractile component of the muscle, the sarcomere). These grab onto each other and pull together, cumulatively shortening the muscle and causing muscle contractions.

Muscle fibers respond to training, developing more type I or type II fibers based on the forces imposed on them. For example, a weightlifter will likely generate more slow-twitch muscles (heavy weights, repetitions), whereas a boxer will develop more fast-twitch (acceleration, speed). These fibers are further compared in the table below.

Muscle Fiber Types		
Muscle type	Slow Twitch (Type I)	Fast Twitch (Type II)
Energy	Oxidative metabolism	Anaerobic glycolysis
Fatigue	Resistant	Susceptible
Physical activity	Prolonged (marathon)	Forceful (sprinting)

Reference: Ørtenblad N, Nielsen J, Boushel R, Söderlund K, Saltin B, Holmberg HC. The Muscle Fiber Profiles, Mitochondrial Content, and Enzyme Activities of the Exceptionally Well-Trained Arm and Leg Muscles of Elite Cross-Country Skiers. Front Physiol. 2018;9:1031. Published 2018 Aug 2. doi:10.3389/fphys.2018.01031

56. (Content: I-A-4) A 66-year-old female presents to the clinic for worsening vision. She states that this has been progressing for the past six months, but recently nearly caused a car accident. She has also had daily headaches, which she attributes to the vision changes, and reports she always feels hungry. Her vital signs are normal except for her BMI, which has increased from 31 to 33 kg/m² since last year. Physical exam reveals bilateral loss of the lower peripheral visual fields. Laboratory work reveals a TSH is 0.1 µU/mL (reference range: 0.5–5.0 µU/mL) and a T$_4$ is 2 µg/dL (reference range: 5–12 µg/dL). Prolactin levels are normal. Which of the following is the most appropriate next step?

A. **Brain imaging**
B. Levothyroxine replacement
C. Ophthalmology referral
D. Radioactive iodine scan of the thyroid
E. Growth hormone and ACTH levels

(A) This patient is presenting with bilateral hemianopsia, central hypothyroidism, and hyperphagia concerning for hypothalamic obesity. One likely cause is a craniopharyngioma, a rare, slow-growing cystic lesion that develops from the remnants of Rathke's pouch. Compression and damage of the pituitary, hypothalamus, and optic chiasm lead to symptoms. An **MRI of the pituitary** is the most important next step if this condition is suspected.

Hypothalamic obesity occurs due to damage of the ventromedial hypothalamus (VMH), leading to loss of homeostatic inputs, and thus causing decreased energy expenditure, hyperphagia, and subsequent obesity.

Craniopharyngioma is the most common tumor to cause hypothalamic obesity, with other etiologies including brain radiation, trauma, intracranial surgeries, increased intracranial pressure, or other brain tumors. Most patients will have concurrent vision changes, headaches, nausea, and endocrine pathology, including diabetes insipidus, central hypothyroidism, and deficiencies of growth hormone and adrenocorticotropic hormone. Amenorrhea and erectile dysfunction are also common.

Memory aid: Masses in the ventromedial hypothalamus lead to more weight, whereas lesions in the lateral hypothalamus lead to less weight.

Reference: Up To Date: "Craniopharyngioma" and "Obesity in adults: Etiologies and risk factors"

57. (Content: I-B-3) A double-blinded study is performed with patients who have a body mass index between 25-30 kg/m^2. They receive either a placebo or an intravenous medication theorized to increase brown adipose tissue (BAT) activation. At the end of the infusion, patients undergo a positron emission tomography (PET) scan to evaluate the presence of BAT. After the trial, there was an 11% increased tracer uptake, as evidenced by the PET scan, in those receiving the medication compared to the placebo group. Which of the following most accurately describes the studied adipose tissue?

    A. Its brown color is due to increased lysosomes
    B. It couples oxidative phosphorylation, increasing ATP production
    C. It is stimulated by acetylcholine of the parasympathetic system
    D. Resting metabolic rate is inversely proportional to BAT levels
    E. It utilizes glucose and free fatty acids to increase lipolysis

(E) BAT is different from white adipose tissue, as it contains numerous large mitochondria (giving its brown color) and serves as a warming mechanism for vital organs by uncoupling oxidative phosphorylation, thereby generating heat, instead of energy (ATP) via non-shivering thermogenesis. This process increases the resting metabolic rate proportionately to levels of BAT by **utilizing glucose and free fatty acids to increase lipolysis**.

Although thought to be present in infants only and decreasing until no longer present in adulthood, a study published in the New England Journal of Medicine in 2009 revealed that BAT (biopsy-confirmed) could be activated by cold exposure, as displayed on a PET scan. The cold tended to increase BAT activation more in women over men, young more than older, higher in those who are lean, and decreased in those with obesity.

Studies are underway to evaluate pharmacotherapy that could activate brown fat. Most recently, mirabegron was shown in a small study (n=14) to increase BAT with an increased resting metabolism by 6% and improved insulin sensitivity. However, it did not change their weight or body composition.

Beiging is another theory in which white adipose tissue can act like brown adipose tissue (upregulating an uncoupling protein seen in brown fat), leading to increased energy expenditure. Beige is indistinguishable from BAT on scans.

Reference: Chronic mirabegron treatment increases human brown fat, HDL cholesterol, and insulin sensitivity. O'Mara et al. J Clin Invest. 2020 Jan 21. pii: 131126. doi: 10.1172/JCI131126. [Epub ahead of print]. PMID: 31961826.
Reference: Virtanen et al. NEJM 4/9/2009; 360:1518-1525; DOI: 10.1056/NEJMoa0808949

58. (Content: I-D-4) A 29-year-old health-conscious female is discussing her diet with a nutritionist. Although not focused on weight loss, she is interested to see if her diet matches the recommendations based on the acceptable macronutrient distribution range, as set forth by the United States Department of Agriculture (USDA). Which of the following would meet that criteria if the macronutrient was listed as a percentage of her total calories?

    A. Protein 45%
    B. Carbohydrate 60%
    C. Fat 40%
    D. Linoleic acid (Ω -6 fatty acid) 15%
    E. α-Linolenic acid (Ω-3 fatty acid) 5%

(B) Acceptable macronutrient distribution ranges (AMDR) are the percentage of energy intake associated with a reduced risk of chronic disease yet providing adequate amounts of essential nutrients. Of the options, only **carbohydrates are within AMRD for adults, which is 45-65%.**

Note: The AMRD references are not often followed by those attempting weight loss, which may differ drastically from these recommendations.

There is no AMRD for alcohol, but it contains 7 kcal/gm, whereas water contains 0 kcal/gm.

Acceptable Macronutrient Distribution Ranges			
Macronutrient	% of Total Calories for Adults	Kcal/gm	Recommended Daily Allowance (Grams/day)
Protein	10-35%	4	56 (men) 46 (women)
Carbohydrate	45-65%	4	130
Fat[1]	25-35%	9	NA

[1]AMDR of polyunsaturated fatty acids: linoleic acid (Ω -6 fatty acid) is 5-10%, and α-linolenic acid (Ω-3 fatty acid) is 0.6-1.2%. AMDR of saturated fat, cholesterol, and trans-fat are not determined.

Reference: Dietary Reference Intakes for Energy, Carbohydrate, Fiber, Fat, Fatty Acids, Cholesterol, Protein, and Amino Acids (2005)

59. (Content: I-B-8) A 29-year-old female presents for a follow-up appointment with her primary care physician. Over the past year, she has lost 40 lbs (18.1 kg), which she attributes to meal replacements and an effective exercise regimen. A recent body composition scan revealed a 3% reduction in adipose tissue. However, she has regained 5 lbs (2.3 kg) over the past two months. She denies changing her diet or exercise regimen but admits to "sneaking a few extra snacks here and there," as she states her hunger has increased. Which of the following neurohormonal changes is most likely contributing to her increased weight gain?

A. Increased leptin levels
B. **Loss of inhibition of the NPY/AgRP pathway**
C. Melanocortin 4 receptor activation
D. Orexin A and B hormone suppression
E. Inhibition of neurotrophic factor

(B) Adipose tissue is hormonally active, with one of its primary secreted hormones being leptin. Therefore, a decrease in adipose through weight loss would lead to decreased leptin levels. Because leptin is an inhibitor of the orexigenic (i.e., weight-gaining) pathway, this reduces **the inhibition of the NPY/AgRP (orexigenic) pathway,** leading to increased hunger, decreased energy expenditure, and ultimately weight gain.

Leptin hormone is an anorexigenic hormone secreted by white adipose tissue. Its two main functions include:

- Stimulating the anorexigenic neuron system (POMC/CART)
- Inhibiting the orexigenic neuron system (NPY/AgRP)

Note: Decreased leptin is a strong contributor to the weight plateau and regains often seen in patients who lose significant weight.

Reference: Erin E. Kershaw, Jeffrey S. Flier, Adipose Tissue as an Endocrine Organ, The Journal of Clinical Endocrinology & Metabolism, Volume 89, Issue 6, 1 June 2004, Pages 2548–2556, https://doi.org/10.1210/jc.2004-0395

60. (Content: I-A) A poster presentation by medical students compares different exposures that occur both in utero and childhood that may affect weight in order to promote healthy habits and reduce risk factors for children. Which of the following is protective for developing childhood obesity?

 A. **Authoritative parenting style**
 B. Treatment of recurrent ear infections
 C. Low birth weight
 D. In utero exposure to tobacco
 E. Untreated attention deficit disorder

(A) Parenting styles may contribute to the weight of their children. The **authoritative style** is described as responsive and warm but with high expectations. Parents generally respond to their child's hunger and satiety cues, which is protective against excess weight. This style of parenting is associated with eating healthier foods and being more physically active compared to other parenting styles. Other parent styles described below are associated with increased BMIs, likely due to interfering with the child's ability to self-regulate their intake:

- Authoritarian: not responsive, but with high expectations
- Negligent: not responsive with minimal rules
- Permissive or indulgent: responsive and warm but few rules

All of the other answer options are risk factors for developing childhood obesity. Both low and high birthweights increase the risk of future obesity compared to normal-weight infants. In utero tobacco exposure leads to a dose-dependent increased risk of excess weight. Untreated attention-deficit/hyperactivity disorder contributes to weight gain due to impulsivity and poor planning leading to increased caloric intake, in addition to its associations with other psychiatric comorbidities (e.g., depression, anxiety, circadian rhythm disturbances, etc.) that are risks for obesity.

Studies also indicate early and repetitive use of antibiotics pose a slightly increased risk of childhood obesity, likely related to altering a developing gut microbiome, which plays a role in energy balance. This effect seems to be more prominent in males.

Reference: Hampl, S. E., Hassink, S. G., Skinner, A. C., Armstrong, S. C., Barlow, S. E., Bolling, C. F., ... Okechukwu, K. (2023). Clinical Practice Guideline for the Evaluation and Treatment of Children and Adolescents With Obesity. Pediatrics, 151(2), e2022060640. https://doi.org/10.1542/peds.2022-060640.

61. (Content: I-B-1) A 26-year-old entered a hot dog-eating contest at the fair. In preparation for this event, he has fasted since the night prior. If hormone levels were checked at the completion of the event, which of the following would be suppressed the most?

A. Glucagon
B. Cholecystokinin
C. Glucagon-like peptide 1
D. Peptide-YY
E. **Growth hormone-releasing peptide**

(E) Ghrelin, or **Growth hormone-releasing peptide,** is the only orexigenic (i.e., hunger) hormone produced in the gastrointestinal tract that peaks before mealtime and decreases after consumption of food. In this person undergoing a hot dog-eating contest, levels would have been highest just prior to the contest, in the fasting state, but would be suppressed in the fed state after the contest.

Importantly, hormone levels are improved after a Roux-en-Y gastric bypass (RYGB), with baseline GLP-1 levels increasing significantly leading to improved glucose control immediately after surgery. Note that ghrelin significantly declines after a sleeve gastrectomy, as the hormone is produced primarily by the gastric fundus.

The hormonal changes in different states are summarized in the table below:

Alteration in Hormones in Different States			
Hormone	RYGB	Fed	Fasting
Ghrelin	↔	↓	↑
Glucagon	↑		
Insulin	↑ Post-prandial		
CCK	↔		
GIP	↑ Post-prandial		
GLP-1	↑↑	↑	↓
PYY	↑		
Amylin	↑		
Oxyntomodulin	↑		

Reference: Bliss ES, Whiteside E. The Gut-Brain Axis, the Human Gut Microbiota and Their Integration in the Development of Obesity. Front Physiol. 2018 Jul 12;9:900. doi: 10.3389/fphys.2018.00900. PMID: 30050464; PMCID: PMC6052131.

62. (Content: II-B-4) A 34-year-old female with a BMI of 29 kg/m^2 presents to her primary care physician with overeating concerns. She states that she often eats a large amount of food and lacks control while eating during these episodes. She hides this behavior from her roommate as she feels intense embarrassment and guilt. What other finding would most likely be expected?

A. Eating more rapidly than normal
B. Compensatory purging
C. Consuming > 25% of calories after dinner
D. Repetitive behaviors
E. Eating small, unplanned amounts of food

(A) This patient's diagnosis is most consistent with binge eating disorder (BED), the most common eating disorder, affecting up to 3.5% of the general population and up to 50% of individuals with severe obesity. It is associated with **eating more rapidly than usual.**

BED is a compulsive eating disorder that should be treated as part of a comprehensive approach to obesity management.

Diagnostic Criteria for Binge Eating Disorder
Recurrent episodes of binge eating marked by:
• Eating large amounts of food in a discrete amount of time
• A sense of lack of control with eating during these episodes
Associated with 3 or more of the following:
• Eating more rapidly than normal
• Eating until uncomfortably full
• Eating large amounts of food when not physically hungry
• Hiding eating behaviors due to embarrassment
• Feeling disgusted, depressed, or guilty after episodes
Marked distress about binge eating
Occurs on average at least 1 time per week for 3 months
Not associated with compensatory purging behaviors

Reference: DSM-5: Diagnostic and Statistical Manual of Mental Disorders, Fifth Edition
Reference: Up to Date: "Eating disorders: Overview of epidemiology, clinical features, and diagnosis"

63. (Content: II-D-3a) A 43-year-old female is presenting with increased thirst and urination. She states that over the past 2-3 months, she has woken up multiple times in the night to urinate and feels like she cannot "drink enough water." She has a past medical history of autoimmune hemolytic anemia and obesity class II. In addition to other age-appropriate screenings, which laboratory test is most sensitive to diagnose her with the most likely condition?

A. Hemoglobin A1c
B. Fasting glucose levels
C. HOMA-IR levels
D. Oral glucose tolerance test
E. Fructosamine levels

(D) The **oral glucose tolerance test** is the most sensitive test to diagnose diabetes mellitus. This consists of consuming a glucose load followed by subsequent serum glucose levels 2 hours after the glucose ingestion. It is more likely to diagnose diabetes and pre-diabetes but is less commonly done due to the inconvenience compared to hemoglobin A1c (HbA1c) levels. Importantly, HbA1c levels are most accurate in patients with a red blood cell life span of 3 months. If shorter, such as this patient with hemolytic anemia, the test will underestimate the true hemoglobin A1c values.

The American Diabetes Association defines the criteria for diabetes as follows:

- Hemoglobin A1c ≥ 6.5%
- Fasting glucose levels of ≥ 126 mg/dL
- Classic symptoms of diabetes with a random glucose of ≥ 200 mg/dL
- Oral glucose tolerance test (OGTT) displaying a glucose level of ≥ 200 mg/dL two hours after ingestion of 75 grams of glucose

Note: The HOMA-IR can be calculated by obtaining a fasting glucose insulin and glucose level to determine insulin resistance. Its clinical utility is controversial.

Diabetes affects over 30 million Americans (9.4% of the U.S. population), with over 90% of those having a BMI ≥ 25 (having overweight or obesity). Broken down further, 34% had pre-obesity (overweight) and an additional 60% of those with type 2 diabetes had a BMI ≥ 30.

Reference: Daousi C, Casson IF, Gill GV, MacFarlane IA, Wilding JP, Pinkney JH. Prevalence of obesity in type 2 diabetes in secondary care: association with cardiovascular risk factors. Postgrad Med J. 2006 Apr;82(966):280-4. doi: 10.1136/pmj.2005.039032. PMID: 16597817; PMCID: PMC2579635.
Reference: Up to Date: "Clinical presentation, diagnosis, and initial evaluation of diabetes mellitus in adults"

64. (Content: II-C-5) A 3-year-old male is brought into the pediatric office, as the mother has recently noticed increased weight gain and an insatiable appetite that was not previously present. After reviewing the growth chart, it is noted that his height has maintained the 60th percentile. However, his weight has increased from the 50th percentile to the 90th percentile in the past 1.5 years. A speech therapist has seen him for delayed speech, and he is scheduled to see a therapist for late motor development. Which of the following would most likely be seen on physical examination?

A. Short 4th and 5th metacarpals
B. Hepatosplenomegaly
C. Polydactyly
D. Macroglossia
E. Almond-shaped eyes

(E) This patient with neurodevelopmental delays and apparent intellectual disability with excessive weight gain, most likely has Prader-Willi syndrome, a paternal chromosome 15q partial deletion (i.e., under-expressed gene). Physical examination findings include thin upper lips and **almond-shaped eyes.** They are often smaller at birth, with bitemporal narrowing of the head, hypotonia, and characteristic "floppiness."

Other characteristics of Prader-Willi syndrome are discussed below:

- **Diagnosis:** DNA methylation studies.
- **Age of obesity:** Onset between 2-5 years of age
- **Treatment:** Calorie restriction and behavioral therapy are the mainstays for obesity, with growth and sex hormone replacement at puberty.

Note: Other conditions causing some of the above findings include Beckwith-Wiedemann syndrome (macroglossia and hepatosplenomegaly), Albright Hereditary Osteodystrophy (shortened 4th and 5th metacarpal bones), and Bardet-Biedl syndrome (polydactyly).

Reference: Cassidy SB, Driscoll DJ. Prader-Willi syndrome. Eur J Hum Genet. 2009;17(1):3-13. doi:10.1038/ejhg.2008.165
Reference: Up to Date: "Clinical features, diagnosis, and treatment of Prader-Willi syndrome"

65. (Content: II-C-2) A 33-year-old Caucasian female is presenting to her primary care physician for an annual exam. She is up to date on her preventative screenings and immunizations. Although she exercises and avoids eating at fast-food restaurants, she is concerned about her cardiovascular risk, as her father had a heart attack at age 42. At what BMI is it recommended to measure waist circumference for additional cardiovascular risk stratification?

A. 18 kg/m^2
B. 24 kg/m^2
C. **33 kg/m^2**
D. 40 kg/m^2

(C) In patients with a **body mass index between 25-34.9 kg/m^2**, the abdominal circumference is recommended to provide additional information on cardiovascular risk. In those with a BMI ≥ 35 kg/m^2, waist circumference is unlikely to add further risk stratification.

Abdominal obesity indicates excess adiposity and infers an increased risk of cardiometabolic risks such as diabetes, metabolic syndrome, hypertension, etc. Cut-off values for abdominal obesity in the U.S. and Canada are as follows:

- Males: > 102 cm (> 40 in)
- Females: > 88 cm (> 35 in)

Note: A BMI cut-off value of ≥ 23 kg/m^2 should be used for screening and confirmation of excess adiposity in South Asian, Southeast Asian, and East Asian adults. Waist circumference cut-offs of ≥ 85 cm for men and ≥ 74-80 cm for women are consistent with abdominal obesity in these populations. These ethnic populations have similar cardiovascular and diabetes risks at these lower BMIs compared to Caucasians at higher thresholds.

For the most accurate results, abdominal waist circumference should be obtained at the level of the iliac crest (highest point). The measuring tape should be snug but not compress the skin and be kept parallel to the floor. The measurement taken at the end of normal expiration is most precise.

Reference: AACE/ACE Guidelines: AMERICAN ASSOCIATION OF CLINICAL ENDOCRINOLOGISTS AND AMERICAN COLLEGE OF ENDOCRINOLOGY COMPREHENSIVE CLINICAL PRACTICE GUIDELINES FOR MEDICAL CARE OF PATIENTS WITH OBESITY (2016). Recommendation 6-7, and Figure 2.

66. (Content: II-D-2) Researchers are performing a study on obesity and the effects on the associated comorbidities as weight fluctuates over two years. They desire the most accurate fat composition measurements at a molecular level, regardless of cost. Which of the following measurement modalities would meet these criteria?

    A. Skinfold calipers
    B. Deuterium dilution hydrometry
    C. Bioelectric impedance analysis
    D. Dual-energy x-ray absorptiometry
    E. Body mass index

(B) For research purposes, **isotope dilution hydrometry** is considered the most accurate test to determine body fat composition at the molecular level, although this method is not utilized in clinical practice. The principle behind this test is that all cells in the body will take up an administered water isotope tracer, except body fat. Therefore, measurement of the isotope dilution allows for the calculation of non-fat mass, which can be subtracted from total body weight, resulting in fat mass.

Note: Percent body fat can assist in diagnosing patients with obesity, defined as ≥ 25% percent body fat in males and ≥ 32% in females. Caucasian males and Hispanic females generally have higher percent body fat.

Body Fat Measurements		
Method	**Pros**	**Cons**
Calipers	Inexpensive	-User-dependent/variable -Not accurate at ↑ BMI
DXA	-Accurate -Relatively inexpensive -Considered the gold standard	-May not accommodate those with extreme BMI
BIA	-Relatively accurate -Inexpensive -Commonly used	-Hydration dependent -Avoid if the patient has electrical cardiac devices
Underwater densitometry	Very accurate	-Time-consuming -Cumbersome
CT/MRI	Very accurate	-Expensive -Radiation exposure (CT) -MRI spectroscopy is best for determining the quantity of visceral fat

DXA: Dual-energy x-ray absorptiometry; **BIA:** Bioelectrical impedance analysis.
Reference: Obesity Medicine Association: Obesity Algorithm (2023)

67. (Content: II-B-3) A 23-year-old healthy female presents for an annual examination at her family practice physician's clinic. She has decided to pursue a vegan diet in place of the pescatarian diet she had previously consumed. She wants to ensure she does not become malnourished and asks about vitamin supplementation. What deficiency will most likely be present if supplementation is not initiated within the next year?

   A. Vitamin C
   B. Cyanocobalamin
   C. **Vitamin D**
   D. Folate
   E. Vitamin K

(C) Patients consuming a vegan diet (no animal products) are most likely to become deficient and require supplementation of vitamin B_{12}, vitamin D, and omega-3. Of those, **vitamin D** will most likely be deficient within a year, as vitamin B_{12} takes years to deplete stores in the absence of pernicious anemia.

Note: Other vitamin deficiencies vegans are at risk for include iron, zinc, calcium, and the essential amino acid lysine.

There are many benefits of vegetarian and vegan diets, which are considered low fat by definition, as < 20% of total calories come from fat. Some benefits include weight loss, lower risk of certain cancers, cardioprotection, improved lipid profile, and decreased diabetes risk.

Variants of this diet include the following:

- Lacto-ova: Consume dairy and eggs
- Pescatarian: Eat fish (no red meat or poultry)
- Vegans: Consume absolutely no animal products
- Vegetarians: May eat animal products (milk, eggs), but not meat

Reference: Up to date: "Vitamin supplementation in disease prevention"

68. (Content: II-D-3a) A 61-year-old male diagnosed with hypertension and obesity class II presents to his sleep specialist to discuss his overnight polysomnography results. His primary care physician referred him after he was experiencing unrefreshing sleep and waking up holding his breath. His spouse also had concerns about loud snoring with pauses in his breathing. Given this patient's history, what is the minimal apnea-hypopnea index (AHI) needed to diagnose obstructive sleep apnea?

A. **5 per hour**
B. 15 per hour
C. 30 per hour
D. 60 per hour

(A) This patient is presenting with severe symptoms of obstructive sleep apnea, **requiring an AHI ≥ 5 episodes of apnea or hypopnea per hour** to meet diagnostic criteria for obstructive sleep apnea.

OSA severity and diagnosis are based on the apnea-hypopnea index (AHI), which is the summation of the following events per one-hour period (total events/total hours of sleep):

- **Apnea:** Respiratory pauses that last ≥ 10 seconds
- **Hypopnea:** Shallow breathing leading to oxygen desaturation of ≥ 4%

An additional diagnostic criterion is the respiratory disturbance index (RDI), which adds respiratory effort-related arousals (RERA) to hypopnea and apnea. RDI, therefore, is more sensitive.

Diagnostic Criteria for Obstructive Sleep Apnea	
1. AHI or RDI > 15/hr **or**	
2. AHI or RDI > 5/hr with severe symptoms (≥ 1 of the following):	
• Daytime sleepiness	• Fatigue
• Unrefreshing sleep	• Insomnia
• Waking up breath-holding, gasping, or chocking	• Witnessed apneic episodes
	• Loud snoring
Severity (AHI): Mild (5-15); Moderate (15-30); Severe > 30	

AHI: Apnea-hypopnea index; **RDI:** Respiratory disturbance index

Reference: Up To Date: "Clinical manifestations and diagnosis of OSA in adults"

69. (Content: II-A-1) A physician is working in an obesity medicine clinic and seeing a patient with inadequate insurance coverage. The patient meets criteria for pharmacologic therapy and is interested but cannot afford name-brand combination medications. Therefore, the physician discusses the off-label use of medications, including emulating the newer combination medications by prescribing the two medications separately. The patient comes back one month later with no weight loss. He explains that he lost one of the two prescriptions. Which medications did he most likely take for the past month?

A. Topiramate
B. Phentermine
C. Bupropion
D. Liraglutide
E. Naltrexone

(E) Of the options above, the only medication that is used in a combination anti-obesity medication for its synergistic effect, but is ineffective alone in causing weight loss, is **naltrexone.**

Bupropion and naltrexone are used for their synergistic effects in weight loss. Bupropion works by stimulating the cleavage of POMC, while increasing the agonism of melanocortin-4 receptors, by releasing α-MSH, assisting the anorexigenic pathway. However, another cleavage product from POMC, β-endorphin, causes a negative feedback loop within the POMC neuron when it binds the μ-opioid receptor, thereby decreasing the neuronal activity. This opioid receptor and subsequent downstream effects of β-endorphin are blocked by naltrexone, thus amplifying the α-MSH effects and reducing further food intake. Without the effects of bupropion, the counter effects are not present, and therefore naltrexone, by itself, is ineffective.

Reference: The burden of obesity in the current world and the new treatments available: focus on liraglutide 3.0 mg Marcio C. Mancini1,2,3 and Maria Edna de Mel. Mancini and de Melo Diabetol Metab Syndr (2017) 9:44 DOI 10.1186/s13098-017-0242-0

70. (Content: II-C-7) A 9-year-old female is brought to her pediatrician for a well-child check. A few years ago, she was diagnosed with depression. Although the medications prescribed have helped with her mood symptoms, her appetite has significantly increased. She eats approximately 3500 kcal/day and admits to playing on the computer and watching more television than previously. Lab work including thyroid hormone levels are normal. Her weight is displayed on the growth chart below. Which stature curve would best correlate with her height?

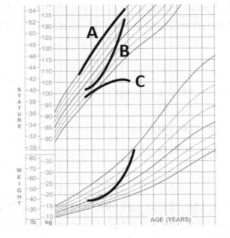

A. Line A
B. Line B
C. Line C

(B) Children consuming excess calories leading to weight gain would have an upward trajectory on both the height and weight curves in a proportional manner, consistent with **line B**. In contrast, those with endocrinopathies such as hypothyroidism or Cushing's disease would develop increased weight with decreased growth velocity, leading to flattening of the growth curve (line C).

Exceptions to the generalized statements above occur in various genetic etiologies of obesity:

- **Tall stature:** Melanocortin 4 receptor deficiency leads to persistently tall stature with increased weight. This would likely cause a growth curve similar to line A.
- **Short stature:** Turner syndrome, Down syndrome, Prader-Willi, and Albright Hereditary Osteodystrophy would cause a patient to be persistently on a lower percentile growth curve.

Reference: Styne DM, Arslanian SA, Connor EL, Farooqi IS, Murad MH, Silverstein JH, Yanovski JA. Pediatric Obesity-Assessment, Treatment, and Prevention: An Endocrine Society Clinical Practice Guideline. J Clin Endocrinol Metab. 2017 Mar 1;102(3):709-757. doi: 10.1210/jc.2016-2573. PMID: 28359099; PMCID: PMC6283429.

71. (Content: II-C-3) A 27-year-old female with a history of hypertension and recently diagnosed obstructive sleep apnea (OSA) presents for evaluation after having failed many name-brand diets. She states she has always been "on the heavier side," but needing a CPAP machine for OSA motivated her to lose weight. Physical examination reveals a rounded face and truncal obesity with widened abdominal striae. Laboratory work reveals a hemoglobin A1c in the pre-diabetes range. What other finding would most likely be present on physical exam?

    A. Scalloped tongue
    B. Hirsutism
    C. Decreased deep tendon reflexes
    D. Periumbilical hernia
    E. Superficial ecchymosis

(E) This patient presenting with hypertension, OSA, wide (> 1 cm) abdominal striae, and moon facies has physical exam findings consistent with the diagnosis of Cushing's syndrome. Facial acne and **easy bruising** are also commonly seen. Clinical and physical findings are related to hypercortisolism.

Cushing's syndrome is a rare cause of secondary obesity, but essential to consider in the right clinical scenario. Clinical pearls are listed below:

- **Clinical manifestations:** Facial plethora, moon/round face, dorsal fat pad (buffalo hump), hypertension, truncal obesity (thin extremities), proximal muscle weakness, osteoporosis, glucose intolerance, acne, and ecchymosis.
- **Etiology:** The most common cause of hypercortisolism is iatrogenic, although central (excess ACTH secretion), peripheral (adrenal adenoma), and paraneoplastic etiologies are possibilities.
- **Initial screening:** 24-hour urinary-free cortisol excretion (x2), overnight 1 mg dexamethasone test, or late-night buccal salivary swab (x2).

Reference: Up to Date: "Establishing the diagnosis of Cushing's syndrome"

72. (Content: II-D-1) A female sprinter undergoes indirect calorimetry to determine her respiratory quotient (RQ), which is obtained by measuring carbon dioxide eliminated divided by oxygen consumed. When the athlete is slowly jogging, it is determined that her body mostly utilizes lipids for energy. However, during sustained sprinting, her RQ would be expected to be near which of the following values?

A. 0.5
B. 0.7
C. 1.0
D. 1.3

(C) The respiratory quotient (RQ) equals eliminated carbon dioxide divided by oxygen consumed, measured on indirect calorimetry. The RQ can determine which macronutrients are being metabolized (energy utilized by the body). If energy consumption is only from lipids, the RQ will be 0.7, whereas if solely from carbohydrates, it will be closer to 1.0.

The respiratory quotient allows you to determine which macronutrients are being consumed for energy in a steady state.

- If low-energy but sustainable exercise is being performed (jogging in a marathon), then the RQ will be closer to 0.7, as stored fats are primarily being used for energy. In addition, inactivity tends to be closer to 0.7.
- If high-intensity, high-energy exercise is being performed (sprinting), carbohydrates are mainly used for energy, and the **RQ is near 1.**

In summary, the more intense the workout, the more carbohydrates are utilized for energy. The longer the duration of exercise, the more lipids (fats) are utilized for energy.

Note: This topic will likely be tested in a simple form; memorizing the RQs in the table below and having a basic understanding will be sufficient.

Respiratory Quotient	
Carbohydrates	1
Proteins	0.8
Fats	0.7
Mixed	0.8

Reference: Patel H, Kerndt CC, Bhardwaj A. Physiology, Respiratory Quotient. 2020 Sep 16. In: StatPearls. Treasure Island (FL): StatPearls Publishing; 2021 Jan–. PMID: 30285389.

73. (Content: II-C-6) A 44-year-old female presents for a follow-up three years after undergoing a Roux-en-Y gastric bypass. She is pleased with her results, having lost nearly 55% of her total body weight, and she states she continues to lose weight despite no longer following the dietician's recommendations or exercising. She denies depression and says she feels well but admits to diarrhea. Preoperative BMI was 47.3 kg/m^2, and today it is 22.7 kg/m^2. Physical exam is normal except for excess skin in the abdomen and arms. She has not followed up with her surgeon after the first year. Which of the following may explain her weight loss?

    A. Vitamin deficiency
    B. Anastomotic stricture
    C. Small intestinal bowel overgrowth
    D. A shorter common intestinal channel
    E. Expected post-surgical weight loss

(D) The common channel is the portion of the intestine after the digestive and alimentary tracts connect. A shorter channel (as seen in biliopancreatic diversion with a duodenal switch) leads to decreased absorption of nutrients. This otherwise asymptomatic patient has lost an excessive amount of weight (35% expected after Roux-en-Y gastric bypass) in the setting of not adhering to dietary or physical activity recommendations. This is concerning for an anatomical cause, most likely **a shorter common channel** leading to malabsorption, which also explains this patient's persistent diarrhea. Other causes of excess weight loss are discussed below:

- Eating disorders such as bulimia or anorexia nervosa
- Underlying malignancy, which is usually associated with increased fatigue, night sweats, and potentially localizing symptoms
- Small intestinal bowel overgrowth of which symptoms would include bloating, nausea, early satiety, abdominal discomfort, and diarrhea
- Anastomotic stricture with symptoms including localized abdominal pain, food aversion, and possible dysphagia
- Depression or other psychiatric conditions

Reference: Akusoba I, Birriel TJ, El Chaar M. Management of Excessive Weight Loss Following Laparoscopic Roux-en-Y Gastric Bypass: Clinical Algorithm and Surgical Techniques. Obes Surg. 2016 Jan;26(1):5-11. doi: 10.1007/s11695-015-1775-7. PMID: 26105983.

74. (Content: II-D-3a) A 14-year-old female with a BMI of 39 kg/m^2 presents to her family practitioner for recurrent headaches. She states the headaches are pulsatile and occasionally cause loss of appetite. In addition, she now has difficulty seeing the board during school and must sit toward the front of her class. She has intermittent loss of vision and diplopia when standing up. Which of the following would be the best test to determine the cause of her headaches?

A. Orthostatic vital signs
B. Overnight sleep study
C. Ophthalmologic evaluation
D. Brain imaging
E. Cerebral spinal fluid studies

(E) This adolescent female with obesity class II has intermittent headaches, vision changes, and positional diplopia. She likely has a diagnosis of idiopathic intracranial hypertension (IIH), also known as pseudotumor cerebri. Although many options are valid, only a **lumbar puncture displaying elevated opening pressure** will definitively diagnose this patient with IIH.

Note: Imaging may be necessary to exclude secondary causes for headaches, while an ophthalmology examination is necessary to document the degree of papilledema. Although sleep apnea can cause headaches, it should not cause vision changes.

IIH is most commonly seen in women with excess weight and is characterized by vision loss, papilledema, and headaches caused by elevated intracranial pressures with otherwise normal cerebral fluid studies.

Treatment options should include weight loss of >5-10% (lifestyle modifications and/or medical and surgical options) with a low-sodium diet. In addition, carbonic anhydrase inhibitors such as acetazolamide or topiramate (which also helps with weight loss) lower cerebral fluid pressure.

Surgical interventions such as optic nerve sheath fenestration and shunting procedures should be pursued for deteriorating vision or intractable headaches.

Reference: Up to Date: "Idiopathic intracranial hypertension (pseudotumor cerebri): Clinical features and diagnosis & prognosis and treatment"

75. (Content: II-C-7) A mother brings her 9-year-old son to his pediatrician for evaluation, as she is concerned that his height and weight are increased in comparison to his peers. The mother states that her son does tend to watch 4-5 hours of television daily and is "constantly snacking." The son has no known health concerns, and overall appears happy. Physical examination reveals a BMI of 19.75 kg/m^2, which is the 86th percentile for his age and gender. Which of the following most accurately describes his weight categorization?

    A. Underweight
    B. Healthy weight
    C. Overweight
    D. Class 1 obesity
    E. Class 2 obesity

(C) Unlike adults, in which absolute BMI is used to categorize weight, in children aged 2-20, weight status is based on a <u>percentile</u> range of BMI, taking into consideration gender and age. For this patient, who is in the 86th percentile range for BMI, this places him in the **overweight category.**

Importantly, BMI is not used until children reach 2 years of age. Instead, weight for length is used in those ages 0-2 years of age.

Childhood Obesity Classification (Age 2-19 years)	
Classification	**Percentile Range[1] (% BMI)**
Underweight	Less than 5%
Healthy weight	5 to < 85%
Overweight	85 to < 95%
Obesity	95 to < 99%
Severe Obesity	≥99th percentile
Expanded Definition (Splits Obesity into Class I, II, and III)	
Class 1 Obesity	≥ 95th percentile to < 120% of the 95th percentile
Class 2 Obesity[2]	≥ 120% to < 140% of the 95th percentile or BMI ≥ 35 to ≤ 39 kg/m^2
Class 3 Obesity[2]	≥ 140% of the 95[th]percentile or BMI ≥ 40 kg/m^2

[1]Percentile range based on age and gender.
[2]Criteria can be made based on BMI **or** percentile, whichever meets the criteria

Reference: Obesity Medicine Association: Pediatric Obesity Algorithm (2023-2024)

76. (Content: II-A-3) A 19-year-old male presents to his primary care physician for an annual physical evaluation. He admits to eating significantly more since he started college. He relates this to stress and a change in sleep habits since moving to the dormitories. He states he has gained approximately 20 lbs (9.1 kg) over the past five months. His BMI is 29 kg/m². Laboratory findings include a hemoglobin A1c of 5.9% (reference range: < 5.7%), and his fasting cholesterol panel is consistent with dyslipidemia. To diagnose him with metabolic syndrome, what additional finding is necessary?

A. Abdominal circumference of 100 cm (39 inches)
B. Diagnosis of obstructive sleep apnea
C. Diastolic blood pressure of 82 mmHg
D. Being treated with amlodipine

(D) This patient with pre-diabetes (HbA1c 5.7-6.5%) and dyslipidemia nearly meets the criteria for metabolic syndrome. Of the answer options, the additional **presence of hypertension, with or without treatment**, would meet the National Cholesterol Education Program (NCEP) Adult Treatment Panel III (ATP III) criteria for metabolic syndrome. Diagnostic criteria for metabolic syndrome requires 3 of the following 5 to be present:

- Abdominal obesity, defined as a waist circumference ≥ 102 cm (40 in) in men and ≥ 88 cm (35 in) in women
- Serum triglycerides ≥ 150 mg/dL or drug treatment for elevated triglycerides
- Serum high-density lipoprotein (HDL) cholesterol < 40 mg/dL in men and < 50 mg/dL in women, or drug treatment for low HDL cholesterol
- Blood pressure ≥ 130/85 mmHg, or drug treatment for elevated blood pressure
- Fasting plasma glucose (FPG) ≥ 100 mg/dL, or drug treatment for elevated blood glucose

Metabolic syndrome is associated with increased levels of resistin and inflammatory cytokines and a decrease in adiponectin, leading to dysfunctional adipose tissue. This adiposopathy increases the risk of cardiovascular complications, fatty liver disease, and insulin resistance leading to the diagnostic findings.

Reference: Up to Date: "Metabolic syndrome (insulin resistance syndrome or syndrome X)"

77. (Content: II-B-5) A 14-year-old female presents to her pediatrician's office for an annual examination. She denies any concerns but appears withdrawn. She states school is "going okay." When asked about diet, she says she hardly eats because she is "fat and ugly." Physical examination reveals a BMI of 17 kg/m^2, with a global cachectic appearance. Which of the following is most associated with her underlying condition?

    A. Tachycardia
    B. Urinary phosphate wasting
    C. Increased osteoblast activity
    D. Decreased luteinizing hormone
    E. Respiratory alkalosis

(D) This patient is presenting with a low BMI and restricted calorie intake due to a distorted body image, consistent with the diagnosis of anorexia nervosa. This condition is associated with many findings, including:

- Central hypogonadism (functional amenorrhea) with **low luteinizing hormone (LH)** and follicular stimulating hormone (FSH)
- Bradycardia
- Electrolyte disturbances, especially hypomagnesemia, hypokalemia, and metabolic alkalosis
- Osteoporosis (decreased osteoblast and osteoclast activity)

Diagnostic Criteria for Anorexia Nervosa[1]	
Restriction of energy intake relative to requirements leading to ↓ weight	
Intense fear of gaining weight or becoming overweight or persistent behavior that interferes with weight gain	
Body image distortion/lack of recognition of the seriousness of ↓ weight	
Specifiers • Restricting type (i.e., diet) • Binge eating/purging type	**Severity** • Mild: BMI ≥ 17-18.5 kg/m^2 • Moderate: BMI 16-17 kg/m^2 • Severe: BMI 15-16 kg/m^2 • Extreme: BMI < 15 kg/m^2

[1]Amenorrhea is no longer a diagnostic criterion

Reference: DSM-5: Diagnostic and Statistical Manual of Mental Disorders, Fifth Edition

78. (Content: II-C-7) A 4-year-old child experiences a decline in BMI during the first few years of life, reaching a minimum point. However, instead of a gradual increase in BMI typical for this age, there is an early onset of BMI increase before the age of 5. This phenomenon places the patient at risk for an

A. early growth spurt
B. adiposity nadir shift
C. **early adiposity rebound**
D. accelerated BMI normalization

(C) **Early adiposity rebound (EAR)** refers to a phenomenon in childhood growth patterns where a child's body mass index (BMI) reaches its lowest point and then begins to increase again at an earlier age than usual.

In typical growth patterns, a child experiences a decline in BMI during the first few years of life, reaching a minimum point known as adiposity nadir. After this point, BMI usually increases gradually until puberty, when another growth spurt occurs. However, in the case of early adiposity rebound, the increase in BMI begins earlier than expected, often before the age of 5.

Early adiposity rebound is considered a risk factor for the development of obesity later into adolescence and adulthood. It also is associated with an increased likelihood of developing health risks, such as cardiovascular disease, diabetes, and other obesity-related conditions.

Several factors may contribute to early adiposity rebound, including genetic predisposition, early feeding practices, dietary habits, physical activity levels, and environmental factors. Understanding and identifying early adiposity rebound in childhood can be important for implementing preventive measures and interventions to promote healthy growth and reduce the risk of obesity-related health issues later in life.

Summary: BMI rapidly increases in the first year, then slows down and reaches nadir. At age 5-7 years of age, the BMI increases again as adiposity increases. This is the second rise of the BMI, which is normal. An early rebound before age 5 increases the risk of overweight/obesity.

Reference: Kang MJ. The adiposity rebound in the 21st century children: meaning for what? Korean J Pediatr. 2018 Dec;61(12):375-380. doi: 10.3345/kjp.2018.07227. Epub 2018 Dec 6. PMID: 30585060; PMCID: PMC6313085.

79. (Content: II-C-6) A 22-year-old female presents to the emergency department with persistent nausea, vomiting, and lack of nutrition for the past week since her discharge from the hospital after undergoing a Roux-en-Y gastric bypass. She has skin tenting and dry mucous membranes. Which of the following physical exam findings is most likely to be present?

A. Night blindness
B. Positive Romberg sign
C. Jaundice
D. **Nystagmus**

(D) This patient is presenting with a clear lack of nutrition due to nausea and vomiting with dehydration (i.e., skin tenting and dry mucous membranes). Compared to other vitamin deficiencies, symptoms of thiamine deficiency can occur rapidly without proper oral intake, within days to weeks, and is a medical emergency. Thiamine deficiency can lead to Wernicke's and includes ataxia and **nystagmus.** Other nutritional deficiencies take more time to manifest including vitamin A (night blindness) and vitamin B_{12} (positive Romberg sign).

Nutritional deficiencies leading to neurologic findings are high-yield for boards. Important associations include:

- B_1 (thiamine): Occurring days to weeks after surgery. Often presenting with ascending weakness mimicking Guillain–Barré syndrome.
- B_{12} (cyanocobalamin): Occurring months to years after surgery with myeloneuropathy including loss of proprioception and vibration sense.
- Copper: Occurring months to years after surgery. Myelopathy (similar to B_{12}) with anemia and neutropenia are common. A spastic gait, ataxia, and paresthesias in a stocking-glove configuration may also be seen.

Neurological Findings in Nutritional Deficiencies	
Finding	**Associated Deficiency**
Confabulation	Thiamine (B_1): Korsakoff's
Dementia/memory issues	Niacin (B_3), folate (B_9), or cyanocobalamin (B_{12})
Neuropathy	Thiamine (B_1), cyanocobalamin (B_{12}), pyridoxine (B_6), or copper
Ophthalmoplegia/ nystagmus	Thiamine (B_1)
Myelopathy	Copper

Reference: Kushner, R. (2020). Primary Care: Evaluation and Management of Obesity. United States: Wolters Kluwer Health.

80. (Content: II-C-3) A 13-year-old male presents to urgent care with hip and knee pain. His weight is in the 95th percentile and his height is in the 80th percentile. He takes no multivitamins and avoids meat. Imaging is completed, as shown below.

Which of the following is the most appropriate recommendation at this time?

A. Encourage increased vitamin D supplementation
B. **Urgent surgical evaluation**
C. Discuss weight loss options
D. Rest, ice, compression, and elevation
E. Endocrinopathy testing

(B) This patient with excess weight is presenting with hip and knee pain, with the x-ray of the pelvis showing a right-sided slipped capital femoral epiphysis (SCFE). This radiographic finding appears as ice cream falling off the cone (arrow). Although the most common risk factor is obesity which must be addressed, the priority is to refer to an **orthopedic surgeon immediately** to stabilize the joint with pinning.

Reference: Up to Date: "Evaluation and management of slipped capital femoral epiphysis (SCFE)"
Image reference: Marquez D, Harb E, Vilchis H. Slipped capital femoral epiphysis and hypothyroidism in a young adult: a case report. J Med Case Rep. 2014 Oct 10;8(1):336. doi: 10.1186/1752-1947-8-336. PMID: 25304936; PMCID: PMC5011917.

81. (Content: II-F) A researcher is planning to initiate a study evaluating the effectiveness of four different dietary plans compared to an unrestricted eating plan. There are 100 volunteers that will be split into each of the five study arms and will be followed for six months. Prior to being placed into their groups, the dietician overseeing the study discusses her personal success with intermittent fasting. Which research bias is being demonstrated?

    A. Measurement bias
    B. Recall bias
    C. Response bias
    D. Sampling bias
    E. Observer bias

(E) This dietician discussed her personal preference with the study candidates, thus displaying **observer bias,** also known as researcher or interviewer bias. This type of bias occurs when a researcher unintentionally influences study outcomes through their observations, data collection, or interactions with participants due to their expectations or beliefs. Other research biases include:

- **Selection:** When the sample of study participants is not representative of the target population, leading to nongeneralizable results
- **Sampling:** When the method used to select study participants is flawed, leading to a non-random/unrepresentative sample
- **Non-response:** When participants who do not respond to a survey or research request are significantly different than those who do
- **Recall:** Awareness of a disorder alters recall by subjects, or they do not remember important information from past exposures
- **Measurement:** Inaccuracies in how data is measured (e.g., noncalibrated blood pressure cuff), recorded, or interpreted
- **Publication:** Studies that have more favorable or statistically significant results are more likely to be published leading to an overrepresentation of positive results. This is common with weight-loss supplement studies.
- **Response:** Where participants provide inaccurate information due to misinterpreting questions or wanting to represent themselves positively
- **Confirmation:** Interpreting results in a way that confirms to pre-existing beliefs while ignoring contradictory information

Reference: Pannucci CJ, Wilkins EG. Identifying and avoiding bias in research. Plast Reconstr Surg. 2010 Aug;126(2):619-625. doi: 10.1097/PRS.0b013e3181de24bc. PMID: 20679844; PMCID: PMC2917255.

82. (Content: II-D-1) A sports medicine physician is working with athletes to optimize their performance. He has them undergo testing to determine the VO_2 maximum, in order to calculate their cardiorespiratory fitness level. Which of the following statements is most accurate regarding VO_2 max?

    A. VO_2 max increases with age
    B. Professional athletes have low levels of VO_2 max
    C. Decreasing body fat percentage improves VO_2 max
    D. VO_2 max is similar among genders

(C) The volume of oxygen consumed (VO_2) is a marker of oxygen utilization, with higher levels indicating increased efficiency. Efficiency includes oxygen absorption (lungs), oxygen distribution (heart), and oxygen utilization (muscles). Pathology or inefficiency of any of these systems would decrease VO_2 max.

VO_2 max is measured by cardiopulmonary exercise testing. Patients breathe through a closed loop system containing a mask and tubing, with the tubes connected to an oxygen and carbon dioxide analyzer. Measurements of oxygen consumption are in mL/kg/min.

Generalizations about VO_2 max include:

- Levels decrease with age (approximately a 30% decrease at age 65 compared to age 20).
- Athletes have higher levels
- **Decreasing body fat percentage increases levels**
- Males generally have higher VO_2 levels when compared to females

VO_2 max is often looked at as a marker of cardiorespiratory fitness and endurance, with some of the fittest athletes having levels in the 90 mL/kg/min range. In contrast, the average female and male are in the 35 and 45 mL/kg/min range, respectively.

Reference: Lundby C, Montero D, Joyner M. Biology of VO2 max: looking under the physiology lamp. Acta Physiol (Oxf). 2017 Jun;220(2):218-228. doi: 10.1111/apha.12827. Epub 2016 Nov 25. PMID: 27888580.

83. (Content: II-D-3a) A 34-year-old male presents to the clinic after attending a bariatric seminar. He is interested in weight loss surgery. He takes amlodipine for hypertension and is adherent with continuous positive airway pressure (CPAP) for his obstructive sleep apnea. He denies any tobacco or alcohol history. Which of the following would be the most appropriate initial screening test for metabolic-associated fatty liver disease at this time?

    A. History
    B. Physical exam findings
    C. Laboratory work
    D. Right upper quadrant ultrasound
    E. Liver biopsy

(C) All patients diagnosed with overweight or obesity, type 2 diabetes mellitus, or metabolic syndrome should be screened for metabolic-associated (nonalcoholic) fatty liver disease (MAFLD). Screening should be completed with a **liver enzyme (AST/ALT) evaluation.** ALT is the most specific enzyme for MAFLD in adults and children.

Although the physical examination is essential, it is not sensitive nor specific for diagnosing MAFLD. Therefore, initial laboratory testing with a complete metabolic panel is indicated, followed by imaging modalities such as a liver ultrasound or transient elastography if liver transaminases are elevated.

MAFLD includes a spectrum of fatty liver diseases as follows:

- Hepatosteatosis is fatty liver
- Hepatosteatitis is fatty liver with inflammation
- Metabolic-associated steatohepatitis (MASH) is the presence of > 5% hepatic fat, with inflammation and hepatocyte injury, +/- cirrhosis

No FDA drugs are explicitly approved to treat MAFLD, although GLP-1 receptor agonists and PPAR (i.e., thiazolidinediones) have shown some potential.

Update: Recent changes to nomenclature have changed nonalcoholic fatty liver disease (NAFLD) to metabolic-associated liver disease (MAFLD) to better describe the underlying physiology of this condition.

Reference: AACE/ACE Guidelines: AMERICAN ASSOCIATION OF CLINICAL ENDOCRINOLOGISTS AND AMERICAN COLLEGE OF ENDOCRINOLOGY COMPREHENSIVE CLINICAL PRACTICE GUIDELINES FOR MEDICAL CARE OF PATIENTS WITH OBESITY (2016). Recommendation 16.
Reference: Obesity Medicine Association: Obesity Algorithm (2023)

84. (Content II-C-1) A 22-year-old male is frustrated by his recent diagnosis of "overweight," which was made at an insurance screening exam. He weight-lifts for 3-4 hours daily and competes at the state and national level for body-building. Prior testing reveals an 18% body fat composition. What other condition would act similarly to this patient in terms of an increased BMI with a discordant obesity-related risk association?

    A. **Congestive heart failure**
    B. Increased age
    C. Southeast Asian ethnicity
    D. Sarcopenia
    E. Osteoporosis

(A) **Congestive heart failure** or any condition that increases excess water through third spacing (e.g., cirrhosis, nephrotic syndrome) tends to overestimate body mass index (BMI) but not increase adiposity-related risk factors that are usually associated with an increased BMI. The other listed choices tend to underestimate the adiposity risk associated with a particular BMI.

Note: Body mass index does not consider body composition, which is a better measurement for obesity in those with fluid overload or extremes of muscle mass (e.g., bodybuilders or those with sarcopenia).

BMI is generally the first step in determining the degree of excess weight to estimate adiposity. However, this does not always accurately determine cardiovascular risks, as this may be better predicted by waist circumference, waist-to-hip ratio, or body-mass composition in certain populations.

Regardless, BMI is overall easy to obtain, reproducible, cheap, and for the general population, it correlates with adiposity. Therefore, many insurance companies (and the FDA) rely on this almost exclusively to determine the inclusivity of bariatric surgery and anti-obesity medications.

Reference: Obesity Medicine Association: Obesity Algorithm (2023)
Reference: Up to Date: "Obesity in adults: Prevalence, screening, and evaluation"

85. (Content: II-C-6) A 63-year-old female presents to her primary care physician's office for follow-up after starting methotrexate with complaints of a sore tongue and irritability. She was diagnosed with polymyalgia rheumatica two years ago and was placed on 15 mg of prednisone daily. However, she had gained nearly 60 lbs (27.2 kg) while on prednisone. Eight months ago, she was transitioned to methotrexate for glucocorticoid-sparing therapy. Her BMI is 35 kg/m^2. Which of the following is most responsible for her current condition?

A. Vitamin B_1
B. Vitamin B_2
C. Vitamin B_3
D. Vitamin B_9
E. Vitamin B_{12}

(D) This patient, who is on methotrexate without mention of folate supplementation, presenting with glossitis and irritability, most likely has developed **functional folic acid deficiency (B_9)**. Although the intention to treat secondary obesity was appropriate, the lack of proper vitamin supplementation was not. B_9 deficiency can also be seen in patients with alcohol use disorder and other medications such as phenytoin, sulfasalazine, and TMP-SMX.

Water Soluble B Vitamin Deficiencies		
$B_\#$	Name	Deficiency
B_1	Thiamine	Wernicke's encephalopathy, Korsakoff syndrome, Beriberi: wet (cardiovascular) and dry (neurologic)
B_2	Riboflavin	Sore throat, cheilitis, stomatitis, glossitis, itchy eyes
B_3	Niacin	Pellagra (dermatitis, diarrhea, dementia, death)
B_5	Pantothenic acid	Rare! Paresthesia, restlessness, apathy, hypoglycemia
B_6	Pyridoxine	Peripheral neuropathy, microcytic anemia
B_7	Biotin[1]	Facial dermatitis, neurologic findings (depression, neuropathy, hallucinations)
B_9	Folate	Macrocytic anemia without significant neurologic findings, mouth ulcers, irritability. Fetal neuro tube defects in pregnancy.
B_{12}	Cyanocobalamin	Subacute combined degeneration, macrocytic anemia, glossitis, neurologic manifestations

[1]Consumption of large quantities of raw egg whites can bind to biotin, preventing its absorption, leading to a deficiency.

Reference: Up to Date: "Overview of water-soluble vitamins"

86. (Content: II-C-4) A 14-year-old male presents to his family practice physician for his annual physical examination. He is in the 105th percentile for weight and the 65th percentile for height. His upper arm circumference is 37 cm. Which of the following would likely cause an inaccurately elevated systolic blood pressure?

  A. Using a large adult-sized cuff (16x36 cm)
  B. Sitting in a chair with back support
  C. **Having the patient rest his arm by his side**
  D. Telling the patient not to talk during inflation
  E. Deflating the cuff at 5-10 mmHg per second

(C) Understanding blood pressure monitoring is vital to ensure accurate results and avoid overtreatment and overdiagnosing hypertension. Systolic blood pressure may appear artificially elevated if the patient is supine, the patient's legs are crossed, **the arms are allowed to rest unsupported by the patient's side**, or when using an undersized blood pressure cuff.

Note: ABOM will ask questions on the appropriate evaluation of comorbidities of obesity, including proper techniques. Expect these questions on test day!

Accurate blood pressure monitoring is essential in determining a disease that often requires medications. Proper techniques are described below:

- Patients should be seated comfortably. The back should be supported, and the legs should be uncrossed.
- The blood pressure cuff should be on bare skin.
- The patient's arm should be supported at the level of the heart.
- The cuff bladder length should encircle 80-100% of the arm circumference, which is taken into account by the posted cuff size (cm).
- There should be no talking while obtaining the measurement.

An appropriately sized blood pressure cuff for the patient's arm size is required. The term "large adult" for a blood pressure cuff is a misnomer, as it should be based on the arm circumference, not a subjective adult size.

References: New AHA Recommendations for Blood Pressure Measurement; Am Fam Physician. 2005 Oct 1;72(7):1391-1398.
Reference: 2017 ACC/AHA/AAPA/ABC/ACPM/AGS/APhA/ASH/ASPC/NMA/PCNA Guideline for the Prevention, Detection, Evaluation, and Management of High Blood Pressure in Adults

87. (Content: II-B-4) A 44-year-old female presents to the office with concerns about weight gain. She rarely eats breakfast but instead eats from the time she gets home from work until bedtime. She occasionally awakens and consumes calories at night. The only medication she takes is zolpidem for insomnia. Which of the following questions would be most helpful to determine if the nocturnal caloric intake is caused by zolpidem versus night eating syndrome?

A. **Are you aware during your nocturnal eating episodes?**
B. What is the dose of your zolpidem?
C. Do you have a prior history of sleep walking?
D. Do you take any other over-the-counter medications?
E. Are you drowsy in the mornings after taking zolpidem?

(A) Night eating syndrome (NES) is often associated with depression and insomnia. One of the characteristic features of NES is waking up in the night to eat. Importantly, **patients are awake and aware they are eating**, which differentiates this from sleep-related eating disorders (SRED) caused by sleep medications (e.g., zolpidem). SRED is a parasomnia where patients unknowingly "sleep-eat" with no memory of this in the morning. SRED are often treated by sleep specialists, as they are sleep disorders, not an eating disorder.

Diagnostic Criteria for Night Eating Syndrome
Increased intake after evening meal: <ul><li>At least 25% of daily caloric intake occurs after the evening meal</li><li>Two episodes of nocturnal eating per week</li></ul>
Three of the following: <ul><li>Lack of desire to eat breakfast (≥4 times per week)</li><li>Increased appetite after supper and/or throughout the night</li><li>Sleep onset and/or sleep maintenance insomnia is present</li><li>Feeling that one must eat in order to fall back to sleep</li><li>Mood is often depressed or worsens in the evening</li></ul>
Awareness of nocturnal episodes present (excludes SRED)
Marked distress or impairment in functioning
Pattern of eating is present for at least 3 months
Findings not attributed to substance use, medication, or other disorders

SRED: sleep-related eating disorder

Reference: Allison KC, Lundgren JD, O'Reardon JP, Geliebter A, Gluck ME, Vinai P, Mitchell JE, Schenck CH, Howell MJ, Crow SJ, Engel S, Latzer Y, Tzischinsky O, Mahowald MW, Stunkard AJ. Proposed diagnostic criteria for night eating syndrome. Int J Eat Disord. 2010 Apr;43(3):241-7. doi: 10.1002/eat.20693. PMID: 19378289; PMCID: PMC4531092.

88. (Content: II-F) A university hospital is working with the Centers for Medicare and Medicaid Services (CMS) regarding billing and repayments. The current system allows for an increased hospital length of stay based on body mass index alone. The new proposal is to establish repayments and recommended appropriate length of stay on obesity-related comorbidities and functional limitations. Which of the following would be the best categorization method to initiate?

    A. New York Heart Association Classification
    B. Edmonton Obesity Staging System
    C. Epworth Sleepiness Score
    D. World Health Organization Obesity Classification
    E. King's Obesity Staging Criteria

(B) **The Edmonton Obesity Staging System (EOSS)** is used to categorize patients based on the severity of obesity-related comorbidities, psychologic symptoms, and functional limitations rather than focusing strictly on anthropometric measurements such as waist circumference and body mass index.

Therefore, this staging system provides better insight into the patient's long-term impact of obesity and may help determine the level of appropriate treatment (along with established metrics).

For example, if there are two patients, both with a BMI of 32 kg/m^2, and one is EOSS stage 0 (asymptomatic with no risk factors), and the other is EOSS stage 2 (moderate, established comorbidities), prioritizing more frequent visits, anti-obesity medication management, dieticians, etc. for the latter patient may have a more substantial health impact, especially if resources are limited.

Note: The King's Obesity Staging Criteria staging system was designed to compare baseline pre-operative and post-operative variables in bariatric surgery patients. Some variables are more subjective (i.e., perceived health status and body image) and thus would be less helpful in this vignette.

Reference: Using the Edmonton obesity staging system to predict mortality in a population-representative cohort of people with overweight and obesity. Raj S. Padwal, Nicholas M. Pajewski, David B. Allison and Arya M. Sharma. CMAJ October 04, 2011 183 (14) E1059-E1066; DOI: https://doi.org/10.1503/cmaj.110387
Reference: "Assessment of obesity beyond body mass index to determine benefit of treatment." E. T. Aasheim, S. J. B. Aylwin, S. T. Radhakrishnan, A. S. Sood, A. Jovanovic, T. Olbers, C. W. le Roux, First published: 05 July 2011 https://doi.org/10.1111/j.1758-8111.2011.00017.x

89. (Content: II-D-2) A physician is discussing the different terminology used in body composition to a rotating internal medicine resident. She describes a term that encompasses muscles, organs, water, bones, ligaments, tendons, and essential fat, but does not include nonessential adipose tissue. Which of the following terms is she most likely describing?

    A. Fat mass
    B. Fat-free mass
    C. Lean body mass
    D. Total body mass
    E. Percent body fat

(C) **Lean body mass** is the total body mass (including muscles, internal organs, water, bones, ligaments, and tendons) excluding nonessential adipose tissue. It slightly differs from fat-free mass because lean body mass includes the <u>essential</u> fat in the bone marrow, central nervous system, and internal organs. Lean body mass makes up approximately 75% of total body mass (40% muscle, 25% organs, and 10% bone).

Note: Fat-free mass does not include **<u>ANY</u>** body fat in its calculation. Fat-free mass is often within 5% of lean body mass given that lean body mass includes only a limited subset of adipose tissue (i.e., essential fat).

Importantly, lean body mass is:

- Less in females
- Less in those who are sedentary
- Decreases as age increases

Higher lean body mass is associated with increased health, whereas increased fat mass is associated with increased health risks.

Although most dual-energy x-ray absorptiometry (DXA) scans measure fat, soft tissue, and bone, more advanced ones will decipher the type of fat, thus allowing for lean body mass calculations. In those that do not, fat-free mass (FFM) is calculated by taking total mass minus fat mass.

Reference: Obesity Medicine Association: Obesity Algorithm (2023)

90. (Content: II-A-3) A 21-year-old female with class II obesity presents to urgent care for periodic headaches and recent vision changes. She states that the vision changes have started to interfere with her collegiate studies. Physical exam shows the following findings on fundoscopic examination. What is the next best step in management for this patient?

A. Request an ophthalmology referral
B. Order a lumbar puncture
C. Initiate therapy with topiramate
D. Order brain imaging
E. Discuss weight loss medications

(D) This patient is presenting with papilledema (as shown in the image), headaches, and vision changes concerning for idiopathic intracranial hypertension (IIH). Although weight loss, medications, and ophthalmology are all indicated for IIH, a definitive diagnosis is needed first. In a patient with papilledema, **brain imaging** to rule out secondary causes of increased intracranial pressures is needed prior to definitive diagnosis with a lumbar puncture (LP) showing increased opening pressure with normal cerebral spinal fluid results.

"Best Next Step" IIH Questions

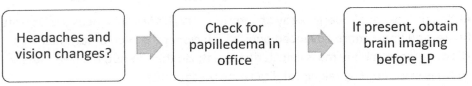

Reference: Up to Date: "Idiopathic intracranial hypertension: Clinical features and diagnosis"
Reference: Retina photo of a right eye, patient with Severe Idiopathic Cranial Hypertension (aka Pseudotumor Cerebri).jpg. (2022, January 1). Wikimedia Commons. Retrieved 02:18, October 11, 2023 from https://commons.wikimedia.org/w/index.php?title=File:Retina_photo_of_a_right_eye,_patient_with_Severe _Idiopathic_Cranial_Hypertension_(aka_Psuedotumor_Cerebri).jpg&oldid=618332774.

91. (Content: II-A-3) A 7-year-old female presents to her pediatrician for a follow-up regarding her blood pressure. On three separate office visits, her blood pressure has averaged in the 90th percentile. She has occasional headaches after reading for long periods of time but otherwise has no complaints. She is performing well at school. Which of the following blood pressure categories for her age does this fall into?

A. Normal
B. **Elevated blood pressure**
C. Stage 1 hypertension
D. Stage 2 hypertension
E. Hypertensive urgency

(B) This patient meets the criteria for **elevated blood pressure** given her blood pressure is persistently at the 90th percentile. It is recommended to evaluate for hypertension at every visit in those ≥ 3 years old with overweight and obesity.

It is vital to ensure accurate blood pressure measurements. Ensuring accurate cuff sizing and repeating measurements allows for confirmation of hypertension. In those with an initially elevated reading:

- Two more readings with auscultation are recommended during the same visit.
- These values should be averaged together to determine the accurate blood pressure and appropriate category.
- In addition, blood pressure measurements must be repeated and confirmed on multiple separate clinic visits to make the diagnosis, as summarized in the visit # column of the table below.

Pediatric Hypertension Diagnostic Criteria			
Category	Children 1-13 years old	Children ≥ 13 years old	#
Normal	< 90th percentile	<120/80 mmHg	NA
Elevated	≥ 90th percentile	120-129/<80 mmHg	3
Stage 1	≥ 95th percentile	130-139/80-89 mmHg	3
Stage 2	≥ 95th percentile + 12 mmHg	≥ 140/90 mmHg	2

Visit # is the number of separate clinic visits required to diagnose the category of hypertension.

Reference: Hampl, S. E., Hassink, S. G., Skinner, A. C., Armstrong, S. C., Barlow, S. E., Bolling, C. F., ... Okechukwu, K. (2023). Clinical Practice Guideline for the Evaluation and Treatment of Children and Adolescents With Obesity. Pediatrics, 151(2), e2022060640. https://doi.org/10.1542/peds.2022-060640. Table 12 and KAS 8.

92. (Content: II-B-4) A 37-year-old mother of two presents to her primary care physician's office for follow-up after recently being diagnosed with binge-eating disorder (BED). She has started cognitive behavioral therapy and has noticed improvements. She states that upon researching BED, she has seen a lot of the same tendencies and characteristics of her condition in her 11-year-old daughter. Her daughter is scheduled to meet with her pediatrician and will likely be diagnosed with which of the following?

    A. Grazing
    B. Anorexia nervosa
    C. Loss of control eating disorder
    D. Night eating syndrome
    E. Bulimia nervosa

(C) This patient's daughter, who has many of the same symptoms of BED, will likely be diagnosed with **loss of control eating disorder (LOC-ED)**. This condition is nearly identical to BED, but is only diagnosed in children < 12 years old. First-line treatment for LOC-ED is interpersonal psychotherapy.

Diagnostic Criteria for Loss of Control Eating Disorder (age < 12 years old)
Recurrent episodes of binge eating marked by: <ul><li>Eating large amounts of food in a discrete amount of time</li><li>A sense of lack of control with eating during these episodes</li></ul>
Associated with 3 or more of the following: <ul><li>Eating more rapidly than normal</li><li>Eating until uncomfortably full</li><li>Eating large amounts of food when not physically hungry</li><li>Hiding eating behaviors because embarrassed by behavior</li><li>Feeling disgusted, depressed, or guilty after episodes</li></ul>
Marked distress about binge eating
Occurs on average at least 1 time per week for 3 months
Not associated with compensatory purging behaviors

Reference: Tanofsky-Kraff M, Marcus MD, Yanovski SZ, Yanovski JA. Loss of control eating disorder in children age 12 years and younger: proposed research criteria. Eat Behav. 2008;9(3):360–365. doi:10.1016/j.eatbeh.2008.03.002

93. (Content: II-C-1) A patient is discussing a news story that was heard earlier in the day with a physician. The report stated patients who have a BMI $\geq$ 25 kg/m^2 have a longer life expectancy than those with a BMI < 25 kg/m^2. The patient now questions the utility of obtaining a BMI at each visit. Which is a true statement regarding the correlation between BMI and obesity-related comorbidities?

A. A BMI of 35 kg/m^2 decreases life expectancy the same as smoking
B. BMI is the best indicator of cardiovascular disease
C. 50% of those with type 2 diabetes have a BMI $\geq$ 25 kg/m^2
D. **A 5-unit increase in BMI increases ischemic stroke risk by 20%**

(D) Despite the well-established health risks associated with obesity, some studies suggest that patients with obesity may experience better outcomes and lower mortality rates in specific scenarios— a phenomenon known as the obesity paradox. Adipose tissue may provide limited protective benefits, like increased energy storage for those with malignancy or increased visceral padding in trauma. However, for the majority of people, the pathogenicity outweighs the benefits.

Both extremes of BMI have increased mortality, although BMI alone does not account for cardiovascular risk in individuals, especially in those with a BMI between 25-35 kg/m^2. In these moderate BMI ranges, visceral (or truncal) obesity better predicts cardiovascular risk; waist circumference or waist-to-hip ratio serve as a proxy for visceral adiposity. Regardless, BMI does have many direct correlations, discussed below:

- **Mortality:** A BMI between 25-35 kg/m^2 reduces life expectancy by 2-4 years, and a BMI of 40-45 kg/m^2 by 8-10 years (similar to smoking).
- **Heart failure:** Risk increases 2-fold with a BMI $\geq$ 30 kg/m^2.
- **Atrial fibrillation:** For every ↑ of 1 unit BMI, risk increases by 4%.
- **Diabetes type 2:** 90% of those with diabetes have a BMI $\geq$ 25 kg/m^2
- **Cerebral vascular accident:** For **every ↑ 1 unit BMI, there is an increase in ischemic stroke by 4%** and hemorrhagic stroke by 6%.
- **Sleep apnea:** BMI > 30 kg/m^2 incurs a 30% risk of sleep apnea.

Note: There are 230 comorbidities associated with obesity, including malignancy.

Reference: Up to Date: "Overweight and obesity in adults: Health consequences"

94. (Content: II-C-5) A 3-year-old female is referred to a geneticist for evaluation after persistent milestone delays and a recent seizure. The child appears very happy, smiling and laughing frequently during the examination. Her movements are spastic and she is only able to pull herself up to a seated position and stand with assistance. She does not talk and only babbles intermittently. What would the genetic workup most likely reveal?

A. **Angelman syndrome**
B. Turner syndrome
C. Borjeson-Forssman-Lehmann syndrome
D. Albright hereditary osteodystrophy
E. Fragile-X syndrome

(A) This patient presents with seizures, speech, and balance issues, and an overly happy affect, consistent with **Angelman syndrome.** This syndrome often occurs de novo due to errors in maternal imprinting. In addition, these patients may have increased appetites leading to obesity (one-third of patients).

Patients with Angelman syndrome have some unique characteristics:

- A very happy personality, with frequent smiling and laughing
- Development delays, including walking
- Minimal talking (often babbling)
- Seizures between 2-3 years of age
- Spastic and jerky movements with microcephaly
- Sleep disorders, including insomnia

This condition is caused by a genetic abnormality of chromosome 15 called the ubiquitin protein ligase E3A (UBE3A), which is normally inherited from the mother (maternal imprinting). However, if the mother's gene is missing or defective, this causes Angelman syndrome. A similar paternal deletion of a gene on the same chromosome causes Prader-Willi syndrome.

Reference: Up To Date "Microdeletion syndromes (chromosomes 12 to 22)"
Reference: https://www.mayoclinic.org/diseases-conditions/angelman-syndrome/symptoms-causes/syc-20355621

95. (Content: II-A-3) A 68-year-old female with a history of type 2 diabetes presents to the clinic following a bariatric seminar. Although she understands there is no definitive age limit to surgery, she elects to undergo medical management. Her current diabetic medication regimen includes a maximum dose of metformin. Her hemoglobin A1c is 9.6%. The risks and benefits of a daily FDA-approved injectable, anti-obesity medication for long-term use is discussed. What medical history would be necessary for the physician to inquire about before starting this medication?

    A. Papillary thyroid carcinoma
    B. Suicidal ideation
    C. History of cholelithiasis
    D. Diabetic gastroparesis

(D) This patient with a history of obesity and diabetes would be a great candidate for liraglutide, a daily FDA-approved long-term-use anti-obesity drug. However, given the mechanism (GLP-1 receptor agonist), it can slow gastrointestinal motility and gastric emptying. Therefore it should be avoided in those with a **history of severe gastroparesis.**

Liraglutide (Saxenda®)	
Dose	Inject 0.6 mg subcutaneously daily. Increase by 0.6 mg daily at weekly intervals to a target dose of 3.0 mg/day
Mechanism	Glucagon-like peptide 1 receptor agonists activate the hypothalamus, reducing food intake, increasing satiety, decreasing caloric intake and improving glucose metabolism (incretin).
Contraindications	Prior hypersensitivity to liraglutide, history of or family history of medullary thyroid carcinoma (black box warning), patients with multiple endocrine neoplasia type 2, and pregnancy. *Relative contraindication: Severe gastroparesis and those at increased risk of pancreatitis[1]
Side Effects	Gastrointestinal distress (abdominal pain, nausea, vomiting), dizziness, and increased lipase (increased risk of pancreatitis[1])

[1]Meta-analysis has shown no increased risk of pancreatitis or pancreatic cancer with GLP-1 use.

Reference: Liraglutide package insert

96. (Content: II-C-3 and I-B-4) An 11-year-old male presents to his pediatrician with right lower extremity pain. He states the pain has worsened over the past month, describing it as a dull ache. There was no preceding trauma. His mother brought him in after she noticed him walking with a limp. His BMI is in the 120th percentile for his age and gender. Physical examination reveals limited internal rotation of his right hip and an antalgic gait. Which of the following is most likely the culprit of his presenting condition?

    A. Blount disease
    B. Slipped capital femoral epiphysis
    C. Osgood-Schlatter disease
    D. Legg-Calve-Perthes disease
    E. Aseptic necrosis

(B) This adolescent patient with excess adipose tissue presents with a new-onset unilateral limp and external rotation (i.e., resistance to internal rotation) of the hip. These findings are most consistent with **slipped capital femoral epiphysis (SCFE).**

SCFE results from the instability of the growth plate of the proximal femur, resulting in a Salter-Harris fracture. This is most commonly from fat mass disease (i.e., mechanical overload), although it can also be from a growth spurt. It requires urgent surgical evaluation.

Other differentials and their characteristics are discussed below:

- Blount disease is the bowing of the tibia (varus) and can be seen in children with obesity.
- Legg-Calve-Perthes disease is idiopathic avascular necrosis of the femoral head and can present similarly to SCFE, including impaired internal rotation; however, it usually affects younger patients (ages 5-6 years old). It may be painless and present only as a limp.
- Osgood-Schlatter disease is seen in young, active patients and presents with a pronounced tibial tuberosity.

Reference: Up to Date: "Evaluation and Management of Slipped Capital Femoral Epiphysis (SCFE)"

97. (Content: II-B-1) A mother of three children presents to her family practitioner for well-child examinations. Two of the children have been diagnosed with obesity. The mother has not followed up with the dietician as recommended, and the children are still consuming high-caloric density packaged food. Which of the following would be the most appropriate question to ask now?

A. **Do you run out of food towards the end of the month?**
B. Is your transportation adequate for making appointments?
C. Do you feel like you are suited to take care of your children?
D. What sweets could be eliminated from your children's diets?
E. How can we incorporate physical activity?

(A) Food insecurity can lead to excessive weight due to poor quality of food intake (calorie-rich food, but poor nutritional value) and food deserts (inadequate grocery stores within a reasonable parameter of home). Screening questions for food insecurity include:

- In the past 12 months, have you been worried about whether food would run out before you got money to purchase more?
- In the past 12 months, **has the food you purchased run out,** and you didn't have the money to buy more?

These two questions can clue you into the potential financial constraints the patient is experiencing and the underlying etiology of childhood obesity. Poorer quality food tends to be less expensive, is packaged (better preservation), and may be preferential to higher-quality foods (increased spoilage and cost).

Nearly 1 out of 5 children meet the definition of food insecurity (75 million families), often related to household poverty, parents' educations (highest correlation), single-parent homes, and larger families.

Having a working knowledge of local and federal resources may bridge the gap and provide improved nutrition leading to long-term benefits.

Reference: Obesity Medicine Association: Pediatric Obesity Algorithm (2023-2024)

98. (Content: II-C-7) An 11-year-old male is presenting for a well-child check with his growth chart below. What is the most accurate criteria this patient met on their first documented visit?

A. Overweight
B. Obesity
C. Obesity class I
D. **Obesity class II**
E. Obesity class III

(D) This patient is currently (farthest right point) presenting with a BMI percentile above 120% of the 95th percentile and BMI > 35 kg/m², both of which meet the criteria for class II obesity. However, even on the first visit (farthest left point), even though the BMI looks to be < 35 kg/m², the patient meets the criteria for **class II obesity**, as the criteria is based on the lowest met criteria, in this case, being ≥ 120% to < 140% of the 95th percentile.

Obesity, defined in children aged 2-19 years old, is classified as a percentile range greater than the 95th percentile based on age and gender. However, it can be further classified into classes, as shown below:

- **Class I obesity:** ≥ 95th percentile to < 120% of the 95th percentile
- **Class II obesity:** ≥ 120% to < 140% of the 95th percentile or BMI ≥ 35 to ≤ 39 kg/m², whichever met criteria is lower.
- **Class III obesity:** ≥ 140% of the 95th percentile or BMI ≥ 40 kg/m², whichever met criteria is lower.

Reference: Obesity Medicine Association: Pediatric Obesity Algorithm (2023-2024)

99. (Content: II-D-3a) A 14-year-old male is being evaluated for excess weight at a family medicine visit. After undergoing a comprehensive physical examination with appropriate testing, he is diagnosed with metabolic syndrome. Which of the following diagnostic criteria is most likely present in this patient?

    A. Diagnosis of obstructive sleep apnea
    B. Low HDL levels
    C. Treatment of hypercholesterolemia
    D. Left ventricular hypertrophy
    E. Family history of coronary artery disease

(B) Although all of the above are risk factors or comorbidities of obesity, only **low HDL levels** are part of the diagnostic criteria for metabolic syndrome. Children at risk for metabolic syndrome include large for gestational age at birth and maternal gestational diabetes or obesity. Diagnosis of metabolic syndrome imposes a significantly increased risk of cardiovascular disease and type II diabetes mellitus.

In addition to advanced obesity treatments for metabolic syndrome, the American Academy of Pediatrics recommends a dietary increase in fruits and vegetables, a reduction in saturated fat intake, and a reduction in carbohydrate consumption.

Metabolic Syndrome Diagnostic Criteria (Requires 3 of 5)		
Criteria	12-19 years of age[1]	≥ 19-years old
Triglycerides[2]	≥ 100 mg/dL	≥ 150 mg/dL
HDL[2]	≤ 10th percentile for age/sex	< 40 mg/dL in men < 50 mg/dL in women
Glucose[2]	Fasting glucose ≥ 100 mg/dL	Fasting glucose ≥ 100 mg/dL
Waist circumference	≥ 90th percentile for ethnicity, age, sex	≥ 102 cm (40 in) in men ≥ 88 cm (35 in) in women
Blood pressure[2]	≥ 90th percentile for age, height, and sex	≥ 130/85 mmHg

[1]Modified NCEP-ATP III
[2] Or treatment for conditions

Reference: Up to Date: "Metabolic syndrome (insulin resistance syndrome or syndrome X)"
Reference: Obesity Medicine Association: Pediatric Obesity Algorithm (2023-2024)

100. (Content: II-A-3) A 27-year-old female was recently diagnosed with polycystic ovarian syndrome after a workup for infertility. The patient is educated on complications and the physiology of this condition. Her chief concern is the development of diabetes, which her mother has. Which is the best test to determine early insulin intolerance in this patient?

    A. Hemoglobin A1c
    B. Fasting glucose level
    C. Oral glucose tolerance test
    D. Homeostasis model assessment of insulin resistance

(C) The most sensitive test to diagnose early type II diabetes or insulin resistance in a patient diagnosed with polycystic ovarian syndrome (PCOS) is the **two-hour oral glucose tolerance test (OGTT).** The risk of diabetes is increased in those with PCOS and significantly increased (2.6x risk) in those with a first-degree relative with diabetes.

Screening for diabetes with fasting blood glucose underestimated the prevalence of diabetes in those with PCOS, as this was not found to adequately diagnose glucose intolerance when compared to the 75 g two-hour OGTT. The American College of Obstetrics and Gynecology and the American Association of Clinical Endocrinologists recommend OGTT screening for insulin intolerance at the time of diagnosis of PCOS, although subsequent interval screening in those with normal values differs across organizations.

Note: Although the homeostasis model assessment of insulin resistance (HOMA-IR) may be utilized by clinicians, the absence of a universally standardized insulin assay and the absence of data confirming that markers of insulin resistance can predict treatment response, make this answer option very unlikely to be a preferred option on obesity medicine boards.

Reference: Al Wattar BH, Fisher M, Bevington L, Talaulikar V, Davies M, Conway G, Yasmin E. Clinical Practice Guidelines on the Diagnosis and Management of Polycystic Ovary Syndrome: A Systematic Review and Quality Assessment Study. J Clin Endocrinol Metab. 2021 Jul 13;106(8):2436-2446. doi: 10.1210/clinem/dgab232. PMID: 33839790; PMCID: PMC8830055.
Reference: Up to Date: "Diagnosis of polycystic ovary syndrome in adults"

101. (Content: II-D-1) A 30-year-old male is being seen in an obesity medicine clinic with a nutritionist who wants to determine his basal metabolic rate. The clinic has no access to indirect calorimetry. He weighs 100 kg and is 5' 11" (180 cm). Which of the following is closest to his resting metabolic rate utilizing the Mifflin – St. Jeor formula?

    A. 1600
    B. 1800
    C. 2000
    D. 2200

(C) This patient's resting metabolic rate (RMR) can be estimated by the Mifflin – St. Jeor formula. For males, this would be (10 x 100) + (6.25 x 180) – (5 x 30) + 5 = 1980 kcal/day, **closest to 2000 kcal.**

Note: The ABOM will require you to know a few equations (confirmed with recent feedback), including the Mifflin – St. Jeor formula. The Mifflin St. Jeor formula is an estimate of RMR and is preferred over the Harris-Benedict formula (approximately 5% more accurate) in those with obesity.

The formula, listed below, also shows the relationship between different factors. For example, as age increases, RMR decreases. In contrast, patients with a higher weight or height and males will have higher basal metabolic rates. In addition, RMR will decrease in those with hypothermia or on mechanical ventilation, and increase in those with sepsis, trauma, organ failure, and extensive burns. These differences are adjusted by a multiplier. For example, a patient with hypothermia could be assessed by multiplying 0.8 x RMR, whereas someone with sepsis would have a multiplier of 1.2 x RMR to decrease or increase, respectively, total caloric needs at rest.

Calculating Resting Metabolic Rate (Mifflin - St. Jeor Formula)	
Male	**Female**
(10 x weight [kg]) + (6.25 x height [cm]) - (5 x age [years]) + 5	(10 x weight [kg]) + (6.25 x height [cm]) - (5 x age [years]) - 161
Multiplier (e.g., 1.2 x RMR in sepsis; 0.8 if hypothermic or on ventilation)	

Reference: Frankenfield D, Roth-Yousey L, Compher C. Comparison of predictive equations for resting metabolic rate in healthy nonobese and obese adults: a systematic review. J Am Diet Assoc. 2005 May;105(5):775-89. doi: 10.1016/j.jada.2005.02.005. PMID: 15883556.

102. (Content: II-A-4) A 25-year-old male presents to his primary care physician's office with the complaint of weight gain. Over the past two years, he has gained nearly 35 lbs (15.9 kg). He states that he first noticed the weight gain once he began to work the night shift. He says he still exercises 30 minutes daily before work but does admit to increased hunger and snacking throughout his shift. Compared to 4 years ago, which of the following would most likely be observed in the patient at this visit?

    A. Decreased orexin
    B. Increased cortisol
    C. Suppressed ghrelin
    D. Increased melatonin
    E. Increased adiponectin

(B) Patients who work rotating or night shifts have circadian misalignment, which increases their risk of obesity, diabetes, depression, hypertension, and hyperlipidemia. Of the list above, these patients have **increased cortisol levels**, as well as the following:

- Decreased energy expenditure
- Increased inflammatory cytokines (IL-6, TNF-α, IL-1β)
- Decreased adiponectin
- Decreased leptin, melatonin, and metabolic rate
- Blunted post-meal suppression of ghrelin
- Increased insulin resistance and risk of diabetes

There appears to be a cumulative effect on circadian misalignment, with those working > 10 years on the night shift having the highest risk of obesity and obesity-related comorbidities.

Options to help with circadian rhythm dysfunction that arise with rotating shifts include incorporating sleep hygiene, using melatonin before sleep and stimulants such as caffeine during work shifts. This allows for a quicker adjustment of sleep/work cycles, mitigating the negative effects above.

Reference: Kim, Tae Won & Jeong, Jong-Hyun & Hong, Seung-Chul. (2015). The Impact of Sleep and Circadian Disturbance on Hormones and Metabolism. International Journal of Endocrinology. 2015. 1-9. 10.1155/2015/591729.
Reference: Peplonska B, Bukowska A, Sobala W. Association of Rotating Night Shift Work with BMI and Abdominal Obesity among Nurses and Midwives. PLoS One. 2015;10(7):e0133761. Published 2015 Jul 21. doi:10.1371/journal.pone.0133761

103. (Content: II-B-2) A 31-year-old male presents as a 2-week follow-up to his weight management clinic. Since being seen previously, he has decreased his soda consumption and has reduced the number of times he eats fast food from three times weekly to once. Also, he has started to briskly walk around his neighborhood for approximately 30 minutes three times weekly. He has lost 4 lbs (1.8 kg) since his last appointment. According to current minimum recommendations, what goal should be set regarding his 30-minute exercise sessions?

A.   Increase to daily sessions
B.   Increase to 5 sessions weekly
C.   Change from walking to jogging
D.   Set a goal in terms of miles, not minutes
E.   No changes necessary

(B) This patient is making significant progress in his lifestyle changes. Per recommendations by many entities, aerobic physical activity should be prescribed to patients who carry a diagnosis of overweight or obesity. **The minimum goal should be ≥ 150 min/week of moderate-intensity exercise, performed during 3-5 sessions per week.**

Other essential recommendations regarding exercise are as follows:

- Resistance training should be prescribed to those undergoing weight-loss therapy to promote fat loss while preserving lean mass (goal 2-3x weekly).
- To reduce a sedentary lifestyle, encourage increasing non-exercise and active leisure activities.
- Exercise should be individualized based on patient capabilities and preferences, considering physical limitations.

Note: Higher levels of physical activity (> 300 minutes/week) are recommended to prevent weight regain in the long term (> 1 year).

Reference: AACE/ACE Guidelines: AMERICAN ASSOCIATION OF CLINICAL ENDOCRINOLOGISTS AND AMERICAN COLLEGE OF ENDOCRINOLOGY COMPREHENSIVE CLINICAL PRACTICE GUIDELINES FOR MEDICAL CARE OF PATIENTS WITH OBESITY (2016): Recommendation 67- 70

104. (Content: II-B-5) A 16-year-old female presents to her family practitioner at the request of her mother after being found to be self-inducing vomiting. The patient states this is something she has done for the past few months, often after she eats more than she intends to, saying it helps with the guilt. She is active in sports, has several close friends, and is getting good grades. Given the underlying diagnosis, which abnormality is most likely to develop in this patient if left untreated?

    A. Anion gap metabolic acidosis
    B. Shortened corrected QT interval
    C. Mallory-Weiss tear
    D. Melanosis coli
    E. Keratoconjunctivitis sicca

(C) This patient is presenting with concerning findings for bulimia nervosa, a predominantly female eating disorder that can lead to esophageal tears **(i.e., Mallory-Weiss tears),** melanosis coli (if laxative-induced), fluid and electrolyte disturbances (metabolic alkalosis in the setting of emesis), arrhythmias, dental erosions, swollen salivary/parotid glands, and loss of the gag reflex.

The diagnostic criteria for bulimia nervosa is summarized below.

Diagnostic Criteria for Bulimia Nervosa

Recurrent episodes of binge eating characterized by BOTH:
  • Eating in a discrete amount of time an amount of food that is larger than most would eat during a similar time/circumstance
  • Sense of lack of control over eating during an episode

Recurrent inappropriate compensatory behaviors, such as:
  • Self-induced vomiting
  • Misuse of laxatives, diuretics, enemas, or other medications
  • Fasting or excessive exercise

Binge eating/compensatory behavior occurs once weekly x 3 months
Self-evaluation is unduly influenced by body shape and weight
The disturbance does not occur exclusively during episodes of anorexia nervosa.

Reference: DSM-5: Diagnostic and Statistical Manual of Mental Disorders, Fifth Edition

105. (Content: II-D-3b) A 26-year-old female is presenting to her family practitioner for an infertility evaluation. She states that although she has unprotected sex approximately three times weekly, she has not become pregnant for the past two years. She says she averages one heavy menstrual cycle every three months. Her BMI is 34 kg/m². Physical examination reveals facial hair stubble. Pelvic examination is unremarkable; however, clitoromegaly is noted. An ovarian ultrasound is unrevealing. Given these findings, which lab test would most likely be present?

A. **Increased luteinizing hormone**
B. Decreased free thyroxine levels
C. Decreased androgen levels
D. Elevated cortisol levels
E. Elevated vitamin D (25-OH) levels

(A) This patient who has findings of hirsutism and virilization (clitoromegaly) with amenorrhea meets the criteria for the diagnosis of polycystic ovarian syndrome (PCOS), the most common endocrine disorder in women (affecting 10%). This condition is an imbalance of hormones characterized by **an increased luteinizing hormone (LH): follicular stimulating hormone (FSH) ratio** and increased androgens.

Notably, nearly 50% of women with PCOS have insulin resistance and are affected by excess weight/obesity. Metformin and anti-obesity medications are effective treatment options for weight and insulin resistance.

Rotterdam Consensus states patients must meet 2 of the 3 for diagnosis:

- Hyperandrogenism (biochemical or clinical)
- Menstrual irregularities (anovulation)
- Polycystic ovaries by ultrasound

Note: A 5-10% decrease in weight increases the chance of ovulation and fertility. It is essential to discuss this with patients.

Reference: Up to Date: "Diagnosis of polycystic ovary syndrome in adults"

106. (Content: II-B-3) A 45-year-old female presents to her internist with concerns of bleeding within her mouth. She states that she has been utterly frustrated with her weight and has decided to go on an "extreme diet" for the past three months. She has been consuming water and only small amounts of protein and carbohydrates. She lost nearly 45 lbs (20.4 kg) during this time. A physical exam shows dried blood on her gums and spiral hair on her arms. Given her most likely deficiency, which of the following is a potential complication?

A. Peripheral neuropathy
B. Hallucinations
C. High-output cardiac failure
D. Dermatitis
E. **Poor wound healing**

(E) Vitamin deficiencies are common after malabsorptive procedures but can also be seen in extreme dieting. Given this patient's lack of fruits or vegetables in her diet, gum disease, and spiral hairs (corkscrew hairs), she has most likely developed scurvy due to severe vitamin C deficiency. Symptoms include anemia, perifollicular microhemorrhages, and weakness. Also, **poor wound healing** can occur as vitamin C is involved in the hydroxylation of collagen.

In addition to poor dietary intake of fruits and vegetables, overcooking these sources of vitamin C can also result in a deficiency. Vitamin C deficiency may also lead to the following:

- Petechia[1]
- Ecchymosis[1]
- Bleeding gums
- Dry skin

[1]Also consider vitamin K deficiency with these findings

Another life-threatening concern in those who are malnourished is refeeding syndrome. This occurs in the setting of prolonged malnutrition leading to depleted phosphate storage. If provided nutrition, especially high carbohydrate loads, insulin release causes phosphate to shift intracellularly. Because phosphate is used for energy in the form of ATP, muscle weakness (including cardiac and diaphragm) and fatal arrhythmias can occur.

Reference: Léger D. Scurvy: reemergence of nutritional deficiencies. Can Fam Physician. 2008;54(10):1403–1406.

107. (Content: II-D-3a) A 63-year-old female presents to her primary care office for a routine evaluation. Her lab results reveal a TSH level of 11.1 mU/L (reference range: 0.4-4.5 mU/L) with a normal T_4 level. She had similar lab values two months prior, completed for insurance screening purposes. She feels well overall and denies fatigue, constipation, or cold intolerance. Which of the following would be the next best step?

A. Start levothyroxine if the patient begins having symptoms
B. Order thyroid peroxidase antibodies
C. **Initiate weight-based synthetic thyroxine replacement**
D. Repeat TSH, T_3, and T_4 levels in 3 months
E. Discuss desiccated thyroid replacement therapy

(C) This patient is presenting with subclinical hypothyroidism, defined as an elevated thyroid stimulating hormone (TSH) with normal thyroid hormone levels (T_4). TSH levels $\geq$ 10 mU/L are an indication to **initiate weight-based levothyroxine** regardless of symptoms. Importantly, desiccated thyroid should not be used for the treatment of hypothyroidism as dosages vary and contain active (T_3) hormone in significant amounts.

Note: T_3 is generally not tested in patients with hypothyroidism. Even in profound hypothyroidism, T_3 levels can be normal.

Subclinical hypothyroidism is common, affecting approximately 5-10% of the general population and 1 out of 5 women older than age 60. Treating with thyroid replacement is indicated in the following situations:

- Primary hypothyroidism (elevated TSH with decreased T_4)
- Central hypothyroidism (decreased or inappropriately normal TSH in the setting of decreased T_4)
- Asymptomatic subclinical hypothyroidism with a TSH $\geq$ 10 mU/L
- Subclinical hypothyroidism with a TSH 4.5-10 mU/L with symptoms (cold intolerance, etc.). Treating in this TSH range if asymptomatic is controversial and, therefore, not testable.

Reference: Hossein Gharib, R. Michael Tuttle, H. Jack Baskin, Lisa H. Fish, Peter A. Singer, Michael T. McDermott, Subclinical Thyroid Dysfunction: A Joint Statement on Management from the American Association of Clinical Endocrinologists, the American Thyroid Association, and The Endocrine Society, The Journal of Clinical Endocrinology & Metabolism, Volume 90, Issue 1, 1 January 2005, Pages 581–585, https://doi.org/10.1210/jc.2004-1231

108. (Content: II-B-3) A 15-year-old male is presenting to a dietician to discuss healthy eating patterns. To get a better idea of what foods the patient is consuming, she had him fill out a 5-day food record prior to this appointment. She noticed more intake of fruits and vegetables on the food record than what the primary care physician had documented. What is the most likely cause of this discrepancy?

A. **Altered eating behaviors**
B. Fraudulent reporting of intake
C. Memory recall bias
D. Tracking weekdays only
E. Parental tracking inaccuracies

(A) There are numerous ways in which dietary information can be obtained to understand the eating habits of patients. This patient was asked to do a 5-day food record which consists of measuring and documenting food for a specific period, with 3-5 days being the most common. This option has been shown to **alter food behaviors** and thus may provide less accurate insight into the dietary patterns, as the patient tends to eat more healthily while tracking food intake. This idea is why one of the behavioral pillars for the treatment of obesity includes monitoring, as most patients will alter their behavior as they keep track of dietary and physical activity.

Two other common methods for measuring dietary intake include:

- Food frequency questionnaire (FFQ): Uses a food list to determine how frequently a patient consumes certain foods
- Food recall: Review all items consumed in the prior 24 or 72 hours during the office visit

Measuring Dietary Intake		
Method	**Advantages**	**Disadvantages**
FFQ	• Research settings • Self-administered	• Requires memory and reading • Does not explain eating behaviors
Food record	• No memory recall • Displays patterns	• Requires writing • May alter eating behavior
Food recall	• No reading/writing • Displays behaviors	• May not display true daily patterns, especially if a special event (eating out, party, etc.)

Reference: Up to Date: "Dietary assessment in adults"

109. (Content: II-A-3) An 8-year-old male with class I obesity is brought into the clinic by his mother for snoring and "holding his breath" in the middle of the night. Upon examination, significant tonsillar hypertrophy is present, however, the mother is resistant to surgery. A sleep study confirms obstructive sleep apnea, and a continuous positive airway pressure machine is prescribed, which the patient does not tolerate and refuses to wear. Which morning lab abnormalities may be seen in this patient?

    A. Decreased bicarbonate
    B. Elevated pH level
    C. Polycythemia
    D. Hyponatremia
    E. Elevated liver enzymes

(C) This patient with untreated obstructive sleep apnea (OSA) may have compensatory metabolic alkalosis due to increased bicarbonate levels to offset the nighttime respiratory acidosis (decreased pH). This finding would only be seen in the early morning, as levels would resolve after the patient is awake. This differs from obesity hypoventilation syndrome which causes persistent daytime pCO_2 elevations. **Polycythemia** may also be seen due to nocturnal hypoxia increasing erythropoietin levels. Polycythemia is supportive of the diagnosis of sleep apnea but is commonly absent in patients.

In addition to snoring and apnea, symptoms of OSA in children can present with daytime sleepiness, nocturia, nocturnal enuresis, and daytime hyperactivity. Tonsillar hypertrophy and obesity are the two most common risk factors for OSA in children. Management differs from adults, in that those who still have adenoids and tonsils should be referred to an otolaryngologist to evaluate for adenoidectomy and tonsillectomy. Watchful waiting (approximately six months) is appropriate in those without severe OSA. In those who do not meet the criteria for surgery or do not want surgery, positive pressure ventilation is the treatment. Weight loss should be pursued if the patient has excess weight.

Reference: Up to Date: "Evaluation of suspected obstructive sleep apnea in children"
Reference: Obesity Medicine Association: Pediatric Obesity Algorithm (2023-2024)

110. (Content: II-C-3) A 27-year-old male presents to a new primary care physician's office for evaluation of fatigue. He has not been seen by a physician "since high school," as he has felt well and has not been seriously ill. He denies alcohol or tobacco use and states that he tries to avoid fast food. Vital signs are within normal limits, besides a BMI of 28 kg/m². Physical examination reveals hyperpigmented skin in his axillary folds and the nape of his neck. Other physical exam findings are unremarkable. A cholesterol panel reveals total cholesterol to be 220 mg/dL (reference range < 200 mg/dL) and HbA1c of 6.0% (reference range: < 5.7%). What other physical examination finding is most likely present?

A. Xanthoma
B. Easy bruising
C. Acrochordons
D. Dry skin
E. Corkscrew hairs

(C) This patient presenting with an elevated hemoglobin A1c within the prediabetic range and acanthosis nigricans (hyperpigmentation of the neck, axilla, or groin) has findings consistent with insulin resistance. Other findings associated with insulin resistance include **acrochordons (skin tags).**

Skin findings associated with obesity are discussed below:

Skin Findings Associated with Obesity-Related Conditions	
Exam Findings	**Associated Condition**
Acanthosis nigricans and skin tags	Insulin resistance/diabetes
Acne	Polycystic ovarian syndrome and Cushing's syndrome/disease
Xanthelasmas or xanthomas	Hyperlipidemia (very elevated)
Moon facies, buffalo hump, wide-based striae, easy bruising, facial plethora	Cushing's syndrome/disease
Dry and cracked skin, thinning of eyebrows, periorbital edema	Hypothyroidism

Note: Flesh-colored striae (i.e., stretch marks) are associated with rapid weight gain. In contrast, Cushing syndrome, associated with hypercortisolism, is associated with wide-based, purple striae.

Reference: Up to Date: "Overweight and obesity in adults: Health consequences"

111. (Content: II-C-7) A mother brings her child to the pediatrician for his 18-month well-child exam. He has met all of his age-appropriate milestones, including starting to walk at 12 months old. She states that he has gained more "rolls" in the arms and legs and seems to be gaining weight faster than she recalls of her other children. Which would be the most accurate way to track this patient's weight parameters?

A. Weight-for-height
B. Body mass index
C. Age-adjusted growth
D. **Weight-for-length**
E. CDC growth charts

(D) Weight assessment in those under 2 years old is done by evaluating **weight-for-length** using the World Health Organization charts, taking into account gender and age. The body mass index percentile is not used until two years of age.

Growth charts are available from 2 different organizations:

- **Centers for Disease Control and Prevention (CDC):** These charts are based on a cohort of primarily non-breastfed, Caucasian American children. The CDC chart cohort data was unavailable for the first three months of age, and the sample sizes were limited for sex and age for the first six months, limiting its utility in those under 2 years of age.
- **World Health Organization (WHO):** This is based on cohorts from more diverse ethnic backgrounds, predominantly breastfed children. These children were breastfed for at least four months, with most still breastfeeding at 12 months.

The recommendations from the CDC are to use the WHO growth standards for infants 0-2 years of age and the CDC growth charts thereafter. The WHO charts more accurately reflect the recommended standards for infant feeding in the early population.

Reference: https://www.cdc.gov/growthcharts/who_charts.htm

112. (Content: II-E and II-A-3) A 46-year-old male with a BMI of 38 kg/m^2 presents for follow-up regarding his diabetes. He is being treated with metformin and empagliflozin; his last HbA1c was 6.8%. He has mild knee pain with prolonged exercise but otherwise feels well. According to the Edmonton Obesity Staging System, he would be classified as which of the following?

A. Stage 0
B. Stage 1
C. **Stage 2**
D. Stage 3
E. Stage 4

(C) The Edmonton Obesity Staging System (EOSS) is a tool that considers comorbidity and functional limitations to better determine obesity cardiometabolic risks and treatment aggressiveness compared to anthropometric-based categorization alone. A patient with a BMI of 38 kg/m^2 (class 2 obesity) with diabetes would be classified as **EOSS stage 2.**

A patient that meets the criteria for obesity but has no risk factors, symptoms, or functional limitations would be EOSS stage 0. The other stages are below:

EOSS Staging System	
Stage 1	**Stage 2**
Subclinical risk factors with **mild** symptoms such as borderline hypertension, pre-diabetes, or mild osteoarthritis	Established comorbidities requiring medical treatment with **moderate** symptoms such as depression, HTN, T2DM, GERD, OSA, and HLD
Stage 3	**Stage 4**
Significant obesity-related comorbidities with **significant** limitations, end-organ damage, or impairment, such as myocardial infarction, suicidal ideation, reduced mobility, stroke, and diabetic complications	**Severe** (i.e., end-stage) disabling symptoms and limitations such as wheelchair or bed-bound, pulmonary hypertension from OHS, end-stage renal disease from DM nephropathy, and decompensated cirrhosis from MAFLD

HTN: Hypertension; **T2DM:** Type 2 diabetes mellitus; **GERD:** Gastroesophageal reflux disease; **OSA:** Obstructive sleep apnea; **HLD:** Hyperlipidemia; **OHS:** Obesity hypoventilation syndrome; **MAFLD:** Metabolic-associated fatty liver disease

Reference: Using the Edmonton obesity staging system to predict mortality in a population-representative cohort of people with overweight and obesity. Raj S. Padwal, Nicholas M. Pajewski, David B. Allison and Arya M. Sharma. CMAJ October 04, 2011 183 (14) E1059-E1066; DOI: https://doi.org/10.1503/cmaj.110387

113. (Content: II-B-4) A 21-year-old male with a past medical history of depression and obesity presents to a dietician for a nutrition evaluation. He states that he has overeaten at night for as long as he can remember. He admits to craving sweets and even sometimes wakes up throughout the night to get a snack. Given his most likely underlying diagnosis, which of the following findings is likely to be seen in this patient?

A. Daytime fatigue
B. Excessive daily protein intake
C. Pica
D. Frequent daytime grazing
E. **Morning anorexia**

(E) This patient's history is most consistent with the diagnosis of night eating syndrome (NES), a condition seen in 1.5% of the general population and approximately 30% of those seeking bariatric surgery. NES is classically characterized by the triad of **morning anorexia**, evening hyperphagia, and insomnia. It is commonly associated with those with low self-esteem or self-image, depression, and those with increased perceived stress. It is also associated with the following:

- Nocturnal awakening and food consumption
- Increased carbohydrate-to-protein ratio (7:1)
- Consumption of 25-50% of daily calories after the evening meal

Treatment for NES is focused on encouraging regular meal consumption earlier in the daytime, with increased protein intake being very effective. Cognitive-behavioral therapy can help with many eating disorders, including NES. Pharmacotherapy may be considered, including selective serotonin reuptake inhibitors, with a very high response rate to sertraline.

Binge Eating Disorder (BED) vs. Night Eating Syndrome (NES)		
Findings	BED	NES
Consume ≥ 25% of calories after dinner at least twice weekly		X
Consume a large amount of food in a discrete time period	X	
Believe that one must eat to sleep		X

Reference: Allison KC, Tarves EP. Treatment of night eating syndrome. Psychiatr Clin North Am. 2011;34(4):785–796. doi:10.1016/j.psc.2011.08.002

Reference: McCuen-Wurst C, Ruggieri M, Allison KC. Disordered eating and obesity: associations between binge-eating disorder, night-eating syndrome, and weight-related comorbidities. Ann N Y Acad Sci. 2018 Jan;1411(1):96-105. doi: 10.1111/nyas.13467. Epub 2017 Oct 16. PMID: 29044551; PMCID: PMC5788730.

114. (Content: II-D-1) An electrophysiology study is being performed, which evaluates the resting metabolic rate of individual organs in an average person without excess body weight. A radiotracer is injected into a patient who is lying still, and a subsequent body scan is performed. The tissue with the highest metabolic rate displays the brightest on body scan imaging, with quantitative data extrapolated. Based on this scan, which tissue would most likely display the brightest on imaging?

A. Kidneys
B. Heart
C. Digestive system
D. Liver
E. Fat

(D) Resting metabolic rate (RMR) refers to energy expended at rest and accounts for 70% of total daily expenditure. Of the components that make up RMR, **skeletal muscle and the liver** comprise the most substantial portion, accounting for 20% of RMR each.

Note: Basal metabolic rate (BMR) is similar to RMR, but requires the individual to be fasting, resting, and be supine in a thermoneutral environment. Thus, RMR is more frequently used due to its ease of obtainability with indirect calorimetry. Both BMR and RMR are increased in the setting of excess weight.

Total energy expenditure is made up of resting metabolic rate, physical activity, and dietary thermogenesis, with contributions of 70%, 20%, and 10%, respectively, for each component.

Note: RMR ≈ 1 metabolic equivalent of task (MET).

Resting Metabolic Rate by Organ System			
Organ	Component	Organ	Component
Skeletal muscle	20%	Digestive system	10%
Liver	20%	Kidneys	5%
Brain	15%	Fat	5%
Heart	10%	Remaining	15%

Reference: **Reference:** Obesity Medicine Association: Obesity Algorithm (2023)

115. (Content: II-A-4) A 33-year-old male presents to his family practice physician at his wife's request for "sleep-eating." He states that his wife has caught him multiple times in the middle of the night eating large amounts of food before returning to bed. He has no recollection of this in the morning but has noticed that he has consistently gained weight despite a relatively healthy diet and exercise. He does admit to working rotating shifts. Given this history, which medication is this patient most likely taking?

A. Diphenhydramine
B. Eszopiclone
C. Ramelteon
D. Trazodone
E. Ginkgo biloba

(B) This patient is experiencing a sleep-related eating disorder, a misnomer as it is not an actual eating disorder but rather a parasomnia. Patients taking sedatives such as **eszopiclone (Lunesta®)** are most likely to experience this.

Sleep-related eating disorder (SRED) is a variant of sleepwalking, affecting approximately 3% of the general population. It most commonly occurs in the first one-third of the sleep period.

Its associations are listed below:

- Occurs with increased frequency in those with high stress
- The majority (80%) have associated restless leg syndrome (RLS), periodic limb movement disorder (PLMD), obstructive sleep apnea (OSA), or somnambulism.
- Medications correlating with incidence are sedative-hypnotics, such as antipsychotics and psychotropic medications.

Treatment is targeted at removing the offending agent and treating any underlying associated disorders (RLS, OSA, PLMD). Topiramate, SSRIs, and trazodone also have some efficacy in treatment.

Reference: Up To Date: "Disorders of arousal from non-rapid eye movement sleep in adults"

116. (Content: II-D-3a) A 51-year-old female is undergoing a preoperative evaluation for a planned Roux-en-Y gastric bypass. She admits to often feeling tired during the day and occasionally falling asleep during conversations. Her spouse has told her that she snores very loudly, sometimes requiring him to sleep in another bedroom. Vital signs are within normal limits. BMI is 39 kg/m^2, and her neck circumference is 17 inches (43.2 cm). What is the next best step in evaluating for obstructive sleep apnea?

A. Inquire if she has stopped breathing during sleep
B. Place a referral for an overnight pulse-oximetry test
C. **Place a referral for polysomnography**
D. Perform a physical exam, focusing on the oral exam
E. Order a daytime arterial blood gas

(C) This patient meets the criteria for a positive screening for obstructive sleep apnea (OSA) via the "STOP-BANG" questionnaire. She scored 5 points (snores, fatigued, increased body mass index, neck circumference, and age), placing her at high risk and warranting further evaluation with **polysomnography**.

The STOP-BANG screening tool was validated in preoperative evaluations, with a score ≤ 2 adequately excluding a diagnosis of OSA, whereas a score of ≥ 5 makes OSA highly likely (specificity 80%).

STOP-BANG Score (1 point for each positive)			
S	Snore loudly	B	BMI ≥ 35 kg/m^2
T	Tiredness (daytime fatigue)	A	Age > 50 years old
O	Observed apnea	N	Neck circumference > 40 cm
P	Pressure (elevated BP)	G	Gender: Male
Risk: Low (0-2), Intermediate (3-4), High[1] (5-8)			

BP: Blood pressure
[1]Some recommendations state that ≥ 3 is considered high risk and warrants further evaluation

Note: Another clinical pretest probability scoring system that may be used for OSA is the Epworth Sleepiness Scale, which includes a series of questions about the likelihood of them falling asleep during certain activities throughout the day.

Reference: AACE/ACE Guidelines: AMERICAN ASSOCIATION OF CLINICAL ENDOCRINOLOGISTS AND AMERICAN COLLEGE OF ENDOCRINOLOGY COMPREHENSIVE CLINICAL PRACTICE GUIDELINES FOR MEDICAL CARE OF PATIENTS WITH OBESITY (2016). Recommendation 21.

117. (Content: II-A-1) A 17-year-old female presents to her family medicine doctor for a sports physical. She has no prior medical history, although she feels more fatigued than usual. Vital signs reveal a heart rate of 60 BPM and a BMI of 22 kg/m². A physical exam reveals parotid gland enlargement and scrapes over the dorsum of her second metacarpal phalangeal joint. She is elusive when asked questions about her eating habits. Which medications is contraindicated given her most likely underlying diagnosis?

A. Trazodone
B. Bupropion
C. Topiramate
D. Sertraline
E. Buspirone

(B) This patient presents with findings of Russell's sign (callouses or cuts on the knuckles due to repetitive self-induced vomiting) and parotid gland enlargement. In the setting of a normal BMI, this is concerning for the diagnosis of bulimia nervosa. **Bupropion is contraindicated in eating disorders**, epilepsy, or other conditions that lower the seizure threshold.

Note: By definition, anorexia nervosa requires a low body weight (BMI < 18.5 kg/m²), which can help differentiate it from bulimia nervosa.

Bulimia affects up to 10% of women over their lifetime, with 16-22 years old being the most common age group affected. The vast majority are females (90%), often with a concurrent mood disorder or history of abuse, especially sexual abuse (25%).

Treatment options for bulimia nervosa should include nutritional rehabilitation and cognitive behavioral therapy. Often these are combined with medications for a synergistic effect. Fluoxetine is FDA-approved for bulimia nervosa, whereas other SSRIs, such as sertraline, are effective but used off-label.

Reference: Bupropion package insert
Reference: Up to Date "Bulimia nervosa in adults: Pharmacotherapy"

118. (Content: II-B-5) A 29-year-old male presents to an internist to establish care. His chief concern is related to his lack of upper body strength, in particular the muscle size. He states despite working out his arms for nearly 3 hours daily, his arms still appear smaller than he would like. He has difficulty focusing on his work as a car salesman, as he feels people notice his arms and admits to being very self-conscious. A physical exam reveals a healthy, muscular-appearing male in no distress. If inquired, the patient most likely would admit to experiencing which of the following?

    A. Compulsive behaviors
    B. Anxiety attacks
    C. Severe calorie restriction
    D. Nocturnal eating
    E. Delayed sleep onset

(A) This patient's preoccupation with his appearance (i.e., arm size) is consistent with the diagnosis of body dysmorphic disorder with muscle dysmorphia. This condition is closely related (and treated similarly) to **obsessive-compulsive disorders**.

Body dissatisfaction responds well to cognitive behavioral therapy, whereas medications (SSRIs, topiramate, lamotrigine) are used off-label.

Diagnostic Criteria for Body Dysmorphic Disorder
Preoccupation with ≥ 1 flaw in physical appearance that is not observable or appears slight to others.

Performed repetitive behaviors:
  • Mirror checking
  • Excessive grooming
  • Skin picking
  • Reassurance seeking
  • Compares his/her appearance with others

Preoccupation causes distress/impairment in areas of functioning
Preoccupation is not better explained by another eating disorder

Reference: DSM-5: Diagnostic and Statistical Manual of Mental Disorders, Fifth Edition

119. (Content: II-D-3b) A university is conducting a research study. The primary objective is to correlate quantitative sex hormone binding globulin (SHBG)) levels with different patient characteristics. In particular, age, weight, and comorbid conditions such as polycystic ovarian syndrome (PCOS) are analyzed. Which of the following patients would have an increased SHBG level compared to their comparative matched cohort?

A. A patient with a BMI of 45 kg/m^2
B. A female with a diagnosis of PCOS
C. A younger individual
D. A male with decreased total testosterone
E. A patient six months status post gastric bypass

(E) Sex hormone binding globulin directly correlates with several conditions, including comorbidities of excess weight. Older patients and those who have lost weight **(through bariatric surgery** or other means) have higher SHBG levels than younger patients or those with a similar BMI who have not lost weight.

Correlations between patient characteristics/comorbidities and corresponding SHBG levels should be understood, as discussed below:

- SHBG is decreased in patients with obesity. However, with weight loss, these levels will increase.
- Patients with PCOS have decreased SHBG levels due to the increased levels of insulin inhibiting hepatic SHBG production.
- Males with obesity have decreased total testosterone levels due to decreased SHBG, although free testosterone is similar amongst variations in BMI in the absence of other conditions.
- SHBG increases proportionally with age.

Reference: Zhu JL, Chen Z, Feng WJ, Long SL, Mo ZC. Sex hormone-binding globulin and polycystic ovary syndrome. Clin Chim Acta. 2019 Dec;499:142-148. doi: 10.1016/j.cca.2019.09.010. Epub 2019 Sep 13. PMID: 31525346.
Reference: Cooper LA, Page ST, Amory JK, Anawalt BD, Matsumoto AM. The association of obesity with sex hormone-binding globulin is stronger than the association with ageing--implications for the interpretation of total testosterone measurements. Clin Endocrinol (Oxf). 2015 Dec;83(6):828-33. doi: 10.1111/cen.12768. Epub 2015 May 11. PMID: 25777143; PMCID: PMC4782930.

120. (Content: II-C-1 and 5) A pediatrician is evaluating a young patient in the office and determines that the growth charts utilized for most children in her practice is inadequate for this patient, and a specialized chart is utilized. Which of the following physical exam findings does the patient most likely have?

A. Bicuspid aorta
B. Macrocephaly
C. Macroglossia
D. Ovarian agenesis
E. Upslanting palpebral fissures

(B) Certain populations have unique pediatric BMI curves, including patients with achondroplasia, which presents with short stature, brachydactyly, **macrocephaly,** and frontal bossing.

Notably, although patients with Down syndrome (presenting with macroglossia and upslanting palpebral fissures) have an increased risk of obesity and use different charts for weight and height, the BMI guidelines from the CDC recommend using charts for normally developing children. This is recommended to provide early detection of excess weight in order to incorporate earlier intervention.

In addition, those with Turner's syndrome (with physical examination findings displaying ovarian agenesis and having a correlation with a bicuspid aorta) commonly have abnormal glucose metabolism and a higher prevalence of diabetes mellitus. Although there are unique BMI charts for this population, they are very specific to the locality (i.e., Turkey and Japan) and are not universally accepted by the CDC.

Note: All of the above conditions have associations with shorter stature and increased weight, as well as complications including obstructive sleep apnea, cardiovascular disease, and potentially early-onset impaired motility.

Reference: Up to Date: "Achondroplasia"
Reference: Obesity Medicine Association: Pediatric Obesity Algorithm (2023-2024)

121. (Content II-C-1) A 41-year-old Caucasian male presents to his primary care physician for an annual health screen. His immunizations are up to date. A recent diabetes and hypertension screening completed through work was within normal limits. His height is 70 inches (178 cm), and his weight is 260 lbs (117 kg). By utilizing the chart below, his weight would best be described as being in which of the following categories?

BMI	28	29	30	31	32	33	34	35	36	37	38	39	40	41	42	43	44	45	46
5'4"	163	169	174	180	186	192	197	204	209	215	221	227	232	238	244	250	256	262	267
5'5"	168	174	180	186	192	198	204	210	216	222	228	234	240	246	252	258	264	270	276
5'6"	173	179	186	192	198	204	210	216	223	229	235	241	247	253	260	266	272	278	284
5'7"	178	185	191	198	204	211	217	223	230	236	242	249	255	261	268	274	280	287	293
5'8"	184	190	197	203	210	216	223	230	236	243	249	256	262	269	276	282	289	295	302
5'9"	189	196	203	209	216	223	230	236	243	250	257	263	270	277	284	291	297	304	311
5'10"	195	202	209	216	222	229	236	243	250	257	264	271	278	285	292	299	306	313	320
5'11"	200	208	215	222	229	236	243	250	257	265	272	279	286	293	301	308	315	322	329

(Note: Weight is in pounds)

    A. Normal weight
    B. Overweight
    C. Class I obesity
    D. Class II obesity
    E. Class III obesity

(D) This patient has a body mass index of 37.3 kg/m², placing him in the range of **class II obesity.** The classification of weight based on BMI is shown in the table below:

Classification of BMI			
Classification	BMI (kg/m²)	Classification	BMI (kg/m²)
Underweight	< 18.5	Class I obesity	30-34.9
Normal weight	18.5- 24.9	Class II obesity	35-39.9
Overweight	25-29.9	Class III obesity	≥ 40

Reference: AACE/ACE Guidelines: AMERICAN ASSOCIATION OF CLINICAL ENDOCRINOLOGISTS AND AMERICAN COLLEGE OF ENDOCRINOLOGY COMPREHENSIVE CLINICAL PRACTICE GUIDELINES FOR MEDICAL CARE OF PATIENTS WITH OBESITY (2016)

122. (Content: II-D-3a) A 49-year-old female with a history of severe obesity is following-up with her pulmonologist regarding her pulmonary hypertension, confirmed with a right-heart catheterization. She has no prior tobacco or occupational exposures, and her polysomnography test was negative. Given this information, which of the following would most likely be seen in this patient?

A. Class 4 Mallampati score
B. Increased Epworth sleepiness scale
C. FVC/FEV$_1$ < 0.70
D. Increased respiratory disturbance index
E. **Arterial blood gas PaCO$_2$ > 45 mmHg**

(E) This patient is presenting with pulmonary hypertension in the setting of severe obesity, with obstructive sleep apnea (OSA) ruled out through polysomnography (the gold standard). Given this, the next most likely diagnosis is obesity hypoventilation syndrome, which requires **an increased carbon dioxide level** on a daytime arterial blood gas for diagnosis.

Obesity hypoventilation syndrome (OHS), also referred to as Pickwickian syndrome, is a restrictive lung disease that carries high mortality rates. Although 90% have concurrent OSA, it can occur independently. It is associated with pulmonary hypertension and right-sided heart failure.

Diagnostic criteria include:

- Obesity (body mass index > 30 kg/m^2)
- PaCO$_2$ > 45 mmHg
- Exclusion of other causes

First-line treatment is non-invasive positive airway pressure, whereas definitive treatment focuses on weight loss.

Reference: Up to Date: "Treatment and prognosis of the obesity hypoventilation syndrome"

123. (Content: II-D-3) A mother brings her previously healthy 10-year-old daughter to her family medicine physician for an annual examination. The patient has been spending more time on the computer and watching television, with decreased physical activity. Her weight has steadily increased. Her body mass index is in the 86th percentile for age and gender. The patient denies any symptoms or concerns. Which test should be ordered for evaluation purposes?

A. **Fasting lipid profile**
B. Aspartate aminotransferase
C. Fasting glucose
D. Creatinine
E. Thyroid-stimulating hormone

(A) The American Academy of Pediatrics Clinical Practice Guidelines for the Evaluation and Treatment of Children and Adolescents with Obesity (2023) provides recommendations on performing laboratory tests evaluating for comorbid conditions:

- Age 2-9 years old: *May* evaluate for dyslipidemia in those with obesity.
- Age ≥ 10 years old:
  - Obesity: **Should** evaluate for lipid abnormalities, abnormal glucose metabolism, and abnormal liver function.
  - Overweight: **Should** evaluate for lipid abnormalities. *May* evaluate for abnormal glucose metabolism and liver function in the presence of risk factors for type II diabetes and metabolic-associated fatty liver disease.

Overweight is defined as BMI ≥ 85th percentile to < 95th percentile, whereas obesity is defined as a BMI ≥ 95th percentile.

In children with obesity, nearly 1/3 will have fatty liver disease, with ALT being the best initial screening test. Although a liver biopsy is considered the gold standard for confirmation, more commonly, imaging is utilized (ultrasound, MRI, transient elastography, etc.). Evaluating for diabetes should be done via fasting plasma glucose, 2-hour post-75-gram oral glucose tolerance test, or HbA1c, whereas evaluating for lipid abnormalities should be obtained via a **fasting lipid panel.**

Reference: Hampl, S. E., Hassink, S. G., Skinner, A. C., Armstrong, S. C., Barlow, S. E., Bolling, C. F., ... Okechukwu, K. (2023). Clinical Practice Guideline for the Evaluation and Treatment of Children and Adolescents With Obesity. Pediatrics, 151(2), e2022060640. https://doi.org/10.1542/peds.2022-060640. KAS 3, 3.1, 5, 6, and 7.

124. (Content: II-C-3 and 5) After injuring his finger, a 6-year-old male with class III obesity presents to the emergency department. The mother states that the child was trying to swing at a local park when his finger became stuck in the chain. The patient has full range of motion but increased swelling of his third digit. An x-ray is shown below. Which other finding is most likely?

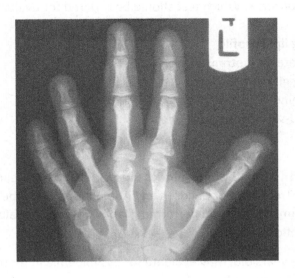

A. **Pseudohypoparathyroidism**
B. History of seizures
C. Almond-shaped eyes
D. Microorchidism

(A) This patient presents with early-onset obesity and shortened 4th and 5th digits (as seen on the hand x-ray) and likely carries the diagnosis of Albright Hereditary Osteodystrophy. This condition is characterized by a shorter stature, round facies, shortened fourth and fifth metacarpals, intellectual disability, impaired olfaction, and **pseudohypoparathyroidism.**

Pseudohypoparathyroidism is characterized by renal resistance to parathyroid hormone (PTH), leading to hypocalcemia, hyperphosphatemia, and elevated PTH levels.

Image Reference: Hasani-Ranjbar S, Jouyandeh Z, Amoli MM, Soltani A, Arzaghi SM. A patient with features of albright hereditory osteodystrophy and unusual neuropsychiatric findings without coding Gsalpha mutations. *J Diabetes Metab Disord.* 2014;13:56. Published 2014 May 22. doi:10.1186/2251-6581-13-56
Reference: Obesity Medicine Association: Obesity Algorithm (2023)

125. (Content: II-C) A 34-year-old female presents to her obstetrician for preconception counseling. She is wanting to become pregnant within the next year and wants to know how much weight gain would be appropriate during pregnancy. Her BMI is 31 kg/m^2. What is the most appropriate answer to her question?

    A. Maintain current weight
    B. 11-20 lbs
    C. 15-25 lbs
    D. 25-35 lbs
    E. 28-40 lbs

(B) This patient with class I obesity prior to pregnancy, should gain **11-20 lbs** during pregnancy. Guidelines recommend certain weight gain during pregnancy based on pre-conception body mass index. Only one-third of women actually gain the recommended weight during pregnancy, with 1 out of 5 gaining too little and nearly 50% gaining too much.

Gaining less weight than recommended increases the risk for a small for gestational age neonate, which may lead to further complications such as not meeting developmental milestones. In contrast, those gaining too much weight have an increased risk of delivery complications, as well as obesity of the child.

Weight Gain in Pregnancy		
Pre-Pregnancy Category and BMI		**Total Recommended Weight Gain During Pregnancy**
Underweight	<18.5	28-40 lbs
Normal weight	18.5-24.9	25-35 lbs
Overweight	25-29.9	15-25 lbs
Obesity (all classes)	≥ 30	11-20 lbs

Reference: CDC: Weight Gain During Pregnancy
https://www.cdc.gov/reproductivehealth/maternalinfanthealth/pregnancy-weight-gain.htm
Reference: Obesity Medicine Association: Obesity Algorithm (2023)

126. (Content: III-H-1) A 7-year-old female and her parents meet with the pediatrician to initiate discussions on treatment options for obesity. The family has tried numerous strategies at home without significant success and is now seeking guidance. Which of the following intensive behavioral lifestyle treatments is most likely to provide the most success?

A. **Providing 30 hours of treatment over a 6-month time frame**
B. Utilizing motivational interviewing focused on patient motivation
C. Encouraging an intense after-school basketball program
D. Initiate pharmacotherapy and follow up in 6 months

(A) Intensive health behavior and lifestyle treatment (IHBLT) is the primary approach to reduce weight gain and improve body mass index (BMI) in children over the age of 6 years old. It is time-intensive, with a direct correlation of effectiveness based on time (hours). Longitudinal care providing ≥ **26 hours over a 3-12 month time period** is the minimum, and interventions ≥ 52 hours provided the most significant reduction in BMI and improvements in cardiometabolic health. IHBLT may be enough for some patients to adequately improve obesity, while others will require advanced therapies.

Incorrect answer choices: Family-oriented activities are more effective in pre-adolescents than individual activities such as camps, afterschool activities, etc. Motivational interviewing in younger patients (pre-adolescent) should focus on parental motivation and transition to patient motivation once an adolescent. Pharmacotherapy should not be used in the absence of close monitoring.

Intensive Health Behavior and Lifestyle Treatment Components	
Who	Patient and family in coordination with primary health care providers and multidisciplinary team (dieticians, behavioral health, etc.), provided in group and/or individual formats
What	Education focused on behavioral modifications of nutritional intake and physical activity
Where	Healthcare setting including medical home and community-based resources
When	Promptly, once overweight or obesity is diagnosed
How Much	≥ 26 hours over a 3–12-month period
How	Face-to-face has the most evidence, but virtual options seem effective and are more readily available

Reference: Hampl, S. E., Hassink, S. G., Skinner, A. C., Armstrong, S. C., Barlow, S. E., Bolling, C. F., ... Okechukwu, K. (2023). Clinical Practice Guideline for the Evaluation and Treatment of Children and Adolescents With Obesity. Pediatrics, 151(2), e2022060640. https://doi.org/10.1542/peds.2022-060640.

Key Action Statements (KAS) with 2023 AAP Guidelines

KAS	Statement
1	Pediatricians/PHCPs **should** measure height and weight, calculate BMI, and assess BMI percentile using age- and sex-specific CDC growth charts annually for all children 2 to 18 y of age.
2	Pediatricians/PHCPs **should** evaluate children 2 to 18 y of age with overweight and obesity for obesity-related comorbidities by using a comprehensive patient history, mental and behavioral health, SDoH evaluation, physical examination and studies.
3	In children 10 y and older, pediatricians/PHCPs **should** evaluate for lipid abnormalities, abnormal glucose metabolism, and abnormal liver function in children and adolescents with obesity and for lipid abnormalities in children and adolescents with overweight.
3.1	In children 10 y and older with overweight, pediatricians/PHCPs may evaluate for abnormal glucose metabolism and liver function in the presence of risk factors for T2DM or NAFLD, and in children 2 to 9 y of age with obesity may evaluate for lipid abnormalities.
4	Pediatricians/PHCPs **should** treat children and adolescents for overweight or obesity and comorbidities concurrently.
5	Pediatricians/PHCPs **should** evaluate for dyslipidemia by obtaining a fasting lipid panel in children 10 y and older with overweight and obesity and may evaluate for dyslipidemia in children 2 through 9 y of age with obesity.
6	Pediatricians/PHCPs **should** evaluate for prediabetes and/or diabetes mellitus with fasting plasma glucose, 2-h plasma glucose after 75-g oral glucose tolerance test, or glycosylated hemoglobin per KAS 3 and 3.1.
7	Pediatricians/PHCPs **should** evaluate for NAFLD by obtaining an alanine transaminase test per KAS 3 and 3.1.
8	Pediatricians/PHCPs **should** evaluate for hypertension by measuring blood pressure at every visit starting at 3 y of age in children and adolescents with overweight and obesity.
9	Pediatricians/PHCPs **should** treat overweight and obesity in children and adolescents, following the principles of the medical home and the chronic care model, using a family-centered and non-stigmatizing approach that acknowledges obesity's biologic, social, and structural drivers.
10	Pediatricians/PHCPs **should** use motivational interviewing to engage patients and families in treating overweight and obesity.
11	Pediatricians/PHCPs **should** provide or refer children 6 y and older (Grade B) and may provide or refer children 2 through 5 y of age (Grade C) with overweight and obesity to intensive health behavior and lifestyle treatment. Health behavior and lifestyle treatment is more effective with greater contact hours; the most effective treatment includes 26 or more hours of face-to-face, family-based, multicomponent treatment over a 3- to 12-month period.
12	Pediatricians/PHCPs **should** offer adolescents 12 y and older with obesity weight loss pharmacotherapy, according to medication indications, risks, and benefits, as an adjunct to health behavior and lifestyle treatment.
13	Pediatricians/PHCPs **should** offer referral for adolescents 13 y and older with severe obesity for evaluation for metabolic and bariatric surgery to local or regional comprehensive multidisciplinary pediatric metabolic and bariatric surgery centers.

AAP: American Academy of Pediatricians; **PHCP:** Primary health care physicians; **CDC:** Centers for Disease Control; **SDoH:** Social determinants of health; **T2DM:** Type 2 diabetes mellitus; **NAFLD:** Non-alcoholic fatty liver disease; **y:** Year; **h:** Hour; **g:** Gram; **Overweight:** BMI ≥ 85th percentile to < 95th percentile; **Obesity:** BMI ≥ 95th percentile; **Severe obesity:** BMI ≥ 120% of the 95th percentile for age and sex

127. (Content: III-D-1) A 39-year-old male presents to the hospital with fatigue and decreased urine output. His past medical history includes obesity class II and prediabetes for which he is on metformin. His New Year's resolution was to lose 25 lbs (11.3 kg) prompting him to initiate high-intensity physical activity. In addition, his physician started him on an anti-obesity medication. During a recent workout, he twisted his ankle and has been taking multiple ibuprofen and naproxen to help with the pain. Recent labs display a creatinine of 2.1 mg/dL (reference range: 0.6–1.2 mg/dL) and a lactate level of 7.1 mmol/L (reference range: 0.5 to 2.2 mmol/L) with an increased anion gap. Which of the following medications was most likely initiated at his recent appointment?

A. Liraglutide
B. Bupropion
C. Orlistat
D. Topiramate
E. Semaglutide

(D) This patient who started taking excessive NSAIDs given his recent ankle injury likely induced an acute kidney injury. His anion gap metabolic acidosis secondary to lactic acidosis was likely caused by his metformin use in the setting of a kidney injury and his new anti-obesity medication containing **topiramate**.

Metformin has a black box warning for lactic acidosis, with risk factors including:

- Renal impairment
- Concomitant use of certain drugs (with the only specifically mentioned medication listed on the black box warning being "carbonic anhydrase inhibitors such as **topiramate**")
- Age ≥ 65 years of age
- Contrasted radiographic studies
- Surgery or other procedures
- Hypoxic states (e.g., acute congestive heart failure)
- Excessive alcohol intake
- Hepatic impairment

Reference: Metformin package insert

128. (Content: III-B-1) A 44-year-old female presents to her primary care physician with dysuria and malodorous urine. She denies abdominal pain. She has type 2 diabetes and was recently started on dapagliflozin to help with weight loss and diabetes control. In addition, she initiated a new diet this week. Her urinalysis dipstick results are below. Given these findings, the diet she has started most likely encourages which of the following components?

Leukocyte	1+	Specific gravity	1.011
Nitrite	2+	Ketone	2+
Protein	Trace	Bilirubin	Not detected
Blood	1+	Glucose	3+

    A. Significant carbohydrate restriction
    B. Avoiding foods with a glycemic index > 70
    C. Increasing omega-3 intake with extra virgin vegetable oil
    D. Limiting fat intake to 20-25% of daily calories
    E. Intake a minimum of 5 servings of fruit daily

(A) A ketogenic diet **significantly restricts carbohydrate** intake, promoting fat for energy and thus placing the patient in a ketotic state. Therefore, her diet is the most likely cause of ketones in her urine. The patient's recent introduction of an SGLT-2 inhibitor may increase her risk of urinary tract infections, cause glucosuria, and may even cause euglycemic diabetic ketoacidosis. However, she has no other symptoms (nausea, abdominal pain, etc.) to indicate ketoacidosis as her cause of ketosis.

The key points of the ketogenic diet are listed below:

- Carbohydrates are generally reduced to 60-90 grams daily in a ketogenic diet. Some may do an initial induction phase (20 g daily).
- A ketogenic diet and Atkin's diet are examples of carbohydrate-restrictive diets (< 45% calories from carbs).
- Fruits, dairy, carbohydrates, and starchy vegetables are restricted.

Note: Extreme caution should be used if a patient is starting a ketogenic diet and is currently taking an SGLT-2 inhibitor due to the risk of ketoacidosis. If the patient is on insulin, it should also be decreased, with hypoglycemic education provided.

Reference: Obesity Medicine Association: Obesity Algorithm (2023)

129. (Content: III-G-4) A 14-year-old male presents for his annual checkup at his pediatrician's clinic. He has no prior medical history. His BMI is 31 kg/m^2. The pediatrician discusses healthy eating choices, exercise, and lifestyle changes to prevent weight-related complications. This discussion is an example of which of the following phases of prevention in chronic obesity?

 A. Primary prevention
 B. Secondary prevention
 C. Tertiary prevention

(B) This pediatrician is trying to prevent future weight gain, as well as weight-related complications of obesity, in a patient that already meets obesity criteria, consistent with the definition of **secondary prevention.**

The three phases of chronic disease prevention apply to obesity, which guides the intensity and modality of disease intervention.

- **Primary prevention:** Prevent the development of overweight and obesity through education, environment, and promoting healthy eating and regular physical exercise.

- **Secondary prevention:** Prevent future weight gain and the development of weight-related complications in patients with excess weight or obesity by initiating lifestyle and behavioral intervention (+/- pharmacologic therapy).

- **Tertiary prevention:** Target weight loss to eliminate or mitigate weight-related complications and prevent disease progression by initiating lifestyle/behavioral interventions, weight-loss medication, and/or potentially considering metabolic surgery.

Reference: AACE/ACE Guidelines: AMERICAN ASSOCIATION OF CLINICAL ENDOCRINOLOGISTS AND AMERICAN COLLEGE OF ENDOCRINOLOGY COMPREHENSIVE CLINICAL PRACTICE GUIDELINES FOR MEDICAL CARE OF PATIENTS WITH OBESITY (2016): Recommendation 2

130. (Content: III-F-2) A patient had a previous bariatric procedure performed ten years ago in which a band was placed around the top of the stomach, creating a small pouch. Although adjustable, the patient has had difficulty following up and thus is interested in a surgical revision. The patient has had three adjustments during the past decade, initially losing 32 lbs (14.5 kg), but has since regained this weight. Which is true of this bariatric procedure?

    A.   It is considered a malabsorptive procedure
    B.   The minimum BMI required for placement is 30 kg/m²
    C.   Mortality rate is similar to other bariatric procedures
    D.   Adjustment requires conscious sedation
    E.   It is the most common weight loss procedure worldwide

(B) Laparoscopic adjustable gastric banding (LAGB) is a restrictive procedure in which a stomach pouch is created by placing an adjustable band around the upper portion of the stomach ❶, allowing for decreased food intake. Also, the increased pressure on the stomach prolongs the sensation of fullness, thus helping suppress appetite. A subcutaneous port ❷ is available and allows for fluid to be added, allowing for increased restriction. It has the lowest mortality rate and is considered the least invasive surgical option. It is approved in those with a **BMI of 30 kg/m² with an obesity comorbidity.**

Image citation: Image created by Charu G. Copyright owned by Kevin Smith, DO
Reference: Suter M, Giusti V, Worreth M, Héraief E, Calmes JM. Laparoscopic gastric banding: a prospective, randomized study comparing the Lapband and the SAGB: early results. Ann Surg. 2005;241(1):55-62. doi:10.1097/01.sla.0000150071.86934.36

131. (Content: III-H-4) A healthy 6-year-old female presents to her primary care physician with her father for an annual exam. She has no prior medical conditions and is up to date on immunizations. Her father has no concerns about her current health but is concerned about preventing weight gain, as her sibling has excess weight. The patient's BMI is in the 50th percentile, with consistent height and weight in the 55th and 60th percentile, respectively. Which of the following is the most appropriate recommendation for this child?

A. Consume 3 or more fruits and vegetables daily
B. Minimize screen time to < 3 hours daily
C. Allow the child to self-regulate meals
D. Encourage at least 8 hours of sleep nightly
E. Eat as a family at least 3 times weekly

(C) This patient with a healthy weight is encouraged to maintain healthy eating and lifestyle choices to continue her current projectile (i.e., primary prevention). There is consistent evidence that allowing children under 12 years old **to self-regulate their meal quantities**, in contrast to promoting restrictive feeding behaviors, is preferred and leads to better weight outcomes. Importantly, this self-regulating applies to meals, not snacking.

In addition to the above recommendation, healthy lifestyle habits for children include healthy eating and decreasing sedentary time, as discussed below:

- Limit screen time to 2 hours daily
- Encourage sleeping 11-14 hours nightly (ages 5-9 years old) and 10-12 hours (ages 10-14 years old)
- Intake ≥ 5 servings of fruits and vegetables daily
- Minimize or eliminate (preferred) sugar-sweetened beverages
- Prepare meals at home when possible
- Eat at the table with family at home frequently
- Consume a healthy breakfast every morning
- Perform at least 60 minutes of moderate to vigorous physical activity daily

Reference: Obesity Medicine Association: Pediatric Obesity Algorithm (2023-2024)
Reference: Hampl, S. E., Hassink, S. G., Skinner, A. C., Armstrong, S. C., Barlow, S. E., Bolling, C. F., ... Okechukwu, K. (2023). Clinical Practice Guideline for the Evaluation and Treatment of Children and Adolescents With Obesity. Pediatrics, 151(2), e2022060640. https://doi.org/10.1542/peds.2022-060640.

132. (Content: III-F-4) A 53-year-old male is presenting for evaluation for weight loss. He has started the bridge-to-transplant program, which requires a BMI of 35 kg/m² or less in order to be listed on the kidney transplant list. His current BMI is 44 kg/m². Both medication and surgical options are discussed. He prefers to undergo bariatric and metabolic surgery. Which of the following surgical options is most preferred?

A. Single anastomosis duodeno-ileal bypass
B. Roux-en-Y gastric bypass
C. Vertical sleeve gastrectomy
D. Gastric balloon
E. Adjustable gastric band

(C) In this patient wishing to undergo a renal transplant, the best choice is a **vertical sleeve gastrectomy (VSG).** Temporary measures such as a gastric balloon may not provide enough time for weight loss and being accepted for a transplant, as they have a maximum duration of 8 months. Other malabsorptive procedures should be avoided in those who will require immunosuppressants, due to absorption issues, and those likely to need frequent steroids, due to the increased risk of anastomotic or marginal ulcers. In addition, a VSG mitigates intrabdominal scar tissue which is important for the subsequent transplant.

Selecting an appropriate surgery will ultimately be up to the surgeon to discuss. However, understanding why specific procedures should be avoided or encouraged is helpful. Other patients who may benefit from a VSG include:

- Ill-patients: Patients who are more chronically ill, including those with obesity-related comorbidities such as pulmonary hypertension and heart failure with preserved ejection fraction may benefit from a sleeve gastrectomy due to shorter anesthesia times.
- Recurrent renal stones: Malabsorptive procedures increase oxalate absorption.
- Risk of severe nutritional deficiencies
- Organ transplant patients, including those on chronic immunosuppressants or those requiring critical medications that require adequate absorption.

Reference: Veroux M, Mattone E, Cavallo M, Gioco R, Corona D, Volpicelli A, Veroux P. Obesity and bariatric surgery in kidney transplantation: A clinical review. World J Diabetes. 2021 Sep 15;12(9):1563-1575. doi: 10.4239/wjd.v12.i9.1563. PMID: 34630908; PMCID: PMC8472502.

133. (Content: III-H-4) A mother presents to her pediatrician with her breastfed 6-month-old daughter to discuss healthy habits to initiate over the next year. The mother is concerned given the family history of obesity that her child will gain excess weight. What recommendations should be given to the parents over the next year?

A. Limit television to less than 1 hour daily
B. Reward good behavior with healthy foods
C. Stop breastfeeding and transition to solid food now
D. Allow the child to feed themselves complementary foods
E. Ensure the child finishes food/milk during each feeding

(D) Recommendations for children less than 24 months of age are to avoid any screen time, exclusively breastfeed for as long as possible (ideally 6-12 months), and **delay introducing complementary foods until 6 months of age.** Food should not be used as a reward, and **children should be allowed to feed themselves,** which promotes self-regulation. They also should not be forced to finish their food when they are refusing. In addition, no fast food or desserts should be given at this age.

General Recommendations for Children (0-4 years of age)		
Conditions	Age 0-24 months	Age 2- 4 years
Screen time[1]	None	<1 hour/day
Sleep time	12-18 hours	11-14 hours
Fast food	None	None
Dessert	None	Only special occasions
Sugary-sweetened beverages or juice	None	None
Activity	Encourage activity and exploring the environment	Constant active play (minimize sedentary time)
Parent's role	Encourage lots of direct interaction with parents	-Parents are role models -Avoid being over-controlling
Other	-Do not force foods -Infants to feed themselves	-Meals at a table/ highchair -Avoid over-controlling -Praise for trying new food

[1]Screen time may replace physical activity and interfere with sleep. Sleep restriction is associated with increased caloric consumption.

Reference: Obesity Medicine Association: Pediatric Obesity Algorithm (2023-2024)

134. (Content: III-H-1 and III-D-6) A mother brings her 6-year-old daughter, who is in the 95th percentile for weight, to her pediatrician's office due to persistent constipation despite increased water intake. They have been using over-the-counter stool softeners without relief. The mother states that the child is not picky regarding food and eats "whatever is available." The physician recommends increasing whole grains. What effect will this indirectly have on the child?

A. Reduces HDL and triglyceride levels
B. Increases risk of irritable bowel syndrome
C. Increases nutrient-rich food intake
D. Increases saturated fat consumption
E. Cause diarrhea and potential fecal incontinence

(C) Increased fiber intake (including whole grains) has been shown to have several positive effects in both children and adults, including decreased energy-dense food intake and **increased desire for nutrient-rich foods.**

Fiber is preferred to come from the diet, such as fruits, legumes, whole grains, and vegetables, rather than supplementation when feasible. Fiber has many benefits, including:

- Improving blood glucose levels
- Reducing total cholesterol
- Reducing LDL cholesterol
- Improving satiety
- Decreasing constipation (via stool-bulking)

In addition, psyllium (a water-soluble fiber) has been shown to improve the above parameters and abdominal pain in those with irritable bowel syndrome. It is recommended at 6 g/day in those aged 6-12 and 12 g/day in those ≥12 years old in combination with low saturated fat to improve lipids and possibly help with weight.

Recommended Dietary Allowance of Fiber	
Men (14- 50 years old)	38 grams per day
Women (19-50 years old)	25 grams per day

Reference: Expert Panel on Integrated Guidelines for Cardiovascular Health and Risk Reduction in Children and Adolescents Full Report. Published Oct 2012.

135. (Content: III-F-5c) A 57-year-old male presents to the emergency department two weeks after a Roux-en-Y gastric bypass for dehydration, nausea, and vomiting. His spouse has also noted some confusion recently. Vital signs reveal a heart rate of 110/min and a blood pressure of 89/58 mmHg. Physical exam reveals dry mucus membranes, nystagmus, and difficulty walking. He is alert but oriented to person only. Given his most likely nutritional deficiency, what other clinical sequelae may be seen if left untreated?

A. Macrocytic anemia
B. Dermatitis (pellagra)
C. Seizure disorder
D. Glossitis and cheilitis
E. **Peripheral neuropathy**

(E) This patient is presenting in the acute post-bariatric surgery period with significant vomiting, confusion, and nystagmus, consistent with Wernicke's encephalopathy from thiamine (B_1) deficiency, a water-soluble vitamin. B_1 deficiency can cause many symptoms, including **symmetric peripheral polyneuropathy.**

Thiamine deficiency presentations vary by chronicity. Some of the more common presentations are discussed below:

- **Wet beriberi:** High-output congestive heart failure, including cardiomegaly, cardiomyopathy, peripheral edema, and tachycardia
- **Dry beriberi:** Symmetric peripheral polyneuropathy (sensory and motor deficits), primarily affecting the distal extremities
- **Wernicke's encephalopathy:** Ataxia, nystagmus, ophthalmoplegia, and confusion; considered reversible
- **Korsakoff syndrome:** Irreversible, a chronic neurological condition characterized by impaired short-term memory and confabulation

Note: It is imperative to give thiamine before glucose to prevent the risk of precipitating Wernicke's encephalopathy.

Reference: Up to Date: "Overview of water-soluble vitamins"

136. (Content: III-D-2) A 59-year-old male presents to his internist with the desire to start anti-obesity pharmacotherapy. The physician is interested in starting a particular combination medication but first inquires about a history of calcium phosphate stones, as this medication should be avoided in those with a history of renal nephrolithiasis. Given the most likely medication eluded to, what is a contraindication of this medicine?

    A. Chronic malabsorption syndrome
    B. Family history of medullary thyroid cancer
    C. Concurrent history of glaucoma
    D. History of epilepsy or risk of seizures
    E. Uncontrolled hypertension

(C) The medication being described is phentermine/topiramate, which should be avoided in those with a history of renal calculus. One contraindication is a diagnosis of **glaucoma.**

Phentermine/Topiramate ER (Qsymia®)[1]	
Dose	-AM dose 3.75/23 mg x 14 days, then 7.5/46 mg daily. -If weight loss < 3% after 12 weeks, increase to 11.25/69 mg x 14 days, then 15/92 mg (full strength). -D/C if < 5% weight loss after 12 weeks at max dose
Mechanism	-**Phentermine:** This sympathomimetic amine stimulates the hypothalamus to release norepinephrine, resulting in decreased appetite and food intake. -**Topiramate ER:** Potential mechanism: Enhances GABA neurotransmitter activity and Na^+ channels, leading to appetite suppression and increased satiety.
Contraindications	Hypersensitivity to phentermine or other formulary components, concurrent MAOI use, hyperthyroidism, glaucoma, and pregnancy. *Avoid in those with renal calculus history, coronary artery disease, and severe anxiety
Side Effects[2]	Paresthesia, insomnia, constipation, dysgeusia, xerostomia, lightheadedness, increased heart rate

[1]As of 2022, phentermine/topiramate ER is now approved for pediatric patients ≥ 12 years old with a BMI of ≥ 95th percentile for age and sex.

[2]Qsymia® does not have any warnings for use in those with increased blood pressure but rather has a warning of causing hypotension in those who achieve weight loss. In contrast, bupropion should be avoided in those with uncontrolled hypertension.

Reference: Phentermine/topiramate ER package insert

137. (Content: III-F-7) A 36-year-old female with diabetes mellitus type 2 presents to her primary care physician's clinic for a bariatric surgery evaluation. Her diabetes has been poorly controlled despite being on metformin, semaglutide, empagliflozin, and now high-dose insulin. She exercises 250 minutes weekly and has been on a low glycemic index dietary plan for the past nine months. Despite this, her hemoglobin A1c is 8.9% (reference range: 4.2-5.7%). Her body mass index is 32 kg/m². Regarding her bariatric surgery eligibility question, would she be a good candidate?

    A. No: Her body mass index is not in an appropriate range
    B. No: She only has one obesity-related comorbidity
    C. No: She should pursue an insulin pump instead
    D. Yes: Her diabetes is difficult to control
    E. Yes: She meets the criteria for Roux-en-Y gastric bypass only

(D) Even as early as 2016, a joint statement from 45 professional societies, including the American Diabetes Association, recommended bariatric surgery in those with a **body mass index (BMI) between 30-34.9 kg/m² and type 2 diabetes with inadequate glycemic control,** despite optimal medical therapy and lifestyle changes.

In 2022, the American Society for Metabolic and Bariatric Surgery (ASMBS) and the International Federation for the Surgery of Obesity and Metabolic Disorders (IFSO) updated bariatric surgery criteria, which includes the following key changes regarding metabolic and bariatric surgery (MBS):

- MBS is recommended for patients with a BMI ≥ 35 kg/m² regardless of comorbidities
- MBS should be considered for individuals with metabolic disease with a BMI 30-34.9 kg/m². A trial of nonsurgical management is recommended prior to pursuing surgical options in this population.
- BMI thresholds should be adjusted in the Asian population, allowing those with a BMI ≥27.5 kg/m² to be offered MBS
- Appropriate children and adolescents should be considered for MBS

These changes are based on numerous studies showing the long-term improvement of mortality and obesity-related morbidities.

Reference: 2022 American Society for Metabolic and Bariatric Surgery (ASMBS) and International Federation for the Surgery of Obesity and Metabolic Disorders (IFSO): Indications for Metabolic and Bariatric Surgery. Published: October 20, 2022 DOI: https://doi.org/10.1016/j.soard.2022.08.013

138. (Content: III-G-7) A 52-year-old male presents to his primary care physician with concerns of decreased libido. He states he has no current sexual desire and does not wake up with a morning erection. A physical exam reveals small testicles, gynecomastia, and a BMI of 52 kg/m². Morning testosterone levels are low on two occasions, while a prostate-specific antigen is within normal limits. What effect would starting testosterone likely have in this patient?

A. Increase HbA1c
B. Decrease fertility
C. Increase weight
D. Worsening lipid panel
E. Increasing blood pressure

(B) In patients with confirmed hypogonadism, testosterone replacement and lifestyle modifications should be considered in those not seeking fertility. Appropriate testosterone replacement is associated with weight loss, **reduced fertility,** decreased waist circumference, and improved glucose, HbA1c, and cholesterol panel. If patients who are taking testosterone lose a significant amount of weight, the dosing may need to be reduced.

The etiology of reduced fertility is shown below.

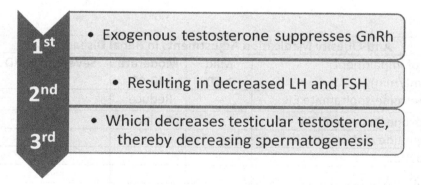

GnRH: Gonadotropin-releasing hormone; **LH:** Luteinizing hormone; **FSH:** Follicular stimulating hormone

Reference: AACE/ACE Guidelines: AMERICAN ASSOCIATION OF CLINICAL ENDOCRINOLOGISTS AND AMERICAN COLLEGE OF ENDOCRINOLOGY COMPREHENSIVE CLINICAL PRACTICE GUIDELINES FOR MEDICAL CARE OF PATIENTS WITH OBESITY (2016): Recommendation 54

139. (Content: III-D-2) A 47-year-old male with end-stage renal disease is presenting to his primary care physician's office with the desire to lose weight. To be considered for a renal transplant, he must lose an additional 22 lbs (10 kg). Although he has incorporated lifestyle modifications, he has failed to meet his weight loss goals. He is interested in bariatric medications. Which of the following would be the most appropriate medication to prescribe?

A. Phentermine/topiramate ER
B. Naltrexone/bupropion ER
C. Liraglutide
D. Phentermine monotherapy
E. Metformin

(C) All FDA-approved anti-obesity medications used for long-term weight loss should be avoided in the setting of end-stage renal disease, except for GLP-1 receptor agonists **(liraglutide or semaglutide),** orlistat, or cellulose and citric acid hydrogel (considered a medical device, not a medication). In addition, metformin is contraindicated if GFR is <30 mL/min.

The use of pharmacologic weight loss treatments in chronic kidney disease is limited and should be used with caution. Significant limitations are summarized below:

Anti-Obesity Medication Adjustments in Renal Disease			
Level of Impairment: GFR (mL/min):	Mild ≥ 50	Moderate 30-49	Severe to ESRD <30
Phentermine/topiramate ER	--	Reduce[1]	AVOID
Naltrexone/bupropion ER	--	Reduce[2]	AVOID
Semaglutide and liraglutide	--	--	--
Tirzepatide	--	--	--
Orlistat[3]	--	--	--
Cellulose and citric acid hydrogel[4]	--	--	--

GFR: Glomerular filtration rate; **ESRD:** End-stage renal disease
[1]Max dose: Phentermine 7.5 mg/topiramate 46 mg once daily
[2]Max dose: Naltrexone 8 mg/bupropion 90 mg twice daily
[3]Caution in the setting of oxalate nephropathy
[4]Not systemically absorbed
-- indicates no dosage adjustment necessary

Reference: AACE/ACE Guidelines: AMERICAN ASSOCIATION OF CLINICAL ENDOCRINOLOGISTS AND AMERICAN COLLEGE OF ENDOCRINOLOGY COMPREHENSIVE CLINICAL PRACTICE GUIDELINES FOR MEDICAL CARE OF PATIENTS WITH OBESITY (2016): Recommendation 83-85

140. (Content: III-D-6) A patient presents to her internist with concerns about supplements she has been taking. She was started on L-carnitine and green tea extract at the recommendation of an herbalist. However, since starting, she has noticed increased anxiety, palpitations, and a slight tremor. Both of these supplements theoretically work by which mechanism?

    A. Energy expenditure
    B. Satiety
    C. Carbohydrate metabolism
    D. Blocking fat absorption
    E. Increase fat oxidation

(E) Both supplements mentioned above have mechanisms of action that include decreasing fat synthesis and **increasing fat oxidation.** Green tea extract in high amounts causes anxiety, tremors, and palpitations.

Note: No legal dietary supplement ingredient has been demonstrated to be effective for weight loss, and these should not be recommended in place of other proven, effective therapies. Also, supplements are often not in a pure form (not regulated) and may contain substances such as stimulants, diuretics, or laxatives that may cause adverse medical effects. Finally, drug-herb interactions are possible.

The table summarizes the mechanism for many different supplements:

Supplement Mechanisms	
↑ Energy expenditure	Yerba mate, ephedra, guarana, Yohimbe, country mallow, bitter orange
↑ Satiety	Guar gum, psyllium, prebiotic fiber
↑ Fat oxidation	L-carnitine, green tea, DHEA, pyruvate, raspberry ketone, hydroxycitric acid, conjugated linoleic acid
↓ Dietary fat absorption	Chitosan
↑ Carbohydrate metabolism	Chromium, ginseng, white kidney bean extract

Reference: Up to Date: "Overview of herbal medicine and dietary supplements"

141. (Content: III-A-1) A 52-year-old female has presented for a follow-up visit to the obesity clinic. A rotating resident is interviewing the patient and is asking questions such as "What weight-loss techniques have worked for you in the past?" and "So, swimming was an exercise you could do long-term?" After further discussions, the resident expresses hope stating, "It sounds like you are ready to pursue and maintain weight loss." He summarizes the visit, and the patient leaves the office. Which skill did this resident utilize?

    A. **OARS**
    B. FRAMES
    C. SMART goals
    D. RULE

(A) OARS is an acronym commonly used as a motivational interviewing skill that leads to higher levels of patient engagement and ownership, while decreasing resistance/barriers leading to improved overall outcomes. **OARS** stands for the following:

- **Open-ended questions:** Avoid yes/no answers. This helps explore the patient's reasoning for the change.
- **Affirmations:** Recognize strengths and how these can be applied to future goals to implement change.
- **Reflection:** Careful listening followed by facilitating evocation, developing discrepancy, resolving ambivalence, offering collaboration, and supporting self-efficacy.
- **Summarize:** Recap of discussion, setting realistic future goals, and plans to follow up.

Other acronyms used in motivational interviewing include:

RULE is an acronym focused on the motivation interview principles, and stands for **R**esist the righting reflex, **U**nderstand your patient's motivation, **L**isten to your patient, **E**mpower your patient.

FRAMES is a structural framework for conducting motivational interviewing and stands for **F**eedback about personal risk, **R**esponsibility of patient, **A**dvice to change, **M**enu of strategies, **E**mpathetic style, and **S**elf-efficacy.

Reference: Obesity Medicine Association: Obesity Algorithm (2023)

142. (Content: III-F-4) An obesity medicine specialist is working with an internal medicine resident and discusses ways to improve surgical outcomes in those undergoing metabolic and bariatric surgery, including decreased hospitalization and recovery times. Which of the following should routinely be performed to improve outcomes?

A. **Preoperative carbohydrate loading**
B. Intraoperative low-molecular-weight heparin
C. Nasogastric nutritional supplementation
D. Intraoperative high ventilator tidal volumes
E. Postoperative intravenous opioid administration

(A) Preoperative enhanced recovery after bariatric surgery (ERABS) clinical pathways should be implemented in all patients undergoing bariatric surgery to improve postoperative outcomes. This includes allowing the patient to have **oral nutrition with carbohydrates up to 2 hours preoperatively** to decrease insulin resistance, decrease protein catabolism, decrease hospital length of stay, and experience a faster return of bowel function.

A summary of additional recommendations are below:

ERABS Summary for Improved Surgical Outcomes	
Preoperative	Prehabilitation: Deep breathing exercises, CPAP, incentive spirometry, leg exercises, H_2 blocker/PPI, carbohydrate loading, pre-anesthesia medication
Intraoperative	Opioid-sparing multi-modal analgesia, pulmonary recruitment maneuvers, protective ventilation strategies, silent bleeding detection, avoiding excess fluid administration (goal-directed fluid management), anti-emetic prophylaxis, regional blocks
Postoperative	Thromboprophylaxis (early ambulation, etc.), early return of oral intake, multimodal analgesia regimen

CPAP: continuous positive airway pressure; **PPI:** Proton pump inhibitors

Reference: AACE/TOS/ASMBS/OMA/ASA 2019 Guidelines: CLINICAL PRACTICE GUIDELINES FOR THE PERIOPERATIVE NUTRITION, METABOLIC, AND NONSURGICAL SUPPORT OF PATIENTS UNDERGOING BARIATRIC PROCEDURES – 2019 UPDATE. Recommendation 34, 35, 36, 40. Table 8.

143. (Content: III-F-5a) A surgeon consults an obesity medicine specialist after a 39-year-old female develops a provoked lower extremity deep venous thrombosis (DVT) extending to the femoral artery on post-operative day three from a Roux-en-Y gastric bypass. Post-op complications included persistent nausea and vomiting, which have now subsided. The surgeon requests assistance with anticoagulation therapy. What is the most appropriate recommendation to provide?

A. Initiate rivaroxaban and check anti-Xa levels in 3 days
B. Bridge anticoagulation with fondaparinux and warfarin
C. Start an unfractionated heparin drip and place an IVC filter
D. Consult vascular surgery for mechanical thrombectomy
E. Discharge patient with weight-based enoxaparin

(E) This patient, who is otherwise ready for discharge, develops a DVT in the post-operative setting after a malabsorptive procedure. Due to studies suggesting increased bleeding risk with warfarin, a vitamin K antagonist (VKA), and decreased absorption of direct oral anticoagulants (DOACs), **weight-based enoxaparin or parenteral options are preferred**.

Bariatric surgery either reduces the stomach volume or bypasses the absorbable intestinal area, leading to unreliable anticoagulation bioavailability.

Recommendations for perioperative VTE treatment is as follows:

- Use parenteral anticoagulation in the early/subacute phase after bariatric surgery (<4 weeks).
- Transitioning to a DOAC or VKA can be considered after at least four weeks of parenteral therapy. Monitoring INR (VKA) closely to verify absorption and bioavailability is recommended.

The bioavailability of DOACs are least likely to be affected in a sleeve gastrectomy, but the guidance above should still be followed. A recent study suggested that DOACs are non-inferior to VTE prevention compared to parenteral options, but this has not been studied in VTE treatment.

Reference: Martin KA, Beyer-Westendorf J, Davidson BL, Huisman MV, Sandset PM, Moll S. Use of direct oral anticoagulants in patients with obesity for treatment and prevention of venous thromboembolism: Updated communication from the ISTH SSC Subcommittee on Control of Anticoagulation. J Thromb Haemost. 2021 Aug;19(8):1874-1882. doi: 10.1111/jth.15358. Epub 2021 Jul 14. PMID: 34259389.

144. (Content: III-E) A recently published study has shown weight-loss success and diabetes improvement with a subcutaneous injectable medication undergoing continued clinical testing. The medication contains GLP-1 and another hormone that is endogenously secreted by the pancreatic beta-islet cells. This dual medication has been shown to have more significant effects on weight than with a GLP-1 alone. The described medication combined with a GLP-1 is

A. gastric inhibitory peptide
B. oxyntomodulin
C. glucagon
D. **amylin**
E. peptide YY

(D) **Amylin** is co-secreted with insulin from the beta-islet cells in the pancreas and plays a role in glucose metabolism by regulating blood sugar levels by slowing down the rate at which glucose is released into the bloodstream after a meal. A long-acting amylin analogue, cagrilintide, in combination with semaglutide is currently being studied for use in patients with diabetes and excess weight. Results published 8/2023 displayed improvements in diabetes, as well as more weight loss with this combination (CagriSema®) than with semaglutide 2.4 mg alone. It is expected to begin phase III trials soon.

Combination medications with different mechanisms of action are continually being explored, as synergistic properties and sometimes improved tolerability are often seen. Tirzepatide (Zepbound®) is the most recent to be FDA-approved for obesity. A few other trials that are advancing and showing significant weight loss include:

- Bimagrumab: An activin type II receptor blockade monoclonal antibody used to treat inclusion body myositis has shown benefits in reducing fat mass, while increasing lean mass.
- Retatrutide: Triad of GLP-1, glucagon, and gastric inhibitory peptide

Reference: Frias, J. P., Deenadayalan, S., Erichsen, L., Knop, F. K., Lingvay, I., Macura, S., Mathieu, C., Pedersen, S. D., & Davies, M. (2023). Efficacy and safety of co-administered once-weekly cagrilintide 2·4 mg with once-weekly semaglutide 2·4 mg in type 2 diabetes: a multicentre, randomised, double-blind, active-controlled, phase 2 trial. The Lancet, 402(10403), 720-730. https://doi.org/10.1016/S0140-6736(23)01163-7
Reference: Effect of Bimagrumab vs Placebo on Body Fat Mass Among Adults With Type 2 Diabetes and Obesity: A Phase 2 Randomized Clinical Trial. JAMA Netw Open. 2021 Jan Heymsfield SB, Coleman LA, Miller R, Rooks DSdoi: 10.1001/jamanetworkopen.2020.33457.

145. (Content: III-D-9) A 44-year-old female with a history of ovarian cancer recently completed chemotherapy. During cancer treatment, she lost substantial weight and currently has a BMI of 20 kg/m². She states she does not have a significant appetite and must force herself to remember to drink protein shakes, although she has no nausea. Her diabetes mellitus type 2 initially had improved with the unintended weight loss and she quit all of her medications during treatment. Her most recent hemoglobin A1c is 7.4% (reference range: ≤5.7%). Which is the most appropriate medication to initiate at this time?

    A. Semaglutide
    B. Sitagliptin
    C. Tirzepatide
    D. Insulin
    E. Dapagliflozin

(B) This patient, who has lost a significant amount of weight in the setting of chemotherapy and has a persistently decreased appetite, would benefit from a weight-neutral diabetes medication. Of the options, only **sitagliptin** is weight-neutral. Besides insulin, which is obesogenic, the other options are weight-negative.

Sitagliptin (Januvia®)	
Dose	Take 100 mg daily orally. *Renal impairment:* Reduce to 50 mg daily if GFR ≥30 to <45 mL/minute, and 25 mg daily if GFR <30 mL/minute (including if on dialysis).
Mechanism	Dipeptidyl Peptidase 4 (DPP-4) inhibitors prevent the breakdown of incretins glucagon-like peptide 1 and gastric inhibitory peptide, increasing pancreatic insulin synthesis and decreasing glucagon.
Contraindications	Prior serious hypersensitivity reaction to sitagliptin
Side Effects	Gastrointestinal distress (diarrhea or nausea), nasopharyngitis (5%), and pancreatitis[1]

[1]A meta-analysis (TECOSS Study) revealed the incidence of pancreatitis with sitagliptin was similar to placebo

Reference: Sitagliptin package insert

146. (Content: III-G-7) A 26-year-old male is presenting for psychiatric evaluation as part of a multi-disciplinary team approach before bariatric surgery. He admits that he eats until he feels uncomfortably full, even eating large amounts when he doesn't feel hungry. This is something that has caused significant guilt and depression. He eats much more over a short period compared to his friends. He states it feels "like I lose control when food is around." Which of the following classes of medications is FDA-approved to treat his underlying condition?

A. **Central nervous system stimulant**
B. Anticonvulsant
C. Atypical antipsychotic
D. Selective serotonin neuromodulator
E. Glucagon-like peptide analog

(A) This patient presents with findings consistent with the diagnosis of binge eating disorder (BED), the most common eating disorder. **Lisdexamfetamine dimesylate, a central nervous system stimulant,** is the only FDA-approved medication to treat this condition.

Cognitive behavior therapy is recommended as first-line therapy to treat BED. While the only FDA-approved pharmacotherapy for BED is lisdexamfetamine dimesylate (brand name Vyvanse®), there are many medications commonly used off-label and have good efficacy, as listed below:

- Topiramate
- Phentermine/topiramate ER
- Selective serotonin reuptake inhibitors
- Bupropion
- GLP-1 receptor agonists

Importantly, BED should be treated before you address obesity with metabolic and bariatric surgery.

Note: Lisdexamfetamine dimesylate is only FDA-approved for BED in adults and attention-deficit/hyperactivity disorder in children and adults.

Reference: Up To Date "Binge eating disorder in adults: Overview of treatment"

147. (Content: III-A-1) A 14-year-old male presents for a sports physical for the upcoming football season. He has always been at the 95th-100th percentile of his weight compared to his peers. His weight today is 204 lbs (92.5 kg). He has unhealthy eating habits and consumes multiple sodas daily. The concern about his weight is discussed, including the health risks. He seems perplexed by this, as he feels he is at a good weight for football. After further discussion, he agrees to a focused follow-up visit regarding dietary modifications. Which of the following stages of change is this patient experiencing?

A. Pre-contemplation
B. Contemplation
C. Preparation
D. Action
E. Maintenance

(B) Although this patient presented in pre-contemplation related to obesity (unaware of the issue), after further discussion with the practitioner, he is not only aware that the problem exists, but he is interested in hearing about potential solutions, moving him into the **contemplation stage.**

Stages of change are a vital component of the transtheoretical model, a framework for understanding the dynamic process of behavior change.

Stages of Change		
Stage	**Definition**	**Intervention**
Pre-contemplation	Unaware of issue or unwilling to change	MI: Build awareness, discuss risks/benefits
Contemplation	Interested in changing within the next 6 months	MI: Assess/provide info, encourage/support
Preparation	Willing to change in the next 30 days (planning)	CBT: Set SMART[1] goals, and develop an action plan
Action	Initiation of change (approx. 6 months)	CBT: Reward and encourage small changes
Maintenance	Continued change for > 6 months	CBT: Positive reinforcement, lapse/relapse coaching
Relapse	Returning to undesirable behaviors	Normalization and assessing which stage they are in

MI: Motivational interviewing; **CBT:** Cognitive behavioral therapy
[1]**SMART:** Specific, Measurable, Achievable, Relevant, and Timing

Reference: Obesity Medicine Association: Obesity Algorithm (2023)

148. (Content: III-C-1) A 57-year-old business executive returns to his primary care physician for follow-up regarding his exercise prescription. Although the prescription clearly states 300 minutes of exercise weekly in the form of brisk walking, he does not have that amount of time to devote to exercise and did not fulfill his prescription. His current BMI is 31 kg/m². What would be the most appropriate modification to his exercise prescription?

    A. Change to water walking
    B. Increase exercise intensity
    C. Change to resistance training
    D. Focus on dietary components instead
    E. Confront him on his priorities

(B) Although this patient was prescribed an appropriate exercise prescription, it did not consider his time constraints. One alternative that would still meet the physical activity guidelines would be to **increase the intensity of exercise from moderate (3-6 METS) to vigorous (> 6 METS),** thereby decreasing exercise time from 150-300 minutes/week to only 75-150.

The recommended level of physical activity to maintain 'active status' consists of 150 - 300 mins of moderate-intensity activity per week or 75-150 mins of vigorous-intensity exercise weekly. Adults should also do weight training or resistance exercise ≥ 2 days weekly.

Important: You can estimate the number of calories burned per minute by the formula: kcal/min = METS x 3.5 x (weight in kg)/200.

Levels of Physical Activity		
Levels	Moderate Intensity	Vigorous Intensity
Inactive	None	None
Insufficient	< 150 mins/ week	<75 mins/week
Active	150-300 mins/week	75- 150 mins/week
Highly active	>300 mins/week	> 150 mins/week

Note: To meet the criteria for each activity level, it is the amount of moderate activity <u>or</u> vigorous activity

Note: Additional health benefits are gained by engaging in physical activity beyond 300 minutes of weekly moderate-intensity exercise.

Reference: Physical Activity Guidelines for Americans: 2nd Edition: https://health.gov/sites/default/files/2019-09/Physical_Activity_Guidelines_2nd_edition.pdf
Reference: CDC: Target Heart Rate and Estimated Maximum Heart Rate. https://www.cdc.gov/physicalactivity/basics/measuring/heartrate.htm

149. (Content: III-F-5c) A general surgeon is discussing one potential bariatric surgical option with a patient in which 80% of the greater curvature of the stomach is resected laparoscopically, allowing for 2-3 ounces (60-90 mL) of volume intake. Which of the following is true regarding the described procedure?

    A. Dumping syndrome is a common complaint
    B. It is the second most common bariatric procedure
    C. The procedure does not affect hunger hormones
    D. Patients are prone to experience vitamin B$_{12}$ deficiency
    E. This surgery is most effective for treating diabetes

(D) Sleeve gastrectomy is the most common bariatric procedure performed worldwide. Due to the removal of 80% of the stomach ❶, many gastric parietal cells (which make intrinsic factor and ghrelin) are removed, thus making patients **more prone to B$_{12}$ deficiency.** Importantly, the pylorus remains intact ❷ without concerns of gastric motility issues.

Note: Patients who underwent a Roux-en-Y gastric bypass had more significant weight loss, slightly higher diabetes remission with decreased relapse, and better long-term glycemic control compared to sleeve gastrectomy[1].

Image citation: Image created by Charu G. Copyright owned by Kevin Smith, DO
[1]**Reference:** McTigue KM, Wellman R, Nauman E, et al. Comparing the 5-Year Diabetes Outcomes of Sleeve Gastrectomy and Gastric Bypass: The National Patient-Centered Clinical Research Network (PCORNet) Bariatric Study. JAMA Surg. Published online March 04, 2020. doi:10.1001/jamasurg.2020.0087

150. (Content: III-F-3) A 39-year-old female with a history of type 2 diabetes and sleep apnea is presenting to her general surgeon after undergoing a Roux-en-Y gastric bypass six months ago. She has noted a weight loss of 47 lbs (21.3 kg) and is happy with the results. She regularly meets with her dietician. Her only complaint is that after she eats certain meals, she experiences facial flushing and lightheadedness. Given the most likely etiology of these symptoms, what other associated finding is she likely to encounter?

    A. Intermittent constipation
    B. Excessive belching
    C. Wheezing
    D. Reactive hypoglycemia
    E. Bacterial overgrowth

(D) Dumping syndrome is a complication most commonly seen after Roux-en-Y gastric bypass (typically within 18 months postoperatively), as the pyloric mechanism is bypassed. Thus, high carbohydrate loads can rapidly empty into the small bowel, leading to symptoms of abdominal pain, cramping, tachycardia, diarrhea, and facial flushing. Although rapid glucose absorption initially leads to hyperglycemia, the subsequent **exaggerated insulin release can cause symptomatic hypoglycemia.** It can be prevented by avoiding excess simple carbohydrates.

Other complications of Roux-en-Y include:

- **Internal hernia:** A small bowel obstruction (SBO) can be caused by a mesenteric defect. Prior to an SBO, intermittent symptoms can be seen in the absence of computed tomography abnormalities.
- **SIBO:** Small intestine bacterial overgrowth can occur due to a blind loop that allows excess bacteria to grow, causing abdominal pain, bloating, diarrhea, and D-lactic acidosis.
- **Gallstone complications:** Rapid weight loss, generally considered > 15 lbs/month, for any reason can lead to the mobilization of cholesterol from adipocytes. In the absence of sufficient bile salts to emulsify and solubilize cholesterol in the bile, there is an increased risk of cholesterol crystal precipitation, contributing to gallstone formation. Prophylactic cholecystectomy during Roux-en-Y surgery is not recommended, although 8% will require it at some point after surgery.

Reference: Up to Date: "Laparoscopic Roux-en-Y gastric bypass"

151. (Content: III-F-3) A rapid response is called on a 33-year-old female 12 hours after undergoing a Roux-en-Y gastric bypass. She complains of progressively worsening mid-epigastric pain with radiation to her left chest and mild dyspnea. Vital signs reveal a heart rate of 120 BPM, respirations 24/min, and oxygen saturation of 99% on room air. A portable chest x-ray shows a new left-sided pleural effusion. A complete blood count reveals a white blood cell count of 13.4×10^3/mcL (reference range: 4.8-10.8×10^3/mcL). What is the next best step in management?

A. Start empiric ceftriaxone and azithromycin
B. Order a stat CTA of the chest
C. Administer 1 mg/kg low molecular weight heparin
D. Contact the attending surgeon
E. Order an electrocardiogram

(D) This patient has concerning findings for an anastomotic leak causing a reactive pleural effusion and leukocytosis. Therefore, the best next step would be **to contact the surgeon for further evaluation** and possibly return to the operating room (if the leak is not contained).

Note: Tachycardia after bariatric surgery is concerning for an anastomotic leak or a pulmonary embolism. Tachycardia is the most reliable initial sign of an anastomotic leak, presenting in 72% of cases.

Anastomotic leaks usually occur within the first few days of surgery, becoming increasingly rare beyond two weeks. It more commonly occurs at the gastrojejunostomy anastomosis and presents as fever, worsening abdominal or chest pain, tachycardia, and leukocytosis.

Complications with Roux-en-Y Gastric Bypass[1]	
Short-Term (30 days)	**Long-Term**
-Death (1:500)	-Peptic ulcer (3-5%)
-Anastomotic leak (1%)	-Small bowel obstruction (1%)
-Infection (2%)	-Internal (1-2%) hernia
-DVT/PE (1-2%)	-Incisional (0.8%) hernia
-Dehydration (2%)	-Stenosis/stricture (6-17%)
-Mesenteric thrombosis (0.3%)	-Malnutrition (15-40%)

DVT: Deep venous thrombosis; **PE:** Pulmonary embolism
[1]Variability in percentages may be seen across studies

Reference: Up to Date: "Laparoscopic Roux-en-Y gastric bypass"

152. (Content: III-D-5) A 39-year-old female presents to the clinic due to nausea, vomiting, and increased fatigue over the past three weeks. Past medical history includes class II obesity, migraines, and polycystic ovarian syndrome (PCOS). She is on oral combined birth control and phentermine/topiramate ER. She has lost 19 lbs (8.6 kg) over the past four months but has recently started to regain some weight over the past month. Which of the following could have prevented the underlying cause of her symptoms?

A. **Adhering to the Risk Evaluation and Mitigation Strategy program**
B. Referral to a dietician to discuss a low-carbohydrate diet
C. Prophylactic ondansetron to take before anti-obesity medication
D. Cognitive behavioral therapy to prevent anxiety from phentermine
E. Adding metformin to treat the current PCOS symptoms

(A) This patient presents with pregnancy symptoms, including nausea, vomiting, fatigue, and weight gain. Topiramate can increase the metabolism of oral contraceptive birth control, leading to decreased effectiveness and an increased risk of pregnancy. The **FDA created the Risk Evaluation and Mitigation Strategy (REMS) program** to promote the safe use of medications that carry high safety risks, including those that may cause serious birth defects.

Phentermine/topiramate ER (Qsymia®) is included as part of the REMS program due to the increased risk of cleft lips and palate if pregnancy occurs while taking this medication (topiramate). The REMS program recommends specific forms of birth control and monitoring to reduce pregnancy risk.

- Pregnancy test before starting medication and monthly after that
- Effective birth control:
    - Used alone: Tubal ligation, intrauterine device, progestin implant, or male partner vasectomy
    - Barrier addition: Any other hormonal birth control, including progestin injection, OCP, and the transdermal patch, requires an additional barrier method to be considered adequate

Notably, the REMS training program is currently not required to prescribe Qsymia® (as of 3/2022), but these recommendations still stand.

Reference: Risk Evaluation and Mitigation Strategy (REMS) | Qsymia®: https://qsymiarems.com

153. (Content: III-G-3) A 39-year-old male presents to the obesity clinic for a 2-month follow-up appointment. He was started on semaglutide six months ago, and has maintained exercise of 200 minutes weekly. He states he feels well and plans to continue his current treatment regimen. Vital signs are within normal limits. Over the past year, he has lost 34 lbs (15.4 kg), accounting for an 8% total body weight loss. He is now at his lowest weight since being seen at the clinic. If he maintains his current regimen, what can you predict about his weight loss in the future?

 A. He will continue to lose weight but at a slower pace
 B. Eventually he will plateau and regain weight
 C. He will lose weight until he plateaus at his ideal body weight
 D. Eventually he will relapse to his previous weight

(B) Patients who lose weight are often disheartened when they eventually **plateau and experience some weight gain** if their treatment regimen isn't adjusted. This should be discussed early in treatment to prevent frustration, with pre-emptive plans to adapt and intensify their regimen accordingly.

Importantly, patients who lose weight will likely plateau and regain weight to some extent. This is related to decreased caloric utilization at a reduced weight (a 300 lb person burns more calories than a 200 lb person doing the same task) and hormonally-mediated etiologies (e.g., decreased leptin).

The National Weight Control registry looks at patients who have successfully maintained weight loss for extended periods. Common traits shared amongst participants include:

- Maintaining high levels of physical activity by exercising an average of 1 hour daily (90%)
- Eating breakfast every day (78%)
- Watching < 10 hours of TV weekly (62%)
- Weighing themselves at least once weekly (75%)

Reference: The National Weight Control Registry Brown Medical School/The Miriam Hospital. Weight Control & Diabetes Research Center

154. (Content: III-F-3) A 44-year-old male is being evaluated in the intensive care unit after a biliopancreatic diversion with duodenal switch. The surgery was particularly time-consuming due to anatomic variation and significant scar tissue from prior abdominal surgeries. The nurse is concerned as his urine has darkened, and the urine output has decreased to < 40 mL per hour despite adequate fluid hydration. His abdomen is soft, with no bowel sounds appreciated. Which of the following tests will most likely be abnormal?

A. **Urinalysis hemoglobin**
B. Renal parenchymal ultrasound
C. Renal vasculature duplex
D. Urine eosinophil count
E. Urine microscopy

(A) This patient, who is presenting with darkening urine and decreased urine output in the setting of a prolonged surgery, has findings concerning for rhabdomyolysis causing an acute kidney injury. Because urinalysis (dipstick) hemoglobin cannot differentiate between myoglobin, hemoglobin, and red blood cells, **the urinalysis hemoglobin is likely to be positive**. Urine microscopy would be normal because it is myoglobin and not red blood cells.

Rhabdomyolysis can occur in the setting of prolonged surgery, with severe obesity being a risk factor. Muscle breakdown can occur as the patient's body lies on the minimally padded operating room table.

Diagnosis is confirmed with serum creatine phosphokinase (CPK) levels. In order to affect kidney function, levels typically need to be greater than 10,000 IU/L, with decreased urine output being one of the initial findings. Myoglobin can turn the urine dark, as seen in this patient.

Treatment includes supportive care with significant intravenous fluids.

Reference: Up to Date: "Clinical manifestations and diagnosis of rhabdomyolysis"

155. (Content: III-D-5) A 62-year-old female is presenting to her primary care physician's office to discuss semaglutide (Wegovy®) for weight loss and diabetes. Her medical comorbidities include diabetes type II and hypertension. She is currently taking metformin, rosuvastatin, sitagliptin, and chlorthalidone. She drinks two alcoholic beverages nightly and quit tobacco products six years ago. Which of the following is the most appropriate action before starting semaglutide?

    A. Obtain baseline lipase levels
    B. Discontinue one of her current medications
    C. Inquire about a family history of MEN 1 syndrome
    D. Require alcohol cessation due to interactions
    E. Obtain triglyceride levels

(B) This patient is being evaluated for the appropriateness of semaglutide, which was approved in 2021 for chronic weight management. DDP-4 inhibitors **(i.e., sitagliptin) should be discontinued** when GLP-1 receptor agonists (GLP-1 RA) are initiated, as there is no additional benefit, and it is not cost-effective.

Summary: If starting a GLP-1 RA, discontinue DDP-4 inhibitors.

Semaglutide (Wegovy®)	
Dose	Inject 0.25 mg subcutaneously weekly for one month. Increase the weekly dose to 0.5 mg, 1.0 mg, 1.7mg, and 2.4 mg at one-month intervals.
Mechanism	Glucagon-like peptide 1 receptor agonists activate the hypothalamus, reducing food intake, increasing satiety, decreasing caloric intake, and improving glucose metabolism (incretin).
Contraindications	Prior hypersensitivity to GLP-1 agonists, history of or family history of medullary thyroid carcinoma (black box warning), patients with multiple endocrine neoplasia type 2, and pregnancy. *Relative contraindication: Severe gastroparesis and those at increased risk of pancreatitis[1]
Side Effects	Gastrointestinal distress (abdominal pain, nausea, vomiting, constipation), dizziness, and increased lipase (increased risk of pancreatitis)[1]

[1]Meta-analysis has shown no increased risk of pancreatitis or pancreatic cancer with GLP-1 use.

Reference: Semaglutide and sitagliptin package inserts.

156. (Content: III-F-3) A 42-year-old female presents with chronic diarrhea, abdominal pain, and bloating for six months. She underwent a duodenal switch approximately eight years ago and has had minimal follow-up due to losing insurance. She admits to now feeling weak and lightheaded with exertion. Laboratory examination reveals macrocytic anemia with increased folate levels. Which of the following tests is most appropriate at this time?

A. Urea breath test
B. Carbohydrate breath test
C. Stool osmolality
D. Stool cultures
E. Endoscopic evaluation

(B) Patients with small intestinal bacterial overgrowth (SIBO) often present with bloating, abdominal pain, watery diarrhea, B_{12} deficiency (due to competitive absorption with the host), and folate excess (over-synthesized by the excessive bacteria). Diagnosis of SIBO is made by a **carbohydrate breath test.**

Normal defense mechanisms to prevent excessive overgrowth of colonized bacteria in the small intestines aim to destroy excess bacteria through digestive or proteolytic enzymes, including gastric acid and bile salts. If these mechanisms are altered, bacterial overgrowth is more prone to occur. In the setting of a gastric bypass or a duodenal switch, a blind intestinal loop may allow for uncontested microbiota growth.

Overgrowth of bacteria may lead to enterocyte damage, leading to:
- **Decreased absorption of carbohydrates:** This causes fermentation of unabsorbed carbohydrates and subsequent release of carbon dioxide, methane, and hydrogen. This leads to abdominal distention, bloating, and flatulence.
- **Fat malabsorption:** In addition to fat malabsorption causing steatorrhea, fat-soluble vitamin deficiency may occur.
- **Neurologic findings:** The production of toxins such as D-lactic acidosis may cause neurologic changes such as confusion, ataxia, and seizures.

Reference: Up to Date: "Small intestinal bacterial overgrowth: Clinical manifestations and diagnosis"
Reference: Up to Date: "Small intestinal bacterial overgrowth: Etiology and pathogenesis"

157. (Content: III-D-9) A 37-year-old male with type 1 diabetes presents to his primary care practitioner to discuss anti-obesity medication. In particular, he would like to start semaglutide. His last HbA1c was 7.4% (reference range: <5.7%) and he is on 18 units of glargine nightly and dosing the aspart based on carbohydrate counting. His current BMI is 31 kg/m^2, which has increased from 27 kg/m^2 since last year. Which of the following is the most accurate statement regarding his inquiry?

A. Semaglutide is contraindicated in patients with type 1 diabetes
B. **I will discuss this with your endocrinologist**
C. You do not meet the criteria for anti-obesity medications
D. Tirzepatide would be a safer alternative
E. I would like to discuss intermittent fasting or a ketogenic diet today

(B) Certain glucagon-like peptide 1 receptor agonists (GLP-1 RA), such as semaglutide and liraglutide, are approved for both weight loss and diabetes mellitus type II. Although GLP-1 RA are not approved to treat diabetes type 1 (DMT1), they can be used to treat obesity in those with DMT1, although this needs to be done cautiously. Patients may benefit from continuous glucose monitoring due to the need for less insulin. A recent study showed improved weight, less insulin requirements, and no significant increase in hypoglycemia risks. Regardless, this should be orchestrated with his **endocrinologist.**

Note: Semaglutide 2.4 mg weekly has been shown to decrease the risk of major adverse cardiovascular events by 20% per the SELECT trials.

In diabetes, GLP-1 RA work via an incretin effect, increasing pancreatic insulin secretion in the setting of carbohydrate ingestion. However, the central effects of GLP-1 RA provide additional weight loss benefits via activation of the POMC/CART pathway leading to increased satiety and energy expenditure. These latter benefits occur independently of diabetes leading to weight loss. In a patient with T1DM in which the pancreas has undergone auto-immune destruction, patients with excess weight can still have weight improvements with this class of medications.

Importantly, ketogenic diets and intermittent fasting may increase the risk of diabetic ketoacidosis and are generally avoided in those with T1DM or insulin-dependent diabetes type 2, as well as those on SGLT-2 inhibitors.

Reference: Guyton J, Jeon M, Brooks A. Glucagon-like peptide 1 receptor agonists in type 1 diabetes mellitus. Am J Health Syst Pharm. 2019 Oct 15;76(21):1739-1748. doi: 10.1093/ajhp/zxz179. PMID: 31612934.

158. (Content: III-A-2) A 17-year-old female with a history of binge eating disorder meets with her primary care physician to discuss techniques to assist in weight loss. She has numerous allergies and is apprehensive about pharmacotherapy. In addition, she has a meniscus injury that limits her physical activity. The physician discusses meeting with a specialist to begin a structured approach that addresses maladaptive thoughts related to eating and physical activity through systematic tracking of daily habits, thoughts, and emotions. What intervention is being discussed?

A. **Cognitive behavioral therapy**
B. Mindfulness-based therapy
C. Motivational interviewing
D. Psychoanalytic therapy
E. Dialectical behavioral therapy

(A) The intervention being discussed is consistent with **cognitive behavioral therapy** (CBT) with monitoring which is a structured and evidence-based therapeutic approach commonly used in obesity medicine. This intervention addresses the cognitive and behavioral aspects of individuals' relationships with food, physical activity, and weight. It aims to identify and modify maladaptive thoughts and behaviors contributing to weight-related challenges.

The key component of CBT with self-monitoring is the systematic tracking of daily activities, including eating behaviors, exercise routines, and emotional responses, enabling individuals to recognize patterns, triggers, and connections between thoughts, emotions, and behaviors. By fostering self-awareness individuals make informed choices to develop healthier behaviors, promoting sustainable and long-term changes in lifestyle, contributing to successful weight management.

Self-monitoring is only one aspect of CBT, with others listed below:

Components of Cognitive Behavioral Therapy	
Self-monitoring	Enlisting social support
Stimulus control	Relapsing prevention training
Problem-solving	Stress management
Goal setting	Rewards
Contingency management	Ongoing contact

Reference: Dalle Grave R, Centis E, Marzocchi R, El Ghoch M, Marchesini G. Major factors for facilitating change in behavioral strategies to reduce obesity. Psychol Res Behav Manag. 2013;6:101-110. Published 2013 Oct 3. doi:10.2147/PRBM.S40460

159. (Content: III-G-1) A geriatrician notices that many of his patients have lost muscle mass with debility or reduced physical activity but continue to gain excess fat mass. Although some of these patients have certain conditions predisposing them to muscle wasting, including malignancy, fractures, and neurodegenerative conditions, the majority experience frailty independent of any underlying diseases. Which of the following would be an important part of the multidisciplinary treatment plan in regard to preventing sarcopenia and subsequent frailty?

A. Prescribe megestrol acetate
B. Encourage resistance training
C. Target protein intake of 0.8 g/kg/day
D. Consider testosterone supplements (males)
E. Encourage water aerobics

(B) Sarcopenia, or muscle loss, is a predisposing condition to eventual frailty, which is characterized by weight loss (often lean body mass), weakness, and reduced physical activity levels. Both of these conditions are related to aging and are treated with the following:

- Adequate protein intake (1-1.5 g/kg/day)
- **Resistance exercise training**
- Adequate vitamin and mineral supplementation

Resistance training is the most effective manner to induce muscle hypertrophy and improve strength and function in older adults. In addition to improving body composition, resistance training may increase resting energy expenditure. Water aerobics, or non-weight-bearing exercise, has less effect on muscle mass gain and nearly no impact on bone health.

Importantly, patients can increase their weight, without increasing muscle mass, by adding adipose tissue (i.e., sarcopenic obesity). Similarly, weight loss in the setting of malnutrition or debility often reduces lean body mass, including muscle mass, which is disproportionately more difficult to regain. Therefore, in those who are elderly, extra caution should be taken to target the loss of fat mass, not lean body mass.

Reference: Morley JE. Treatment of sarcopenia: the road to the future. J Cachexia Sarcopenia Muscle. 2018;9(7):1196-1199. doi:10.1002/jcsm.12386

160. (Content: III-F-5b) A 26-year-old female presents to the emergency department with a laceration above her right eye from a fall. She underwent a single anastomosis duodeno-ileal bypass with sleeve gastrectomy (SADI-S) six months prior and has not followed up with any providers since the surgery. She states she felt light-headed when getting up to go to the restroom and "passed-out" in the bathroom. Her skin turgor is normal. Which of the following questions will assist in preventing future similar hospital admissions?

A. Have you been drinking sufficient fluids?
B. Are you taking your daily vitamins?
C. Have you discontinued your sitagliptin post-operatively?
D. Did you have any alcohol before the fall?
E. **Are you still taking blood pressure medication?**

(E) This patient likely experienced a fall from orthostatic hypotension, given her light-headedness with standing. After bariatric and metabolic surgery with significant weight loss, frequent follow-up is necessary to adjust medications. Due to the patient's lack of follow-up, she may still be taking the same dose of blood pressure medications, causing hypotension. Therefore, **asking about blood pressure medication** would be most appropriate. Other reasons for an increased risk of falls post-operatively include:

- Dehydration (patient had normal skin turgor)
- Thiamine deficiency causing ataxia or neuropathy (would not be transient or cause pre-syncope as seen in this patient)
- Hypoglycemic agents, with insulin and sulfonylureas being the most common (sitagliptin is an incretin that does not cause hypoglycemia).
- Alcohol is more readily absorbed after bariatric surgery, leading to more rapid intoxication.

At each post-operative follow-up visit, recommendations include reviewing vital signs, making medication adjustments, monitoring dietary adherence (including avoiding NSAIDs and alcohol), ensuring they are taking recommended vitamins, evaluating for complications of weight loss (gallstones or gout), and ordering labs as appropriate. Body contouring surgery and bone density scans are addressed approximately two years postoperatively.

Reference: Kim TY, Kim S, Schafer AL. Medical Management of the Postoperative Bariatric Surgery Patient. [Updated 2020 Aug 24]. In: Feingold KR, Anawalt B, Boyce A, et al., editors. Endotext [Internet]. South Dartmouth (MA): MDText.com, Inc.; 2000-. Available from: https://www.ncbi.nlm.nih.gov/books/NBK481901/

161. (Content: III-G-7) A 26-year-old female was recently diagnosed with polycystic ovarian syndrome (PCOS) following a workup for abnormal menstrual cycles. She has noted worsening hirsutism which is bothersome. She is sexually active and uses barrier protection intermittently. A recent pregnancy test and oral glucose tolerance test were negative. She is interested in treatment for PCOS. Which treatment is most appropriate?

A. **Oral contraception**
B. Metformin
C. Spironolactone
D. Intrauterine device
E. Clomiphene

(A) This patient diagnosed with PCOS who is seeking treatment should be initiated on the first-line treatment which is a **combined estrogen-progestin oral contraceptive (OCP).** The benefits include:

- Endometrial protection in the setting of anovulation (progestin)
- Contraceptive protection for those not seeking pregnancy
- Improvement of hyperandrogenic manifestations

Although lifestyle changes to promote weight loss are first-line, many patients will find this to be insufficient in treating their symptoms. In addition, patients obtaining weight loss will increase fertility, which should be taken into consideration, especially in those not seeking to become pregnant.

Treatment for Polycystic Ovarian Syndrome	
Lifestyle changes	First-line non-pharmacologic treatment. The goal is weight reduction which improves insulin resistance, hyperandrogenism, and reproductive benefits.
Contraceptives	OCP's are first-line pharmacotherapy. See above.
Metformin	Restores ovulatory menses in up to 50% of patients, although it lacks the benefit of endometrial protection. Adjunctive with contraceptives in overweight/obesity.
Spironolactone	If oral contraceptive response is suboptimal, consider spironolactone. Given the concern of feminization of male fetuses, it should be avoided in pregnancy, and thus contraceptives are recommended while using.

Reference: Up to Date: "Treatment of polycystic ovary syndrome in adults"
Reference: Evaluation and Treatment of Hirsutism in Premenopausal Women: An Endocrine Society Clinical Practice Guideline. Martin KA, Anderson RR, Chang RJ, Ehrmann DA, Lobo RA, Murad MH, Pugeat MM, Rosenfield; J Clin Endocrinol Metab. 2018;103(4):1233.

162. (Content: III-H-1) An 8-year-old male is presenting to his family medicine provider as a new patient after moving from another state. Past medical history includes depression, migraines, and asthma. His growth chart has consistently been in the overweight category based on body mass index percentile for the past two years. He denies excess hunger but does admit to being sedentary. Which is the most appropriate intervention at this time?

    A. Recheck weight in three months
    B. Evaluate for weight-promoting medications
    C. Initiate pharmacotherapy
    D. Screen for genetic etiologies of weight gain
    E. Refer for metabolic and bariatric surgery

(B) Primary care providers (PCPs) should screen for obesity and evaluate for and concurrently treat comorbid conditions. In addition, **evaluating for weight-promoting medications** is a foundational therapy of obesity that primary care providers should be comfortable with.

Pediatric patients should be treated with foundational therapies and advanced therapies, simultaneously when indicated.

- **Foundational therapies:** Composed of intensive health behavior and lifestyle treatment and mitigation of weight-promoting medications. In addition, evaluating and addressing environmental, social determinants, and genetic contributions to obesity is vital.
- **Advanced therapies:** These are composed of pharmacologic treatments and procedures/surgeries specifically indicated for obesity management.

Advanced therapies should not be used in the absence of foundational therapies in order to maximize effectiveness. Every encounter with a patient is an opportunity to provide education and evaluate the effectiveness of treatment and modify it as needed, with PCPs having a unique longitudinal role.

New guidelines: There is no evidence to support watchful waiting. Treatment should be "as soon as possible, as intensive as available."

Reference: Obesity Medicine Association: Pediatric Obesity Algorithm (2023-2024)
Reference: Hampl, S. E., Hassink, S. G., Skinner, A. C., Armstrong, S. C., Barlow, S. E., Bolling, C. F., ... Okechukwu, K. (2023). Clinical Practice Guideline for the Evaluation and Treatment of Children and Adolescents With Obesity. Pediatrics, 151(2), e2022060640. https://doi.org/10.1542/peds.2022-060640.

163. (Content: III-H-5) A clinician is going through additional training in order to initiate treatment options for her patients with overweight and obesity. She wants to address the physical, emotional, and behavioral aspects in a personalized way by utilizing follow-up visits, motivational interviewing, and individualized treatment options. Based on this, she is most likely going to offer

    A. intensive health behavioral and lifestyle treatment
    B. pharmacotherapy initiation
    C. comprehensive obesity treatment
    D. metabolic and bariatric surgical assessments

(C) **Comprehensive obesity treatment** (COT) involves a multidisciplinary approach aimed at addressing the physical, emotional, and behavioral aspects of obesity management in children and adolescents. This approach typically includes personalized dietary and nutritional guidance to promote healthy eating habits, the incorporation of regular physical activity to enhance fitness levels, and the cultivation of positive behavioral changes. It incorporates the following:

- Provide intensive, longitudinal treatment in the medical home
- Evaluate/monitor for obesity-related comorbidities
- Identify/address social drivers of health
- Use nonstigmatizing approaches to treatment, honoring individual qualities of each child/family
- Utilize motivational interviewing to address pillars of obesity treatment
- Set collaborative goals not limited to BMI, but ones that reflect improvement in treating comorbidities, quality of life, and improving self-image
- Integrate weight management treatments such as intensive health behavior and lifestyle treatment (IHBLT) with pharmacotherapy and metabolic and bariatric surgery if indicated
- Tailor treatments to the individual based on the community context

COT is ideally delivered by primary care health providers (PCHP) in conjunction with pediatric obesity specialists, community partners, and surgical teams if indicated. Some PHCP may also be able to provide some level of IHBLT and pharmacotherapy options as well.

Reference: Hampl, S. E., Hassink, S. G., Skinner, A. C., Armstrong, S. C., Barlow, S. E., Bolling, C. F., ... Okechukwu, K. (2023). Clinical Practice Guideline for the Evaluation and Treatment of Children and Adolescents With Obesity. Pediatrics, 151(2), e2022060640. https://doi.org/10.1542/peds.2022-060640.

164. (Content: III-E) A patient presents to her nutritionist to discuss an article she read on the internet. It discussed making dietary changes by adding nutrients that have potentially favorable effects beyond basic nutrition. She most likely read an article on which of the following topics?

    A. Supplements
    B. Over-the-counter medications
    C. Functional foods
    D. Prescription medications
    E. Herbal remedies

(C) **Functional foods** are nutrients that have potentially favorable effects beyond basic nutrition, such as oatmeal having positive effects on cholesterol. Other examples are discussed below:

- **Dietary fiber:** This may increase the sense of fullness and marginally decrease percent body fat.
- **Prebiotics:** Indigestible oligosaccharides may stimulate intestinal growth, promoting a microbiome conducive to weight loss.
- **Probiotics:** Bacteria (i.e., lactobacilli) in yogurt, etc., may protect against unfavorable yeast/bacterial overgrowth.
- **Caffeine or green tea** (not extracts): May reduce appetite, increase fat oxidation, and provide antioxidants.

In contrast to functional foods, supplements are substances taken in addition to dietary intake (i.e., herbs, vitamins, etc.), are not approved by the FDA (considered food, not a drug), and cannot be marketed to treat, prevent, or cure disease.

Finally, the FDA considers over-the-counter medications safe and effective but do not require a prescription.

Reference: Obesity Medicine Association: Obesity Algorithm (2023)

165. (Content: III-D-2) A 28-year-old healthy male presents to his primary care physician with frustration about his inability to lose a significant amount of weight. For the past six months, he has changed to a vegan diet and exercises 30 minutes daily. Although he has lost 8 lbs (3.6 kg), he feels he should have lost more. His current BMI is 31 kg/m^2. After reviewing the side effects of medications, he chooses one that he feels will be a safe option. After two months, he returns with no significant weight loss. Which of the following anti-obesity medications was he most likely prescribed?

A. Phentermine/topiramate ER
B. Orlistat
C. Naltrexone/bupropion ER
D. Liraglutide

(B) This patient has healthy eating habits and is a vegan. Therefore **orlistat,** which works by inhibiting gastrointestinal fat reabsorption, would be ineffective in a patient who does not intake fatty foods. The other options are more likely to have some weight-loss effect. In contrast, those consuming significant amounts of fat would have considerable side effects.

Note: Orlistat should not be taken within four hours of levothyroxine due to impaired absorption.

The table below summarizes important pharmacologic information.

Orlistat[1] (Alli®: Over the counter, Xenical® Prescription)	
Dose	-60 mg TID within 1 hour of a fatty meal (Alli®) -120 mg TID within 1 hour of a fatty meal (Xenical®)
Mechanism	-Pancreatic lipase inhibitor (inhibits the absorption of dietary fats by 30%)
Contraindications	Hypersensitivity to orlistat or formulary component, pregnancy, chronic malabsorption syndrome, and cholestasis *Avoid if a history of oxalate nephropathy
Side Effects	Headaches, oily rectal leakage, gastrointestinal pain

[1] Orlistat is approved for those ≥ 12 years old and is available at lower doses over-the-counter.

Reference: Orlistat package insert

312

166. (Content: III-F-3) A 24-year-old male is discussing his concerns about blood clots after his planned sleeve gastrectomy surgery next month. His father died from a pulmonary embolism (PE) one week after undergoing a total hip arthroplasty. The patient has no history of deep venous thrombosis, and besides his father, he knows of no other family history. He denies smoking. Which of the following would be the most appropriate statement regarding venous thromboembolism (VTE) in this patient?

A. Delay VTE prophylaxis until at least 48 hours after surgery
B. Low-molecular-weight heparin 40 mg twice daily is considered standard
C. Failure to wean from ventilator support may indicate VTE
D. He should be on extended chemoprophylaxis upon discharge
E. Given his family history, an IVC filter should be discussed

(C) Prophylaxis against venous thromboembolism is recommended for all patients after bariatric procedures. Prevention may include sequential compression devices in addition to pharmacotherapy, such as unfractionated heparin (UFH) or low-molecular-weight heparin (LMWH). Respiratory distress or **failure to wean from ventilator support postoperatively should prompt a work-up for a pulmonary embolism.**

Important points regarding VTE are discussed below:

- Extended chemoprophylaxis after hospital discharge should be considered in high-risk patients (e.g., personal history of VTE, known hypercoagulable condition, or those who have limited ambulation).
- The use of deep venous thrombosis risk calculators are recommended to guide the length of prophylaxis.
- All patients should be encouraged to ambulate early after surgery.
- IVC filters are associated with increased mortality and VTE risk.

Reference: AACE/TOS/ASMBS/OMA/ASA 2019 Guidelines: CLINICAL PRACTICE GUIDELINES FOR THE PERIOPERATIVE NUTRITION, METABOLIC, AND NONSURGICAL SUPPORT OF PATIENTS UNDERGOING BARIATRIC PROCEDURES – 2019 UPDATE. Recommendation 45, 46

167. (Content: III-G-7) A psychiatrist is evaluating a patient in a psychiatric hospital for a recent episode of mania. The patient has a diagnosis of bipolar type I. The patient states that she has stopped her lithium due to excessive weight gain, leading to this current episode. The patient would like to discuss alternative options that would not cause this adverse effect. Which option should be discussed with the patient?

A. Valproate
B. Sertraline
C. Divalproex
D. Gabapentin
E. Lamotrigine

(E) **Lamotrigine** is indicated for focal and general seizures, mood stabilization in those with bipolar, and trigeminal neuralgia prophylaxis. Of the options, it is the only weight-neutral/negative medication used to treat her condition. Selective serotonin reuptake inhibitors such as sertraline should be avoided as monotherapy in the setting of bipolar disorder. All the other listed options are weight-positive.

Lamotrigine is considered either weight-neutral or weight-negative. This variability may be dependent on dosing. Regardless, it is not considered weight positive.

Mood-Stabilizer Medications		
Weight Positive	**Weight Neutral**	**Weight Negative**
-Carbamazepine	-Oxcarbazepine	-Lamotrigine
-Divalproex		
-Lithium		
-Valproate		
-Gabapentin		

Weight effects are generalizations and may be based solely on observational trials and vary depending on dosing, treatment duration, and medication indications. Weight variability may be seen.
Note: Children/adolescents have more significant weight gain than adults with obesogenic medications

168. (Content: III-B-1) A 48-year-old male presents for follow-up with the dietician. He has been doing research and wants to discuss some dietary plans. He has obesity class I without other obesity-related comorbidities and is currently taking no medications besides a daily multivitamin. He asks for an opinion related to frequently used dietary plans. Which of the following recommendations is most accurate?

A. Intermittent fasting allows for a time of restricted eating followed by unregulated calorie consumption
B. The Dietary Approach to Stopping Hypertension (DASH) diet plan provides significant weight loss with cardiovascular benefits
C. Low carbohydrate diets are more effective long-term for weight loss compared to low-fat dietary plans
D. **Eating low-density foods increases the sensation of fullness and thus promotes weight loss in comparison to high-density foods**

(D) **Intaking low-density, higher-weight foods, such as those high in fiber, including vegetables and fruits, promotes fullness, allowing patients to reduce their overall caloric intake and allowing them to obtain subsequent weight loss.** The volume discrepancy between high-density (often high-fat) foods compared to an equal caloric intake but with low-density foods can be staggering.

Newer dietary plans are always being developed and promoted, but often are 're-inventing the wheel' in terms of new names for similar macro-nutrient restrictions. Depending on their publicity, these fad diets may become very popular, while studies supporting their efficacy are lacking. Importantly, regardless of macronutrient content, a caloric deficit diet that is sustainable to the patient is most important for weight loss in the long term, while macronutrients may provide other benefits (cardiovascular risk reduction or diabetes control).

Several studies have focused on the efficacy of intermittent fasting. This dietary plan consists of fasting periods followed by eating periods. These periods can vary, ranging from 18 hours of fasting to 6 hours eating, to day-long periods of fasting/eating. Most importantly, the idea that completely unrestricted eating can occur during the eating period is not supported.

Reference: Stockman MC, Thomas D, Burke J, Apovian CM. Intermittent Fasting: Is the Wait Worth the Weight? Curr Obes Rep. 2018 Jun;7(2):172-185. doi: 10.1007/s13679-018-0308-9. PMID: 29700718; PMCID: PMC5959807.

169. (Content: III-F-1) A patient is meeting with a bariatric surgeon to discuss potential surgical options. Although she has done a lot of research, she still has not committed to one surgery. She asks about the estimated number of bariatric surgeries performed, including which are popular and which are becoming obsolete. Which of the following statements is accurate regarding bariatric surgery statistics over the past ten years?

    A. The number of bariatric surgeries has declined in the past five years
    B. Gastric banding has persistently made up 5% of bariatric surgeries
    C. Roux-en-Y gastric bypass remains the most common surgery
    D. Sleeve gastrectomy surgeries have nearly doubled in number
    E. Intragastric balloons have been available since 2012

(D) Although bariatric surgeries have increased in the past ten years, there have been some interesting findings. **Sleeve gastrectomy has become the most common bariatric surgery performed (doubling)**, while Roux-en-Y gastric bypass has been cut in half. Also, biliopancreatic diversion with duodenal switch has never exceeded 2%, and laparoscopic bands have nose-dived in popularity.

The table below shows the estimated rates of bariatric surgery per American Society for Metabolic and Bariatric Surgery (ASMBS).

Bariatric Surgery Estimates (2012-2021)					
Year	2012	2014	2016	2018	2021[1]
Total	173,000	193,000	216,000	252,000	262,000
SG	33%	51.7%	58.1%	61.4%	58.1%
RYGB	37.5%	26.8%	18.7%	17%	21.5%
Band	20.2%	9.5%	3.4%	1.1%	0.4%
BPD/DS	1.0%	0.4%	0.6%	0.8%	2.1%
Revision	6%	11.5%	14%	15.4%	11.8%
Balloons	--	--	2.6%	2.0%	1.5%
SADI	--	--	--	--	0.4%
OAGB	--	--	--	--	0.4%
ESG	--	--	--	--	0.8%

[1]Significant decrease in surgeries in 2020 related to covid pandemic so 2021 reported.
SG: Sleeve gastrectomy; **RYGB:** Roux-en-Y gastric bypass; **BPD/DS:** Biliopancreatic diversion with duodenal switch; **SADI:** Single anastomosis duodeno-ileal bypass; **OAGB:** One anastomosis gastric bypass; **ESG:** Endoscopic sleeve gastroplasty

Reference: https://asmbs.org/resources/estimate-of-bariatric-surgery-numbers (Accessed 12/18/2023)

170. (Content: III-D-2) A 29-year-old female with a past medical history of migraine headaches and pre-diabetes is presenting to a local obesity medicine clinic frustrated about her lack of weight loss. She exercises 300 minutes/week, restricts her calories to 1200 kcal/day, and takes no medications. She has been working with a weight-loss coach for the past six months. She is interested in weight-loss surgery. Her BMI is 29 kg/m^2, and her vital signs and physical exam are otherwise unremarkable. Which of the following would be the most appropriate action to take now?

    A. Further intensify lifestyle modifications
    B. Begin weight-loss pharmacotherapy
    C. Referral for bariatric surgery
    D. Referral for dietician
    E. Provide reassurance

(B) This patient who has failed comprehensive and intensive lifestyle modifications with a BMI $\geq$ 27 kg/m^2, meets the criteria **for pharmacologic therapy.** Further intensifying her exercise or diet is unlikely to yield the results she desires, and she does not meet bariatric surgery criteria at this time.

All patients trying to lose weight should undergo comprehensive lifestyle interventions[1] before or concurrently with adjunctive therapy. In other words, pharmacotherapy should not be used without lifestyle interventions. BMI indications for pharmacotherapy or metabolic and bariatric surgery are discussed below:

- **Pharmacotherapy:** In those with a BMI $\geq$ 30 kg/m^2 or $\geq$ 27 kg/m^2 with comorbidities.
- **Metabolic and bariatric surgery:** In those with a BMI $\geq$ 35 kg/m^2 or $\geq$ 30 kg/m^2 with metabolic disease (2022 ASBMS/IFSO update).

[1]High-intensity comprehensive lifestyle changes consist of behavioral strategies, moderately reduced-calorie diet, and increased physical activity.

Reference: 2022 American Society for Metabolic and Bariatric Surgery (ASMBS) and International Federation for the Surgery of Obesity and Metabolic Disorders (IFSO): Indications for Metabolic and Bariatric Surgery. Published: October 20, 2022 DOI: https://doi.org/10.1016/j.soard.2022.08.013
Reference: AACE/ACE Guidelines: AMERICAN ASSOCIATION OF CLINICAL ENDOCRINOLOGISTS AND AMERICAN COLLEGE OF ENDOCRINOLOGY COMPREHENSIVE CLINICAL PRACTICE GUIDELINES FOR MEDICAL CARE OF PATIENTS WITH OBESITY (2016):

171. (Content: III-A-1) You are discussing with a patient their interest in physical activity. After asking the patient to grade their motivation in readiness to initiate a workout plan, the patient states they are at a 6 out of 10. What is the most appropriate reply to their assessment?

    A. Why did you not select a number higher than that?
    B. Great- it seems like you are motivated
    C. Why did you not select a 3?
    D. What can I do to convince you to get it to a 10?
    E. It doesn't seem like you are quite ready yet

(C) 'Change talk' guides the patient to see the need for change. It can be helpful to have them rate their readiness or motivation to make a change. After rating, **asking why it is not a lower number** will allow them an opportunity to convince or reiterate to themselves their motivation. Asking why it is not a higher number, may create and reinforce barriers that may actually decrease their motivation. It is not up to you as a clinician during motivation interviewing to convince them to change, but rather help them channel their motivation and desire to change.

Importantly, once you have helped evoke the change, it is helpful to know their barriers to assist with planning, but doing so in a way that allows them to overcome the barriers, such as "if you have had difficulty getting transportation to the gym in the past, what are ways we can ensure reliable transportation this time?"

Motivational interviewing is all about allowing the patient to come up with solutions to barriers and assisting their internal motivation to move them forward. On board exams, look for the answer that promotes this internal change or revelation.

Reference: Obesity Medicine Association: Obesity Algorithm (2023)

172. (Content: III-F-5c) A patient is six months post biliopancreatic diversion with duodenal switch and has been happy with her weight loss thus far. However, she has noticed that her hair has grown slower and started to fall out. This is very concerning to her. She admits to taking one prenatal vitamin daily and following all food restrictions. Recent thyroid levels and complete metabolic panel were normal. Given these findings, what micronutrient deficiency is the most likely explanation for her symptoms?

A. Selenium
B. Zinc
C. Copper
D. Vitamin K
E. Vitamin A

(B) Micronutrient deficiencies occur most commonly in malabsorptive procedures. **Zinc deficiency** can cause alopecia, anosmia, brittle nails, and chronic diarrhea. In males, it can also cause hypogonadism or erectile dysfunction. Importantly, telogen effluvium is common with rapid weight loss and should be considered in the absence of micronutrient deficiencies.

The table below summarizes high-yield deficiencies and their symptoms.

Micronutrient Deficiencies after Malabsorptive Procedures	
Nutrient	**Symptoms of Deficiency**
Vitamin A	Night blindness, follicular hyperkeratosis, Bitot's spots
Vitamin D	Hypocalcemia, secondary hyperparathyroidism, osteomalacia
Vitamin E	Hemolytic anemia, neuromuscular, or ophthalmologic findings
Vitamin K	Excessive bleeding or bruising
Selenium	Fatigue, persistent diarrhea, cardiomyopathy, or metabolic bone disorder
Zinc	Chronic diarrhea, alopecia, pica, dysgeusia, anosmia, hypogonadism, or erectile dysfunction (males)
Copper	Anemia, neutropenia, myeloneuropathy, or impaired wound healing, subacute combined degeneration
Biotin[1]	Seborrheic dermatitis, alopecia, neurologic manifestations

[1]Can be caused by a large consumption of raw eggs.
Note: Nutritional anemias can occur from Vitamin B12, folate, protein, copper, pyridoxine or iron deficiency

Reference: AACE/TOS/ASMBS/OMA/ASA 2019 Guidelines: CLINICAL PRACTICE GUIDELINES FOR THE PERIOPERATIVE NUTRITION, METABOLIC, AND NONSURGICAL SUPPORT OF PATIENTS UNDERGOING BARIATRIC PROCEDURES – 2019 UPDATE. Recommendation 57, 62, 63-65

173. (Content: III-F-2) A family practice physician sees multiple patients during her dedicated bariatric clinic session. A number of them have approached her regarding evaluation for bariatric surgery. Which of the following patients would be the best current candidate for weight-loss surgery?

A. 29-year-old male (BMI 36 kg/m^2) who is a current tobacco user with a history of hypertension and obstructive sleep apnea
B. 34-year-old female (BMI 33 kg/m^2) with a history of cervical cancer status post hysterectomy with clean margins
C. 52-year-old female (BMI 55 kg/m^2) with a history of hypertension, refusing to undergo mammography and colonoscopy
D. **60-year-old male (BMI 34 kg/m^2) with a history of osteoarthritis, hyperlipidemia, diabetes type 2, and chronic kidney disease stage 2**

(D) Although it is still recommended to trial medication management initially in those with obesity class I, new metabolic and bariatric surgery criteria (2022) include patients with a **BMI ≥ 30 kg/m^2 with metabolic disease** (type 2 diabetes, prediabetes, metabolic syndrome, hypertension, metabolic associated fatty liver disease/metabolic associated steatohepatitis, obstructive sleep apnea, polycystic ovarian syndrome, etc). Bariatric surgery is also recommended in those with a BMI ≥ 35 kg/m^2 regardless of comorbidity.

Other valuable perioperative recommendations are discussed below:

- Age is not a contraindication, although perceived long-term benefits should be considered.
- Patients must quit nicotine products 6-8 weeks before surgery.
- Patients should be up to date on all preventative cancer screenings.
- Avoid pregnancy before surgery and 12-18 months postoperatively.
- Estrogen should be stopped for one cycle of oral contraceptives (premenopausal) or three weeks of hormone replacement therapy (postmenopausal) to reduce the risk of post-procedure thrombosis, per current recommendations.

Reference: 2022 American Society for Metabolic and Bariatric Surgery (ASMBS) and International Federation for the Surgery of Obesity and Metabolic Disorders (IFSO): Indications for Metabolic and Bariatric Surgery. Published: October 20, 2022 DOI:https://doi.org/10.1016/j.soard.2022.08.013
Reference: AACE/TOS/ASMBS/OMA/ASA 2019 Guidelines: CLINICAL PRACTICE GUIDELINES FOR THE PERIOPERATIVE NUTRITION, METABOLIC, AND NONSURGICAL SUPPORT OF PATIENTS UNDERGOING BARIATRIC PROCEDURES – 2019 UPDATE. Recommendation 2, 17, 18, 23, 33

174. (Content: III-B-4) A 48-year-old female with the disease of obesity presents for a follow-up appointment regarding increased liver enzymes. She recently completed a right upper quadrant ultrasound that revealed fatty liver infiltration. She denies any significant alcohol use. Which of the following diets should be recommended to her at this time?

A. **Mediterranean-style**
B. DASH diet
C. Low glycemic index
D. Low fat
E. High protein

(A) Although reducing total calories should be the main component of weight loss intervention, specific dietary compositions may be preferred in certain patient populations. **A Mediterranean-style diet is beneficial in hepatic steatosis independent of weight loss.**

Dietary Plan Benefits	
Diet	**Potential Benefits**
Mediterranean-style	- Decreases certain cancer risks - Improves hepatic steatosis - Reduces cardio-metabolic risk - Improves renal function
Low glycemic index	- Decreases adipocyte diameter - Decreases glycemic variability
DASH diet[1]	- Improves blood pressure - Not necessarily designed for weight loss
High protein[2]	- Improves cardio-metabolic risks - Decreases adipocyte diameter - Less relative loss of muscle mass - Prolongs benefit on waist circumference and percent of fat reduction
Low fat	- Beneficial effect on lipids - Improves renal function

[1]Every 1 lb decrease in weight corresponds to the reduction of systolic and diastolic BP by 1 mmHg
[2]Animal proteins (not plant) are associated with increased inflammation

Reference: AACE/ACE Guidelines: AMERICAN ASSOCIATION OF CLINICAL ENDOCRINOLOGISTS AND AMERICAN COLLEGE OF ENDOCRINOLOGY COMPREHENSIVE CLINICAL PRACTICE GUIDELINES FOR MEDICAL CARE OF PATIENTS WITH OBESITY (2016): Recommendation 47, 65-66.

175. (Content: III-B-3) A 42-year-old male presents to a dietary clinic for his initial consultation. He admits that his work schedule is hectic, requiring him to travel frequently, and thus, he feels his weight gain is most likely due to his fast-food intake. He is not interested in calorie counting. His weight loss goals include losing approximately 10% of his weight within the next year, based on mostly diet changes, as he already exercises every morning. His BMI is 37 kg/m^2, and he has no prior medical history. Given these preferences, which would be the best fit regarding weight-loss management?

    A. Mediterranean diet
    B. Paleo diet
    C. Bariatric surgery
    D. Meal replacement
    E. Pharmacotherapy

(D) This patient who wants significant weight loss, but has time constraints and travels frequently, would be a great candidate for **meal replacement therapy.** Pharmacotherapy would not be a great option, as it doesn't change his poor diet. Also, bariatric surgery requires significant commitment and diet monitoring, which he does not appear to be able to commit to at this time.

Meal replacements are a convenient option that can be taken on trips, as they require no cooking or significant preparation. Preferably, it provides a predictable amount of reduced calories (< 200 calories), high-protein (15-30 g) to suppress appetite, and low carbohydrates (< 10 g) to prevent weight gain. Also, they can be added to any diet and contain appropriate macro and micronutrients.

Note: Meal replacements are commonly used as a meal substitute twice daily for weight loss and once daily for weight maintenance. The Look Ahead trial showed increased use of meal replacement of approximately 2 per day were associated with higher levels of weight loss (11.9%) compared to a lower use of 2 per week (5.9%).

Reference: One-year Weight Losses in the Look AHEAD Study: Factors Associated With Success. Thomas A. Wadden Delia S. West Rebecca H. Neiberg Rena R. Wing Donna H. Ryan Karen C. Johnson John P. Foreyt James O. Hill Dace L. Trence Mara Z. Vitolins. Look AHEAD Research Group. First published: 06 September 2012 https://doi.org/10.1038/oby.2008.637

176. (Content: III-D-2) A 52-year-old male presents for follow-up at the transplant center. He was diagnosed with cirrhosis secondary to long-standing metabolic-associated fatty liver disease. He has minimal ascites and his last hospitalization was three months ago for hepatic encephalopathy. His BMI is currently 38 kg/m^2, and he must lose 25 lbs (11.3 kg) before being placed on the liver transplant list. Which of the following anti-obesity medications is contraindicated in this patient?

A. Setmelanotide
B. **Naltrexone/bupropion ER**
C. Semaglutide
D. Orlistat
E. Cellulose and citric acid hydrogel

(B) Levels of naltrexone can increase 5 to 10-fold in those with cirrhosis and, therefore, should be avoided. Of the FDA-approved anti-obesity medications, both phentermine/topiramate ER and **naltrexone/bupropion ER** should be reduced in moderate hepatic impairment (Child-Pugh class B) and avoided in severe impairment/cirrhosis (Child-Pugh class C).

Anti-obesity medications (AOM) can be a great tool to assist those pursuing weight loss to be placed on a transplant list. Knowing which AOM to avoid in the setting of liver or renal impairment is testable.

Anti-Obesity Medication Adjustments in Liver Disease			
Level of Impairment: Child-Pugh class: Child-Pugh score:	Mild Class A (5-6)	Moderate Class B (7-9)	Severe/Cirrhosis Class C (>9)
Phentermine/topiramate ER	--	Reduce[1]	AVOID
Naltrexone/bupropion ER	--	Reduce[2]	AVOID
Semaglutide and liraglutide	--	--	--
Tirzepatide	--	--	--
Orlistat	--	--	--
Cellulose and citric acid hydrogel	--	--	--

MELD: model for end-stage liver disease
[1]Max dose: Phentermine 7.5 mg/topiramate 46 mg once daily
[2]Max dose: Naltrexone 8 mg/bupropion 90 mg twice daily
-- indicates no dosage adjustment necessary

Reference: 2016 AACE/ACE Guidelines: Comprehensive Clinical Practice Guidelines for Medical Care of Patients with Obesity. American Association of Clinical Endocrinologists and American College of Endocrinology.

177. (Content: III-D-1) A patient returns to the office extremely concerned because she recently found out her grandfather had medullary thyroid carcinoma (MTC). She started on semaglutide at her prior appointment to help with weight loss. Which of the following is the best advice to provide the patient?

A. "It is fine to continue the medication, as MTC is not associated with this class of medications."

B. **"The associated risk of MTC has only been shown in animal studies, not in human trials."**

C. "We must monitor calcitonin levels and order a RET oncogene test while on this medication."

D. "Unfortunately, your risk of developing MTC has increased significantly, given your family history."

(B) Although there is a contraindication to any GLP-1 receptor agonist if there is a family history of medullary thyroid cancer or multiple endocrine neoplasia syndrome type 2 (MEN 2), the increased risk of MTC has only been shown in rat studies (duration and dose-dependent), and the risk to humans is unknown. This patient was likely started on a lower initial starting dose and has not been on the medication for long. The best course of action is to discontinue this medication immediately, but provide reassurance that this **medication has only shown an increased risk of MTC in animal studies**.

GLP-1 receptor agonists, including dual incretins such as tirzepatide, carry a black-box warning against use in those with a family history of MTC or MEN 2 syndromes. The recommendation from the manufacture is to:

- Discuss this risk with patients
- Discuss symptoms of thyroid cancer, including dysphagia, voice hoarseness, dyspnea, or a neck mass
- Routine monitoring (calcitonin, a tumor marker for MTC, or thyroid ultrasound) has no current evidence to support its use

GLP-1 receptor agonists have also been associated with pancreatitis, which through a metanalysis has been shown to unlikely be a true association, although this remains listed in the package insert.

Reference: Cao C, Yang S, Zhou Z. GLP-1 receptor agonists and pancreatic safety concerns in type 2 diabetic patients: data from cardiovascular outcome trials. Endocrine. 2020 Jun;68(3):518-525. doi: 10.1007/s12020-020-02223-6. Epub 2020 Feb 26. PMID: 32103407.
Reference: Semaglutide package insert.

178. (Content: III-F-1) A 37-year-old male presents to discuss bariatric surgical options. He had a friend who underwent a single anastomosis duodeno-ileostomy with sleeve gastrectomy (SADI-S) and has done well. He is wondering about the benefits and risks of this procedure compared to a Roux-en-Y gastric bypass (RYGB). What is the best advice to provide?

A. The SADI-S has more anastomotic sites than the RYGB
B. The SADI-S reduces ghrelin significantly more than RYGB
C. A RYGB requires more frequent monitoring of vitamin levels
D. The RYGB leads to increased remission rates of diabetes mellitus
E. The SADI-S is done through an open abdominal procedure

(B) The SADI-S, used interchangeably with the Stomach Intestinal Pylorus Sparing Surgery (SIPSS), is a malabsorptive procedure that includes performing a concurrent sleeve gastrectomy, **thus reducing ghrelin levels significantly**, as this orexigenic hormone is produced in the gastric fundus.

A SADI-S may be preferred over RYGB in certain patients, including those with a BMI > 50 kg/m². Malabsorptive procedures such as the SADI-S and duodenal switch provide 15% more weight loss than a RYGB, and higher resolution of diabetes. Compared to the duodenal switch, the SADI-S has fewer anastomotic sites, less malabsorption, and fewer overall complications, thus increasing its popularity. Like the duodenal switch, the SADI-S may be used as a revision of a prior surgery or staged procedure in high surgical risk patients.

Comparison of Malabsorptive Procedures			
Surgery	SADI-S	BPD/DS	RYGB
Malabsorptive	++	+++	+
Sleeve gastrectomy	Yes	Yes	No
Common channel	300 cm	75-150 cm	Variable
% intestine bypassed	50%	80%	Variable
Excess weight loss	75-95%	75-95%	65-80%
Anastomosis sites	1	2	2

SADI-S: Single Anastomosis Duodeno-ileostomy with Sleeve; **BPD/DS:** Biliopancreatic diversion with a duodenal switch; **RYGB:** Roux-en-Y gastric bypass

Reference: Sánchez-Pernaute A, Herrera MÁR, Ferré NP, Rodríguez CS, Marcuello C, Pañella C, Antoñanzas LL, Torres A, Pérez-Aguirre E. Long-Term Results of Single-Anastomosis Duodeno-ileal Bypass with Sleeve Gastrectomy (SADI-S). Obes Surg. 2022 Mar;32(3):682-689. doi: 10.1007/s11695-021-05879-9. Epub 2022 Jan 15. PMID: 35032311; PMCID: PMC8760573.

179. (Content: III-D-7) A recently graduated advanced practice nurse is prescribing pharmacologic therapy in the clinic. Although she has received her national provider identifier (NPI) number, she currently does not have her Drug Enforcement Agency (DEA) license. Because of this limitation, which of the following medications can she prescribe?

A. Diethylpropion
B. Phentermine/topiramate ER
C. Phendimetrazine
D. **Naltrexone/bupropion ER**

(D) Of the options above, only **naltrexone/bupropion ER** is not a controlled substance and does not require a DEA license for prescribing. The other FDA-approved long-term medications that are not controlled include liraglutide, tirzepatide, semaglutide, and orlistat.

Despite the lack of evidence in well-controlled animal and human studies that phentermine and other sympathetic amines cause physical dependence (as evidenced by abuse and withdrawals), their structural similarities to other classes of medication (i.e., amphetamines) cause certain medications to be classified as controlled substances.

This includes the following:

- FDA-approved long-term use (2)
  - Lorcaserin (removed from market 2/2020) (Class IV)
  - Phentermine/topiramate ER (Class IV)
- FDA-approved short-term use[1] (4)
  - Diethylpropion (Class IV)
  - Phentermine (Class IV)
  - Benzphetamine (Class III)
  - Phendimetrazine (Class III)

Note: Some obesity medications are approved for adults only. The exceptions are phentermine for those ≥ 16 years old, and semaglutide, phentermine/topiramate ER (Qsymia®), orlistat, and liraglutide (Saxenda®) for those ≥ 12 years old. Criteria includes class I obesity with weight comorbidities or class 2 obesity or greater.

[1]Obesity is a chronic disease, and so even though FDA-approved for short-term use, evidence-based medicine supports long-term use. Verify with your state licensure board if long-term use is supported in your state.

Reference: Up to Date: "Overweight and obesity in adults: Health consequences"

180. (Content: III-A-1) A 29-year-old female affected by obesity is presenting for help with losing and maintaining weight. During discussions, the importance of losing 5-10% of her baseline weight related to her health is reiterated, specifically related to improving current medical conditions and preventing future issues. This discussion falls into which of the following categories of the "5 A's of obesity management"?

    A. Ask
    B. Assess
    C. Advise
    D. Agree
    E. Arrange/assist

(C) This patient is being **advised on the benefits** of modest weight loss related to her health. Advisement can incorporate the health risks, benefits, and the need for treatments, as well as potential long-term options.

The 5 A's of motivational interviewing is a memory aid and technique not limited to obesity medicine but is commonly implemented in obesity practice. The five components are summarized in the table below.

The 5 A's Of Obesity Management	
Ask	-Ask for permission to discuss body weight -Explore readiness to change
Assess	-Assess BMI and waist circumference -Explore obstacles and complications of excess weight
Advise	-Advise about the health risks of obesity -Discuss the benefits of weight loss (even modest amounts) -Present the importance of a long-term strategy -Provide potential treatment options
Agree	-Agree on realistic weight-loss goals and expectations -Document specific details of the agreed-upon treatment plan
Arrange/ Assist	-Assist in identifying barriers to weight loss -Provide resources, including consultations with providers -Arrange regular follow-up

Reference: Obesity Medicine Association: Obesity Algorithm (2023)

181. (Content: III-B-4) A 67-year-old male presents for lifestyle modification education after recently having a cardiac stent placed for unstable angina. In particular, he is wondering about "good fats" that his wife has talked about. Which of the following is the most accurate statement?

    A. Saturated fats are unlikely to be absorbed and thus preferred
    B. Trans fats should only be consumed in moderation
    C. Increasing polyunsaturated fats reduces cardiac risk factors
    D. Coconut oil is preferred instead of vegetable oil
    E. Tilapia is a cheaper alternative to salmon with similar benefits

(C) Polyunsaturated fatty acids include omega-3, which has anti-inflammatory effects, thus having cardiovascular benefits and may help prevent/treat atherosclerosis. In contrast, saturated fats should be limited and trans fats have been removed from the market due to adverse cardiac effects. A good rule of thumb is that fats that are solid at room temperature (coconut oil, butter, etc.) contain higher amounts of saturated fats and should be avoided. This contrasts with polyunsaturated fats such as vegetable and olive oil.

Replacing saturated fats with polyunsaturated fats has been shown by the American College of Cardiology to reduce the risk of cardiovascular disease by 30%, having a quantitative effect similar to statin use.

Alpha-linoleic acid is a form of omega-3 polyunsaturated fatty acid that reduces the risk of fatal coronary heart disease and is recommended by the American Heart Association (AHA). This form can be found in fattier fish such as cod, sardines, tuna, salmon, herring, and lake trout. Other sources include avocados, vegetable oil, flax seed oil, walnuts, soy, spinach, and kale.

Importantly, alpha-linoleic acid is involved with neurologic development in children and to some degree is converted to eicosatetraenoic acid (EPA) and docosahexaenoic acid (DHA). It is preferred to obtain these nutrients through food rather than supplementation if possible.

Reference: Dietary Fats and Cardiovascular Disease: A Presidential Advisory from the American Heart Association. Circulation 2017;Jun 15:
Reference: Up to Date: "Dietary fat"

182. (Content: III-F-5 and III-D-3) A 52-year-old female presents to the emergency room by ambulance after a witnessed seizure. The patient is not on any current medications. She underwent a successful Roux-en-Y gastric bypass nearly 2 years ago, with hypertension currently in remission. Her husband states she has complained of lightheadedness and fatigue 1-2 hours after meals for the past few months. However, this is the first time she has had a seizure. Point of care glucose on arrival is 23 mg/dL (reference range: 74-106 mg/dL). Which of the following daily medications may have prevented her seizure?

    A. Semaglutide
    B. Metformin
    C. Metoprolol
    D. Acarbose
    E. sitagliptin

(D) This patient presents with post-prandial hypoglycemia symptoms more than one year after Roux-en-Y gastric bypass, consistent with postprandial hyperinsulinemic hypoglycemia (PHH). Besides **acarbose,** all of the options above may worsen symptoms (or, as with metoprolol, may initially mask symptoms).

Initial treatment of PHH should focus on dietary modifications with a low carbohydrate, mixed diet. If these conservative measures are ineffective, pharmacotherapy can be considered:

- Acarbose: This complex disaccharide delays the digestion of carbohydrates, resulting in delayed/diminished insulin release.
- Octreotide: This somatostatin analog is a potent insulin inhibitor
- Calcium channel blockers: This class of medications acts directly on the β-cells to inhibit glucose-dependent insulin release.
- Diazoxide: Suppresses insulin secretion via β-cell channels.

In severe cases where the above therapies are ineffective, reversal of the RYGB or conversion to a gastric sleeve should be considered.

Reference: Malik S, Mitchell JE, Steffen K, Engel S, Wiisanen R, Garcia L, Malik SA. Recognition and management of hyperinsulinemic hypoglycemia after bariatric surgery. Obes Res Clin Pract. 2016 Jan-Feb;10(1):1-14. doi: 10.1016/j.orcp.2015.07.003. Epub 2015 Oct 27. PMID: 26522879; PMCID: PMC5688875.

183. (Content: III-F-1) Vagal nerve blockade via laparoscopically implanted electrodes (vBloc®) is being discussed with a patient. Which of the following is accurate regarding this device?

A. It is approved for adolescents
B. It produces 8-10% weight loss
C. It increases ghrelin production
D. It is contraindicated in those on dialysis
E. It is approved for short-term use only

(B) The vBloc® device shows **8% total body weight loss** at 24 months.

- **Indications:** Age ≥ 18 years old with a BMI 40-45 kg/m^2 or 35-39.9 kg/m^2 with ≥ 1 obesity-related co-morbidity, and have failed one supervised weight management program within the past 5 years
- **Contraindications:** Cirrhosis, portal hypertension, esophageal varices, or uncorrected significant hiatal hernia. Not MRI compatible. Anyone with an implanted electrical device (i.e., pacemaker, defibrillator, etc.)
- **Side effects:** Pain at the neuroregulatory site of implantation (28%) and heartburn/dyspepsia (25%) are the most common. Although nausea was reported in 6% of cases, it was mild and did not lead to significant vomiting. Other side effects include belching (9%), dysphagia (8%), abdominal cramps (6%), and constipation (6%).

The vBloc® is a vagal neuromodulating therapy with two laparoscopically placed electrodes attached to the anterior ❶ and posterior ❷ branches of the vagus nerve to interrupt daytime hunger signaling. The leads attach to a subcutaneous, rechargeable battery pack ❸ placed outside the ribcage.

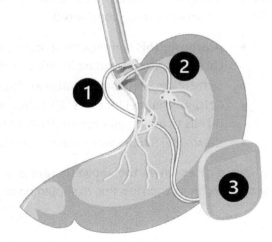

Image citation: Image created by Charu G. Copyright owned by Kevin Smith, DO
Reference: Apovian CM, Shah SN, Wolfe BM, Ikramuddin S, Miller CJ, Tweden KS, Billington CJ, Shikora SA. Two-Year Outcomes of Vagal Nerve Blocking (vBloc) for the Treatment of Obesity in the ReCharge Trial. Obes Surg. 2017 Jan;27(1):169-176. doi: 10.1007/s11695-016-2325-7. PMID: 27506803; PMCID: PMC5187356.

184. (Content: III-C-1) A 50-year-old male has initiated an aerobic training program in preparation for running a half marathon the following year. He would like help determining his target heart rate for high-intensity exercise. He has no prior cardiac history and is asymptomatic. Which recommended heart rate is most appropriate to target?

    A. 115-135 beats per minute
    B. 135-155 beats per minute
    C. 155-175 beats per minute
    D. 175-195 beats per minute

(B) The predicted maximum heart rate is determined by the formula: 220 - age. For this patient who is 50 years old, the maximum heart rate is 220-50 = 170. High-intensity (vigorous) physical activity is determined to be between 77-93% of maximum heart rate:

- 77% is 0.77 x 170 = 131
- 93% is 0.93 x 170 = 158

Thus, for high-intensity (i.e., vigorous) exercise, he should target physical activity that increases his heart rate to a target rate between **131-158 beats per minute.** You will be expected to calculate this on test day. To summarize:

- **Moderate intensity (3-6 METS):** Conversation takes effort. You can talk but not sing. Activity is starting to get challenging. Example: Brisk walking, bicycling < 10 MPH, and recreational swimming.
  - The heart rate should be between 64-76% of the maximum predicted heart rate.
- **High-intensity or vigorous intensity (≥ 6 METS):** Conversation is difficult. Activity is challenging and hard work. Examples: Running, swimming, and playing basketball.
  - The heart rate should be between 77-93% of the maximum predicted heart rate.

Note: In those taking medications affecting heart rate or pulse (e.g., beta-blockers, etc.), the preferred method to assess intensity is the patient's perceived level of exertion with the Borg scale, where 6 is no exertion, 12-14 is moderate intensity, and 20 is maximal exertion.

Reference: CDC: Target Heart Rate and Estimated Maximum Heart Rate.
https://www.cdc.gov/physicalactivity/basics/measuring/heartrate.htm

185. (Content: III-F-5c) A 36-year-old male presents to urgent care with complaints of fatigue, weakness, and numbness in his lower extremities. He underwent a Roux-en-Y gastric bypass 9 years ago but has not had follow-up for the past 5 years. He is taking cyanocobalamin sublingual tabs and calcium. He has a positive Romberg test with diminished vibratory sensations and 4/5 muscle strength in all extremities. Lab work is shown below:

Test	Patient's Value	Reference Range
Hemoglobin	9.4 g/dL	13.5–17.5 g/dL
White blood cells	3100/mm^3	4500–11,000/mm^3
Platelet	200,000/mm^3	150,000–400,000/mm^3
MCV	116 µm^3	80–100 µm^3
LDH	175 U/L	100-280 U/L

Which of the following is the most likely deficiency leading to his findings?

A. Iron
B. **Copper**
C. Folate
D. Vitamin E
E. Pyridoxine

(B) This patient is presenting with subacute combined degeneration, myeloneuropathy, macrocytic anemia, and neutropenia. Of the options, copper deficiency presents with these findings and can mimic severe B$_{12}$ deficiency. **Copper deficiency** presents with the triad of neutropenia, anemia (MCV may vary, but most commonly macrocytic), and myeloneuropathy.

Other nutritional deficiencies that can cause anemia include:

- Pyridoxine (B$_6$): This vitamin deficiency can cause neuropathy, but if it causes anemia, it would be a microcytic anemia.
- Iron: This would cause microcytic anemia without myeloneuropathy
- Vitamin E: Severe deficiency (rare) could cause hemolytic anemia, however, in this patient, the LDH was normal, not elevated.
- Folate: This can cause macrocytic anemia without neurologic findings.
- B$_{12}$: Severe B$_{12}$ deficiency can mimic copper deficiency.

Reference: Wazir SM, Ghobrial I. Copper deficiency, a new triad: anemia, leucopenia, and myeloneuropathy. J Community Hosp Intern Med Perspect. 2017 Sep 19;7(4):265-268. doi: 10.1080/20009666.2017.1351289. PMID: 29046759; PMCID: PMC5637704.
Reference: Up to Date: "Bariatric surgery: Postoperative nutritional management"

186. (Content: III-H-4) An 8-year-old male with excess weight presents to his pediatrician, accompanied by his mother. The patient appears happy, has no other medical conditions, and takes no medications. The mother states the school year has been busy with music lessons and chess tournaments, which he prefers over sports. She says he is physically inactive but has eliminated soda from his diet. Given the mother's work schedule, they often pick up food from restaurants in the evening. Which of the following would be the most effective method to promote weight loss in this patient?

    A. Initiate pharmacotherapy
    B. Wake patient up early to exercise
    C. Restrict dinner portion sizes
    D. Sign the patient up for soccer
    E. Involve the family in weight loss

(E) Pediatric patients tend to have more favorable outcomes **when the family is integrated into the obesity treatment plan**. This is one of the most important steps in treating childhood obesity so the child does not feel singled out.

There are many opportunities for family involvement, including:

- Family recognition of the problem (first step!)
- Increasing the number of family meals together at home
- Limiting eating out
- Incorporating cultural differences and adapting recommendations based on patient and family values, religion, etc.
- Incorporating lifestyle changes within the family unit, including exercise, nutritional changes, and behavioral modification
- Remove televisions and media from the bedrooms and kitchen

Incorporating these changes within a family, thus making it a "new normal" for the family, is much more effective than bestowing these changes on one family member, especially when siblings are present.

Reference: Hampl, S. E., Hassink, S. G., Skinner, A. C., Armstrong, S. C., Barlow, S. E., Bolling, C. F., ... Okechukwu, K. (2023). Clinical Practice Guideline for the Evaluation and Treatment of Children and Adolescents With Obesity. Pediatrics, 151(2), e2022060640. https://doi.org/10.1542/peds.2022-060640.

187. (Content: III-D-1) A 31-year-old female with a body mass index of 36 kg/m^2 presents to her primary care physician after discussing weight loss medications with her friend. She is interested in starting a medication but is unsure of the best option. She denies any tobacco or alcohol abuse. Past medical history reveals a history of recurrent nephrolithiasis and epilepsy. Physical exam reveals truncal obesity with a small reducible umbilical hernia with minimal abdominal striae. Of the options below, which would be her best long-term option?

A. Phentermine/topiramate ER
B. Phentermine monotherapy
C. **Liraglutide**
D. Naltrexone/bupropion ER
E. Orlistat

(C) In patients with or at risk of oxalate nephropathy or nephrolithiasis, orlistat and topiramate, respectively, should be avoided. Bupropion is contraindicated in epilepsy, seizure disorders, or those at risk for seizures (i.e., alcohol use disorder or eating disorders). Although often used long-term with close monitoring, phentermine is less effective than **liraglutide,** which has an FDA approval for long-term weight management and diabetes.

Note: Although GLP-1 receptor agonists (GLP-1 RA) are safe in patients with nephrolithiasis or oxalate nephropathy, gastrointestinal distress is a relatively common side-effect. Therefore, GLP-1 RA should be discontinued if nausea, vomiting, and diarrhea cause hypovolemia or volume contraction, as hypovolemia can increase the risk of nephrolithiasis.

Note: Although phentermine/topiramate ER can be used in those with a history of seizures, all patients should be slowly tapered off this medication if discontinued, especially at higher doses, to decrease the risk of seizures.

Reference: AACE/ACE Guidelines: AMERICAN ASSOCIATION OF CLINICAL ENDOCRINOLOGISTS AND AMERICAN COLLEGE OF ENDOCRINOLOGY COMPREHENSIVE CLINICAL PRACTICE GUIDELINES FOR MEDICAL CARE OF PATIENTS WITH OBESITY (2016). Recommendation 86 and 87.

188. (Content: III-A-1) A 59-year-old female presents to an obesity medicine specialist. She has tried numerous dietary plans and becomes frustrated with the associated restrictions and rules. Since the beginning of the COVID-19 pandemic, she has worked from home, exercises 200-300 minutes weekly, and does resistance training twice weekly. She is interested in anti-obesity medications but also wants to continue working on lifestyle modifications. Which of the following recommendations would be most useful for her?

   A. Recommend increasing her weekly physical activity
   B. Provide resources on mindful eating
   C. Discuss phone-based applications to count calories and macronutrients
   D. Initiate medications and put lifestyle changes on hold
   E. Begin sertraline to help with depression and improve motivation

(B) This motivated patient exercises regularly but struggles with the constraints of dietary plans. Therefore, in addition to continuing her physical activity and discussing anti-obesity medications, a discussion on **mindful eating** may be a great individualized option for her.

Mindful eating is not a dietary plan but an approach to eating that can be applied to any dietary plan or even by itself. The tenants of this approach are being mentally present when eating and focusing on the eating experience including the thoughts and feelings about what you are eating without concern of judgment. Although this approach sounds like it could encourage unhealthy eating, it often leads to the opposite. Some key points are below:

- It promotes knowing your personal hunger signals. In other words, do not eat unless you feel hungry (i.e., homeostatic hunger).
- Paying attention to the food is important, selecting foods they enjoy, but also foods that are consistent with their desired health benefits.
- They are encouraged to examine the food, smell it, focus on the taste, etc. Instead of eating a large bite (or a handful of items), they eat small bites or individual items and enjoy each one.
- It helps avoid stringent rules or calorie counting, which many patients with a history of eating disorders or obsessive-compulsive disorder may struggle with.

Reference: Nelson JB. Mindful Eating: The Art of Presence While You Eat. Diabetes Spectr. 2017 Aug;30(3):171-174. doi: 10.2337/ds17-0015. PMID: 28848310; PMCID: PMC5556586.

189. (Content: III-F-3) A 37-year-old female is following up with her bariatric surgeon after undergoing a successful Roux-en-Y gastric bypass procedure three weeks prior. Overall she is doing well, however, she points to her mid-epigastric region as having increased constant pain, which is not relieved with famotidine. Also, yesterday she noticed nausea, and today she has had two bouts of emesis. She does admit to starting smoking again, but only 4-5 cigarettes daily. Her last bowel movement was three days ago. Which of the following is the most likely diagnosis?

A. Internal hernia
B. Gastric outlet obstruction
C. Mesenteric ischemia
D. Anastomotic stricture
E. **Marginal ulcer**

(E) **Anastomotic or marginal ulcers** are relatively common in gastric bypass, occurring in up to 16% of patients. Patients will classically complain of localized abdominal pain, without alarming abdominal exam findings. Patients often experience nausea and vomiting. Smoking, as seen in this patient, is a strong risk factor.

The table below compares two common postoperative complications:

Anastomotic Ulcer versus Stricture		
Complication	Ulcer	Stricture/Stenosis
Prevalence[1]	Approximately 0.6-16%	Approximately 6-17%
Symptoms	Localized abdominal pain, nausea, vomiting	Dysphagia, solid food intolerance, weight loss
Complications	Perforation, bleeding	Malnutrition, dehydration
Risk factors	NSAIDs, smoking, steroids, *H. pylori*, ischemia	Surgical technique, ischemia, inflammation
Diagnosis	EGD	Upper GI barium, EGD
Treatment	PPI, sucralfate, risk factor reduction (i.e., smoking)	Balloon dilation. Rarely surgical intervention

NSAIDs: non-steroidal anti-inflammatory drugs; **EGD:** esophagogastroduodenoscopy; **GI:** gastrointestinal; **PPI:** Proton pump inhibitor
[1]Variability in percentages may be seen across studies

Reference: Up to Date: "Laparoscopic Roux-en-Y gastric bypass"

190. (Content: III-C-1) A 31-year-old previously healthy male presents to his family care physician for evaluation of his chronic condition of obesity. He started seeing a dietician and is very happy with his progress regarding dietary changes and calorie counting. He has not begun to exercise but is interested. A history and physical is performed, with no limitations to exercise perceived. An exercise prescription is being written. Which of the following is directly part of this prescription?

A. Patient safety
B. Barriers to exercise
C. Motivational interviewing
D. Enjoyment of activity
E. Physical limitations

(D) An exercise prescription should include the following, which can be remembered by the acronym FITTE:

- **Frequency:** The number of days or intervals (e.g., weekdays or every other day) necessary to achieve the total weekly physical activity time goals (listed below).
- **Intensity:** The patient's physical activity and safety should be considered, with moderate to vigorous-intensity exercise preferred.
- **Time:** 150-300 minutes per week of moderate-intensity (or 75-150 minutes of vigorous-intensity) exercise is recommended.
- **Type:** This typically focuses on aerobic/cardiorespiratory and strength/weight training. However, flexibility, functional and balance (safety), speed (competition), and core strengthening can be considered as well, based on goals.
- **Enjoyment:** An individualized exercise regimen based on patient preference (indoor versus outdoor, group classes versus trainer, water versus running) promotes consistent follow-through.

Example: Perform 30 minutes of brisk walking (moderate-intensity) around the park every weekday after dinner. In addition, perform resistance training twice weekly for 20-minute periods.

Reference: Physical Activity Guidelines for Americans: 2nd Edition: https://health.gov/sites/default/files/2019-09/Physical_Activity_Guidelines_2nd_edition.pdf

191. (Content: III-D-1) A 49-year-old female presents to her family practitioner with a complaint of weight gain. She was on fenfluramine in combination with phentermine in the distant past and would like to start on something similar, as it was very effective. She is started on phentermine 15 mg in the morning. What is the most common side effect this patient will likely experience?

A. **Xerostomia**
B. Nausea and vomiting
C. Diarrhea
D. Dysgeusia
E. Headaches

(A) **Xerostomia** (dry mouth) is one of the most common side effects of sympathetic amines like phentermine. Patients are encouraged to increase their water intake to prevent issues such as dental carries. In contrast, topiramate can cause dysgeusia (abnormal taste).

Fenfluramine in combination with phentermine, termed "fen-phen," was taken off the market in 1997 due to an increased risk of valvular heart defects caused by fenfluramine (serotonin 5-HT2B receptor agonist). Importantly, phentermine was never associated with these issues and has never been taken off the market (available since 1959). Lorcaserin (Belviq®), a serotonin 5-HT2C receptor agonist, was marketed to have similar weight loss given the similar serotonergic effects but without the valvular problems. It was removed from the market in February 2020 due to increased incidences of malignancy during a clinical trial.

Phentermine (Adipex®, Lomaira®)	
Formulary	-Capsule/Tabs: 15 to 37.5 mg once daily in morning -Lomaira®: 8 mg TID 30 minutes before meals
Mechanism	Sympathomimetic amines stimulate the hypothalamus to release norepinephrine, resulting in decreased appetite and increased energy expenditure.
Contraindications	Hypersensitivity to phentermine or other formulary components, concurrent MAOI use, hyperthyroidism, close-angled glaucoma, and pregnancy. Avoid in those with coronary artery disease, severe anxiety, or a history of substance use.
Side Effects	Insomnia, constipation, xerostomia, and tachycardia

Reference: Phentermine package insert

192. (Content: III-F-1) A 42-year-old female with a medical history of difficult-to-control diabetes mellitus type 2 and obesity class III presents for a bariatric seminar to learn more about surgical options. She is particularly interested in a more recently endorsed malabsorptive procedure. It is described as having a high diabetes remission rate and causing a significant reduction in hunger due to the removal of a portion of the stomach. Which surgical procedure is she referring to?

A. **Single anastomosis duodeno-ileostomy with sleeve gastrectomy**
B. Vertical sleeve gastrectomy
C. Roux-en-Y gastric bypass
D. Biliopancreatic diversion with a duodenal switch
E. One anastomosis gastric bypass

(A) **Single anastomosis duodeno-ileostomy with sleeve gastrectomy** (SADI-S), also referred to as a stomach intestinal pylorus sparing surgery (SIPSS), is a more recently endorsed metabolic and bariatric surgery (2019).

The SADI-S involves stapling and cutting the duodenum ❷ just distal to the pylorus (pylorus remains intact) and anastomosing a loop of the intestine to the stomach ❸. This procedure has less complications than the duodenal switch including less malabsorption and only one anastomosis. It has increased weight loss and diabetes remission when compared to the RYGB. In addition, a sleeve gastrectomy ❶ is performed, providing an additional restrictive and hormonal (decreased ghrelin) mechanism.

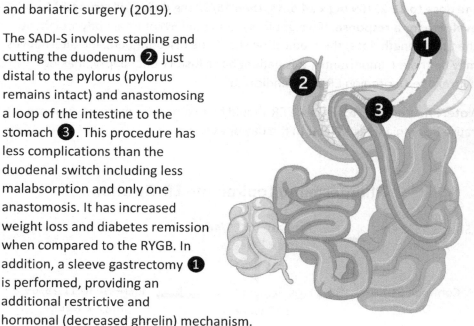

Image citation: Image created by Charu G. Copyright owned by Kevin Smith, DO
Reference: Eichelter J, Felsenreich DM, Bichler C, Gensthaler L, Gachabayov M, Richwien P, Nixdorf L, Jedamzik J, Mairinger M, Langer FB, Prager G. Surgical Technique of Single Anastomosis Duodeno-Ileal Bypass with Sleeve Gastrectomy (SADI-S). Surg Technol Int. 2022 May 27;41:sti41/1571. doi: 10.52198/22.STI.41.GS1571. Epub ahead of print. PMID: 35623034.

193. (Content: III-D-4) A 27-year-old female with a history of epilepsy is returning for a one month-follow up to her primary care physician's office. Three months ago, she was started on phentermine/topiramate ER after lifestyle changes failed to achieve her weight loss goals. Her current dose is 7.5/46 mg phentermine/ topiramate ER daily. She is tolerating the medication well but is unsure of its effectiveness. During the past three months, her weight has decreased from 220 lbs (100 kg) to 216 lbs (98 kg). Which option would be the most appropriate to initiate at this time?

    A. Monitor for weight loss for an additional month
    B. Take an additional phentermine/topiramate ER 3.75/23 mg tab at night
    C. Change the medication to naltrexone/bupropion ER
    D. Titrate up to phentermine/topiramate ER 15/92 mg daily
    E. Titrate off medication, then start liraglutide

(D) This patient, who is tolerating phentermine/topiramate ER, but is not seeing appropriate results (> 3% total body weight loss at 12 weeks), should **increase the dose to 11.25/69 mg x 14 days, then 15/92 mg daily (full strength) to evaluate for a response.** If weight loss is less than 5% of total body weight at the full-strength dose, the medication should be discontinued, and alternatives may be trialed. Importantly, this patient has a history of epilepsy, making naltrexone/bupropion ER contraindicated.

Note: Phentermine/topiramate ER should be taken in the morning, as it can cause insomnia if taken later in the day or evening.

Phentermine/Topiramate ER Titration

Reference: Phentermine/topiramate ER package insert

194. (Content: III-F-5b) A 31-year-old male presents for his initial 1-week post-bariatric surgery (sleeve gastrectomy) follow-up appointment with his dietician. He has continued a liquid diet and has been taking crushed vitamin supplementation. His current vitamin intake includes the following:

- Two adult multivitamins
- Elemental calcium of 1200 mg daily
- 1500 international units of vitamin D
- 65 mg of iron taken on an empty stomach

Which of the following recommendations should be made to this patient?

A. Take iron with calcium for increased absorption
B. Avoid concentrated carbohydrates to prevent dumping syndrome
C. Double the amount of vitamin D intake
D. Decrease the multivitamin to one tablet daily
E. Ensure the multivitamins contain selenium

(C) Except for laparoscopic adjustable gastric banding, all patients status post-bariatric surgery should take two adult multivitamins containing folic acid, thiamine, and vitamin B_{12}. In addition, everyone should **take 3000 international vitamin D units** with dosage titration to maintain dietary vitamin D levels > 30 ng/mL.

Minimum Daily Vitamin and Mineral Intake After Bariatric Surgery				
Procedure	SG	RYGB	BPD/DS & SADI-S	LAGB
Adult MV[1]	2	2	2	1
Calcium	1200-1500 mg		1800-2400 mg	1200-1500 mg
Vitamin D[2]	3000 IU			
Iron[3]	18 mg (men)-60 mg (menstruating females)			
Protein[4]	Minimum of 60 g/day			
Water[4]	At least 50 oz/day to ensure adequate hydration			

LAGB: Laparoscopic adjustable gastric banding; **SG** Sleeve gastrectomy; **RYGB** Roux-en-Y gastric bypass; **BPD/DS:** Biliopancreatic diversion with duodenal switch; **SADI-S:** Single anastomosis duodeno-ileal bypass with sleeve gastrectomy
[1]Multivitamin should contain fat soluble vitamins, copper, zinc, folic acid, thiamine, and vitamin B_{12}
[2]Adequate intake to maintain a vitamin D level ≥ 30 ng/mL
[3]Cannot take with calcium
[4]Individualized

Reference: AACE/TOS/ASMBS/OMA/ASA 2019 Guidelines: CLINICAL PRACTICE GUIDELINES FOR THE PERIOPERATIVE NUTRITION, METABOLIC, AND NONSURGICAL SUPPORT OF PATIENTS UNDERGOING BARIATRIC PROCEDURES – 2019 UPDATE. Recommendation 39.

195. (Content: III-F-5a) A 31-year-old female status post Roux-en-Y gastric bypass is being seen 4 hours postoperatively on the general medical floor by the hospitalist. There were no immediate surgical complications. The patient has type 2 diabetes mellitus and was previously on empagliflozin, tirzepatide, and metformin. She has tolerated a small amount of oral liquid intake. Point-of-care glucose testing reveals a current glucose level of 150 mg/dL. What is the most appropriate management of this patient's diabetes?

A. Decrease empagliflozin by 50%
B. Continue to monitor glucose levels
C. Initiate semaglutide
D. Change metformin to extended-release
E. Start insulin drip to maintain glucose levels of 140-180 mg/dL

(B) After bariatric surgery, patients with diabetes should maintain glucose levels between 140-180 mg/dL to prevent hypoglycemia yet minimize hyperglycemia, which can impair wound healing. Given the patient is in this range in the immediate postoperative period, it would be safe to **continue to monitor glucose levels**, while adding a subcutaneous insulin sliding scale as needed while inpatient. Other important post-bariatric surgery diabetes management include:

- Immediately postoperatively, insulin secretagogues (risk of hypoglycemia), sodium-glucose cotransporter-2 inhibitors (risk for dehydration), and thiazolidinediones should be discontinued.
- GLP-1 RA and tirzepatide could be continued post-operatively, although patients should be closely monitored for adequate fluid and nutritional intake. Given the decreased gastric motility and longer half-life, there is a concern of aspiration due to food remnants in the setting of anesthesia and intubation. Anesthesia likely will stop these one week pre-operatively based on their position statement.
- Incretin-based therapy and metformin can be continued, although metformin should be changed to immediate release.
- Subcutaneous insulin (non-ICU) and insulin drips (ICU) doses should be adjusted to minimize the hypoglycemic risk (goal 140-180 mg/dL).
- Consider an endocrinology consult if the patient with type 1 diabetes or type 2 diabetes has uncontrolled hyperglycemia.

Reference: AACE/TOS/ASMBS/OMA/ASA 2019 Guidelines: CLINICAL PRACTICE GUIDELINES FOR THE PERIOPERATIVE NUTRITION, METABOLIC, AND NONSURGICAL SUPPORT OF PATIENTS UNDERGOING BARIATRIC PROCEDURES – 2019 UPDATE. Recommendation 42

196. (Content: III-A-1) A 34-year-old male is presenting for a 2-week follow-up with his health coach. He had lost 3 lbs (1.4 kg) the first week but has regained that back. He states that work is busy, and he has difficulty avoiding eating fast food, which is convenient. The health coach agrees that losing weight does take effort and then states, "You are showing motivation to lose weight by coming to the office, but yet you continue to eat fast food frequently. How do those two go together?" What motivation interview principle did the coach display?

A. Empathy
B. Avoiding arguments
C. Developing discrepancy
D. Resolving ambivalence
E. Supporting self-efficacy

(C) This health coach uses the principle of developing discrepancy to show the mismatch between what the patient is currently doing and where the patient wants to be by comparing current eating habits to eventual weight loss.

Motivational interviewing uses several principles to explore, nurture, and strengthen the patient's motivation to target behavioral change:

- **Empathy:** Display understanding, collaboration, encouragement, and active listening
- **Avoiding arguments:** "Rolling with resistance" through reflection, shifting the focus, reframing, and siding with the negative
- **Developing discrepancy:** Explore the mismatch from where the patient is today to where they want to be in the future
- **Resolving ambivalence:** Amplify discrepancies and address the uncertainty for motivation to change
- **Supporting self-efficacy:** Affirm favorable results by focusing on patient successes, skills, and strengths

Reference: Obesity Medicine Association: Obesity Algorithm (2023)

197. (Content: III-D-3) A 24-year-old female presents for smoking cessation counseling. She has mild depression symptoms and increased weight gain since starting the night shift. The clinician starts her on a single medication that can treat all of these components. Which of the following parameters may increase once starting this medication?

A. LDL
B. Triglycerides
C. Glucose levels
D. **Blood pressure**
E. Heart rate

(D) Bupropion has several indications, including tobacco cessation, depression, attention deficit disorder, seasonal affective disorder, and the treatment of obesity. This medication is often combined with naltrexone for synergistic weight loss effects. Although this medication improves most cardiovascular parameters, **bupropion may increase blood pressure** and is contraindicated in the setting of uncontrolled hypertension.

Anti-obesity medications on the market improve all cardiovascular parameters via weight loss and weight-independent mechanisms. The exception to this is that bupropion can increase blood pressure despite weight loss, and therefore vital signs must be monitored closely while on this medication.

The table below summarizes the cardiovascular benefits of anti-obesity agents.

Cardiovascular Effects of Anti-Obesity Medications					
Medications	**HDL**	**LDL**	**TG**	**HbA1c**	**BP**
GLP-1 RA and GLP-1 RA/GIP	↑	↓	↓	↓	↓
Bupropion ER/ Naltrexone	↑	↔	↓	↓	↑
Phentermine/ Topiramate ER	↑	↓	↓	↓	↓

HDL: High-density lipoprotein; LDL: Low-density lipoprotein; TG: Triglycerides; BP: Blood pressure (systolic); GLP-1 RA: Glucagon-like peptide 1 receptor agonist; GIP: Gastric inhibitory peptide; ER: Extended-release

Reference: Bupropion package insert
Reference: Vorsanger MH, Subramanyam P, Weintraub HS, Lamm SH, Underberg JA, Gianos E, Goldberg IJ, Schwartzbard AZ. Cardiovascular Effects of the New Weight Loss Agents. J Am Coll Cardiol. 2016 Aug 23;68(8):849-59. doi: 10.1016/j.jacc.2016.06.007. PMID: 27539178.

198. (Content: III-F-5b) A 35-year-old female is following up with her primary care physician two years after undergoing a Roux-en-Y gastric bypass. She has lost and maintained 65% of her excess body weight. Today, her vitamin D (OH-25) is 8 ng/mL (reference range > 30 ng/ml), her parathyroid hormone is slightly elevated, and her corrected calcium levels are normal. She undergoes a bone density scan, which is consistent with osteopenia. Which of the following is the most appropriate treatment at this time?

A. Calcitriol
B. Ergocalciferol
C. Calcium oxalate
D. Oral alendronate
E. Intravenous zoledronic acid

(B) This patient is presenting with findings of severe vitamin D deficiency with secondary hyperparathyroidism and osteopenia. The first step should be to **treat the vitamin D deficiency**, which will normalize the parathyroid hormone and decrease bone reabsorption.

The following recommendations should be followed in post-bariatric surgery, especially malabsorptive procedures:

- Dual-energy x-ray absorptiometry may be indicated two years after surgery to monitor for osteoporosis.
- Baseline and annual vitamin D levels are recommended.
- Daily vitamin D supplementation should be taken after surgery to prevent secondary hyperparathyroidism.
- Antiresorptive agents (bisphosphonates or denosumab) should only be considered after bariatric procedures in those with osteoporosis who have normalized vitamin D and calcium levels.
- Use intravenous bisphosphonates only, as there is a risk of anastomotic ulceration and diminished absorption with oral formulations.

Reference: AACE/TOS/ASMBS/OMA/ASA 2019 Guidelines: CLINICAL PRACTICE GUIDELINES FOR THE PERIOPERATIVE NUTRITION, METABOLIC, AND NONSURGICAL SUPPORT OF PATIENTS UNDERGOING BARIATRIC PROCEDURES – 2019 UPDATE. Recommendation 53, 54, 55, Table 12

199. (Content: III-F-1) A 41-year-old male with a body mass index of 61 kg/m^2 presents for a surgery consultation regarding bariatric surgical options. Comorbidities include well-controlled obstructive sleep apnea, hypertension, and right knee osteoarthritis. Upon discussing goals, he states his primary goal is maximum weight loss. Given his prior medical history and weight loss goals, which of the following would be the most appropriate surgical option for him?

A. Laparoscopic adjustable gastric banding (LAGB)
B. Sleeve gastrectomy (SG)
C. Roux-en-Y gastric bypass (RYGB)
D. **Biliopancreatic diversion with duodenal switch (BPD/DS)**

(D) Given his maximum weight loss goals, a **BPD/DS would provide the most significant total body weight loss (TBWL)**. However, due to the complexity of the surgery, it is not offered by every surgeon.

Bariatric Surgery Options			
Procedure	Weight loss (% TBWL)	Positives	Negatives
LAGB	20-25%	-No anatomic alteration -Removable and adjustable	Erosion, high explant rates, slips
SG	25-30%	-Easy to perform/reproducible -Few long-term complications -No anastomosis -Metabolic effects	Leaks difficult to manage, little data beyond 5 years. GERD (20-30%)
RYGB	30-35%	-Strong metabolic effects - < 5% major complication risk -Effective for GERD -Can be used as 2nd stage	Marginal ulcers, internal hernias, long-term micro-nutritional deficits
BPD/DS	35-45%	-Powerful metabolic effects -Most pronounced weight loss -Effective for high BMI's -Can be used as 2nd stage	Malabsorptive, GERD, protein malnutrition, internal hernia, challenging, duodenal dissection
SADI-S	35-45%	-Similar to BPD/DS, however slightly less malabsorption risks and less complications. -Significant diabetes remission -Can be used as 2nd stage	Malabsorptive, GERD, micronutrient deficiencies

SG: Sleeve gastrectomy; **RYGB:** Roux-en-Y gastric bypass; **BPD/DS:** Biliopancreatic diversion with duodenal switch; **SADI-S:** Single anastomosis duodeno-ileal bypass with sleeve gastrectomy

Reference: AACE/TOS/ASMBS/OMA/ASA 2019 Guidelines: CLINICAL PRACTICE GUIDELINES FOR THE PERIOPERATIVE NUTRITION, METABOLIC, AND NONSURGICAL SUPPORT OF PATIENTS UNDERGOING BARIATRIC PROCEDURES – 2019 UPDATE. Table 6a.

200. (Content: III-D-8) A 43-year-old female presents to the office for increased weight since her last appointment. She was started on amlodipine for blood pressure and has noted a 2.2 lb (1 kg) weight gain despite no other changes to physical activity. What is the most likely explanation for this?

A. **Increased interstitial edema**
B. Increased appetite
C. Decreased energy expenditure
D. Activation of POMC/CART pathway
E. Placebo effect

(A) Amlodipine and nifedipine are dihydropyridine calcium channel blockers (CCBs) used to treat hypertension, vasospastic angina, and Raynaud's phenomenon. It may cause a slight weight gain due to adipose-independent mechanisms described below:

- **Edema:** CCBs cause smooth muscles in the vasculature to relax, leading to vasodilation. This vasodilation leads to an increase in intravascular hydrostatic pressure and therefore **increases gravity-dependent interstitial edema** in the lower extremities.
- **Constipation:** The other most common side effect of CCBs is constipation, leading to increased intestinal stool burden, which may also add minimal weight. Importantly, weight gain is not due to increased adipose tissue deposition.

Both of these common side effects are dose-dependent, with a higher prevalence in females. These effects are less pronounced in non-dihydropyridine CCBs such as verapamil or diltiazem.

In contrast to CCBs, some beta-blockers such as atenolol, propranolol, and metoprolol do increase adipose tissue, leading to increased weight. If patients require beta-blockers, carvedilol is the most weight-neutral option.

Note: Pioglitazone also increases total body weight by adipose-independent means by increasing water retention.

Reference: Amlodipine package insert

201. (Content: III-F-3) A 52-year-old female presents to her primary care physician with intermittent post-prandial fullness, nausea, and occasional vomiting. She underwent a laparoscopic Roux-en-Y gastric bypass two years prior and has been very happy with her weight loss. A barium swallow and subsequent EGD fail to explain her findings. The following week she goes to the emergency department for biliary emesis. The most likely cause of her symptoms is a(n)

A. **mesenteric defect**
B. small intestinal bowel overgrowth
C. *H. pylori* infection
D. marginal ulcer
E. anastomotic stricture

(A) This patient's intermittent abdominal pain and postprandial satiety are concerning for a **mesenteric defect causing an internal hernia.** These symptoms often occur before a small bowel obstruction. It is a difficult diagnosis, as the symptoms tend to be vague early in the course, and contrasted imaging studies are often normal without an acute obstruction.

Note: The most specific CT finding for an internal hernia is a "mesenteric swirl sign," although this may not always be present.

Internal hernias are a late complication of laparoscopic bariatric and metabolic surgery, usually occurring > 1 year postoperatively after the patient has reduced their BMI by 15 kg/m². As the patient loses weight and the intraabdominal adipose tissue regresses, mesenteric defects become more amenable to bowel entrapment. Often this presents with intermittent symptoms initially.

A high clinical indication is necessary for this diagnosis, with colicky abdominal pain, nausea, and early satiety being the most specific findings.

Reference: Internal Hernia after Laparoscopic Gastric Bypass: A Review of the Literature; April 26, 2007 by Louis O. Jeansonne IV, MD; Craig B. Morgenthal, MD; Brent C. White, MD; and Edward Lin, DO

202. (Content: III-F-5b) A 41-year-old female presents to her primary care physician for concerns of diaphoresis, weakness, and tunnel vision approximately two hours after meals. She underwent a Roux-en-Y gastric bypass (RYGB) three years ago and subsequently lost 103 lbs (46.7 kg) with a current BMI of 26.1 kg/m². She denies ever having similar symptoms. She has decreased her carbohydrate intake, which helped minimally. Which of the following conditions most accurately describes her symptoms?

A. Dumping syndrome
B. Insulinoma
C. Postprandial hyperinsulinemic hypoglycemia
D. Nesidioblastosis
E. Noninsulinoma pancreatogenous hypoglycemia syndrome

(C) This patient who is experiencing late (>1 hour) post-prandial neuroglycopenia years after a RYGB surgery is likely experiencing **postprandial hyperinsulinemic hypoglycemia (PHH).** This condition has a female predominance (92%) and can cause mild (lightheadedness, diaphoresis, flushing) to severe (confusion, blurry vision, seizures) transient symptoms.

The etiology of PHH after RYGB is likely multifactorial but thought to be due to a persistent increase in incretins (GLP-1 and GIP) post-operatively, leading to hyperfunctioning/hypertrophied β-islet cells. This, along with improved insulin sensitivity with weight loss, may lead to symptoms.

Causes of Hypoglycemia (After RYGB)			
Conditions:	PHH[1]	Dumping Syndrome	Insulinoma
Hypoglycemia:	Post-prandial	Post-prandial. It may be euglycemic during initial symptoms.	Fasting and post-prandial
Timing:	>1 year post-op. 1-4 hours post-prandial	<1 year post-op. Within 15-30 minutes of a meal	Independent of surgery
Fasting C-peptide	Normal	Normal	Elevated

PHH: postprandial hyperinsulinemic hypoglycemia
[1]Previously referred to as late dumping syndrome

Reference: Honka H, Salehi M. Postprandial hypoglycemia after gastric bypass surgery: from pathogenesis to diagnosis and treatment. Curr Opin Clin Nutr Metab Care. 2019 Jul;22(4):295-302. doi: 10.1097/MCO.0000000000000574. PMID: 31082828; PMCID: PMC6598692.
Reference: Up to Date: "Bariatric operations: Late complications with subacute presentations"

203. (Content: III-G-7) A 39-year-old Caucasian female with a past medical history of obstructive sleep apnea adherent with CPAP and gout presents to her primary care office for follow-up regarding elevated blood pressures. Over the last three months, home and in-office blood pressures have ranged from 150-170/90-105 mmHg. Today, her blood pressure is 164/98 mmHg, and she has a BMI of 34 kg/m². Which of the following is the most appropriate medication to prescribe now?

A. **Losartan**
B. Naltrexone/bupropion ER
C. Chlorthalidone
D. Metoprolol

(A) Renin-angiotensin-aldosterone system (RAS) inhibition (either angiotensin receptor blockers or angiotensin-converting enzyme inhibitors), such as **losartan,** should be considered first-line anti-hypertensive medications to control blood pressure in patients with obesity. Beta-blockers can adversely affect metabolism (metoprolol is weight-positive), and diuretics such as chlorthalidone should be avoided in a patient with gout.

RAAS activation seems to be a primary mediator in hypertension in patients with obesity (especially in children). This is because pro-inflammatory adipokines released by excessive adipose tissue activate the sympathetic nervous system, ultimately activating RAAS, leading to aldosterone-mediated sodium and water absorption within the kidney.

Although weight-loss ultimately will help improve chronic diseases (i.e., diabetes, hypertension, sleep apnea, etc.), medications should be prescribed to control comorbidities and then decreased as able once weight-loss is achieved.

Importantly, naltrexone/bupropion ER should be avoided, as this combination drug is contraindicated in uncontrolled hypertension and should be avoided if other weight-loss medications can be used in the setting of hypertension.

Note: angiotensin receptor blockers or angiotensin-converting enzyme inhibitors must be avoided in pregnancy or those who may become pregnant.

Reference: AACE/ACE Guidelines: AMERICAN ASSOCIATION OF CLINICAL ENDOCRINOLOGISTS AND AMERICAN COLLEGE OF ENDOCRINOLOGY COMPREHENSIVE CLINICAL PRACTICE GUIDELINES FOR MEDICAL CARE OF PATIENTS WITH OBESITY (2016). Recommendation 91-94.

204. (Content: III-F-4) A patient reaches out to her family medicine physician for advice. She was told to discontinue semaglutide one week prior to an elective cholecystectomy. She has had significant weight loss with this medication and has concerns about weight regain. She has been on a stable dose for the past 6 months and has had no adverse effects. The patient was most likely instructed to discontinue this medication due to concerns for

    A. postoperative nausea
    B. perioperative hypoglycemia
    C. reduced wound healing
    D. gastric regurgitation
    E. post-operative ileus

(D) The American Society of Anesthesiologists (ASA) provided pre-operative recommendations in patients taking GLP-1 medications to reduce the risk of aspiration events due to gastric slowing. They recommend holding daily GLP-1 medications (i.e., liraglutide) on the day of an elective procedure, and for those on weekly dosing (i.e., semaglutide), hold one week prior. This is recommended regardless of the indication for the GLP-1 (diabetes or obesity treatment).

The task force that provided the above recommendation was based on anecdotal accounts of increased **gastric regurgitation** leading to pulmonary aspiration, as studies are ongoing on the prevalence of this complication. This, along with fasting durations preoperatively may vary as more data becomes available.

Reference: American Society of Anesthesiologists Consensus-Based Guidance on Preoperative Management of Patients (Adults and Children) on Glucagon-Like Peptide-1 (GLP-1) Receptor Agonists Girish P. Joshi, M.B.B.S., M.D., Basem B. Abdelmalak, M.D., et al. American Society of Anesthesiologists (ASA) Task Force on Preoperative Fasting. June 29, 2023.

205. (Content: III-H-1) A pediatrician working in a rural community wants to provide the highest level of care for her patients. Upon researching the most updated guidelines, the evidence-based approach that will improve the health of her patients with overweight or obesity the most would include

A. discussing surgical options once patients complete puberty
B. evaluating all patients for lipid disorders and insulin resistance
C. starting patients in a staged management approach
D. **familiarizing herself with community-based resources**
E. require lab work evaluating for endocrinopathies

(D) Although the staged or stepped approach was initially considered the standard in the treatment of pediatric obesity, recently-released evidence-based guidelines show that early intervention and access to therapies including surgical, pharmacologic, and intensive health behavior and lifestyle treatment (IHBLT) are appropriate and should be initiated by the primary care clinician based on the patient's disease burden, not their stage of obesity, age, or via a staged approach.

Pediatric healthcare providers should provide comprehensive obesity treatment (COT) by evaluating for obesity and its comorbidities and providing evidence-based physical and dietary guidance. Coordination with subspecialists, nutritionists, and therapist to provide IHBLT is ideal, however, may not be readily available in rural settings or based on family resources. **Utilizing community programs** tailored to family needs augments COT in these settings. Consensus recommendations for primary health care providers include delivering the best available intensive treatment to all children with overweight or obesity and build collaborations with specialists and programs in their communities.

Incorrect answer choices: Patients should only be evaluated for secondary causes such as endocrinopathies based on their targeted history and exam findings, not in a universal manner. Surgical interventions and aggressive weight loss do not affect growth, and therefore should not be delayed for concerns of growth or developmental restrictions. Patients who meet certain criteria should be screened for lipid disorders and diabetes, not all patients. Review the key action statements for more information on who qualifies for these tests.

Reference: Hampl, S. E., Hassink, S. G., Skinner, A. C., Armstrong, S. C., Barlow, S. E., Bolling, C. F., ... Okechukwu, K. (2023). Clinical Practice Guideline for the Evaluation and Treatment of Children and Adolescents With Obesity. Pediatrics, 151(2), e2022060640. https://doi.org/10.1542/peds.2022-060640.

206. (Content: III-G-2) A 48-year-old female started tirzepatide for diabetes and has titrated up to the maximum dose. She has noticed clumps of hair falling out when washing her hair in the shower over the past 2 months and is concerned. She has lost 64 lbs (29 kg) after starting the medication and invoking aggressive lifestyle and behavioral changes. She takes a daily vitamin, and intakes 1400 kcal/day with 82 grams of protein. Which of the following best explains her presenting complaint?

A. **Telogen effluvium**
B. Micronutrient deficiency
C. Perimenopausal status
D. Tinea capitus
E. Protein malnourishment

(A) This patient who is taking daily vitamins, consuming sufficient calories (albeit at a calorie deficit), and protein, has had rapid weight loss and is most likely experiencing **telogen effluvium.** Rapid weight loss can lead to physiologic stress, in addition to potential alterations in hormones (adipokine reduction) that lead to a disturbance in the hair cycle. Stress, illness, and surgery are other risk factors. Although very restrictive diets can cause micronutrient deficiencies, there is no evidence of that occurring in this patient. Most cases self-resolve within 6 months.

One of the difficulties of diagnosing telogen effluvium in the setting of bariatric and metabolic surgery is ruling out secondary causes. Ensuring patients are taking appropriate supplementations to rule out mineral and vitamin deficiencies is important.

Telogen Effluvium	
Findings	Diffuse nonscarring hair loss
Etiology	Shift in follicular cycling (hair cell cycles synchronize when a significant amount of hair cells are pushed into the telogen phase)
Risk factors	Surgery, illness, childbirth, malnutrition, medications, stress, and rapid weight loss
Course	Often reactive and reversible
Management	Given reversibility, may not require treatment. Treatment may include topical or oral minoxidil

Reference: Up to Date: "Telogen effluvium"

207. (Content: III-G-1) A 7-year-old is presenting to his pediatrician for a well-child exam. He overall feels well and his exercise-induced asthma is controlled with an albuterol inhaler. The parents are present with him. Which of the following recommendations is most appropriate at this time?

    A. **Encourage 60 minutes of exercise daily**
    B. Limit bedroom television time to < 1 hour daily
    C. Encourage a sleep duration of at least 8 hours nightly
    D. Dessert should only be given when meal is completed
    E. Limit eating at restaurants to once weekly

(A) This patient who is otherwise healthy should be encouraged to **exercise 1 hour daily** with an additional goal of decreasing sedentary time. In addition, screen time should be minimized to < 1-2 hours daily, with no television being in the child's bedroom. Children in this age group should be getting at least 11 hours of sleep, dessert should be reserved for special occasions, and eating out should be avoided.

Other important recommendations are discussed below:

General Recommendations for Children (5-14 years of age)		
Conditions	**Age 5-9 years old**	**Age 10-14 years old**
Screen time	<1-2 hours/day No TV in the bedroom	1-2 hours/day No TV in the bedroom
Sleep time	11-14 hours	10-12 hours
Fast food	None	None
Dessert	Only special occasions	Only special occasions
Sugary-sweetened beverages or juice	None	None
Activity	-Moderate to vigorous activity ≥ 60 mins/day -Decrease sedentary time	-Vigorous activity ≥ 60 mins/day -Monitor for changes -Decrease sedentary time
Parent's role	-Avoid being over-controlling -Peer groups become more influential	
Other	-Meals at the table with family -OK to leave food on plate	

Reference: Obesity Medicine Association: Pediatric Obesity Algorithm (2023-2024)

208. (Content: III-B-1) A 54-year-old male with a history of gout and class I obesity presents for a 2-week follow-up visit after initiating a ketogenic diet. Per urine ketone strips, he has been in ketosis for the past week. Which of the following lab findings are expected today compared to when he first initiated the diet?

A. **Hyponatremia**
B. Decreased uric acid levels
C. Increased serum pH levels
D. Hyperkalemia

(A) Ketogenic diets were initially created to reduce the risk of seizures in children with epilepsy but have more recently been adopted for weight loss. The idea is that by consuming minimal carbohydrates, adipose tissue is broken down and the ketones are used as a fuel source. Initially, this induces a diuretic effect potentially leading to hypokalemia and **hyponatremia**. This diuretic effect explains the initial rapid weight loss.

Insulin also plays a role in sodium reabsorption in the kidneys. Reduced carbohydrate ingestion causes a decrease in circulating insulin. This reduction in insulin causes a decrease in renal sodium reabsorption and an increase in urinary sodium excretion, thus causing hyponatremia.

Note: A recent meta-analysis showed no changes in uric acid levels, although previously it was thought to cause hyperuricemia and uric acid kidney stones. Other side effects of ketogenic diets include constipation, halitosis, muscle cramps, increased LDL cholesterol, and QTc prolongation.

Reference: Very Low Carbohydrate and Ketogenic Diets and Cardiometabolic Risk, Karen E. Aspry, MD, MS, FACC; Penny M. Kris-Etherton, PhD, RD; Carol Kirkpatrick, PhD.. American College of Cardiology. October 2020
Reference: Gohari S, Ghobadi S, Jafari A, Ahangar H, Gohari S, Mahjani M. The effect of dietary approaches to stop hypertension and ketogenic diets intervention on serum uric acid concentration: a systematic review and meta-analysis of randomized controlled trials. Sci Rep. 2023 Jun 28;13(1):10492. doi: 10.1038/s41598-023-37672-2. PMID: 37380733; PMCID: PMC10307853.
Reference: Muscogiuri, G., El Ghoch, M., Colao, A., Hassapidou, M., Yumuk, V., Busetto, L., & Obesity Management Task Force (OMTF) of the European Association for the Study of Obesity (EASO). (2021). European Guidelines for Obesity Management in Adults with a Very Low-Calorie Ketogenic Diet: A Systematic Review and Meta-Analysis. Obes Facts, 14(2), 222–245.

209. (Content: III-F-4) A 51-year-old female is presenting to her primary care physician with plans to undergo a sleeve gastrectomy. She has a prior diagnosis of polycystic ovarian syndrome and hypertension, for which she is taking metformin and lisinopril. Overall she states she feels well. Her physical activity consists of briskly walking (5 metabolic equivalents) for 45 minutes daily. Physical examination is unrevealing. Her STOP-BANG score is 1. Which would be the most appropriate test to perform before surgery?

A. Pharmacologic stress test
B. **Fasting lipid panel**
C. Thyroid-stimulating hormone
D. Dexamethasone suppression test
E. Overnight polysomnography

(B) A **fasting lipid panel** should be obtained in all patients with obesity, with treatment initiated based on current practice guidelines. A patient that is asymptomatic or lacks suggestive physical exam findings should not be routinely tested for secondary causes of obesity, including hypothyroidism. Also, this patient's STOP-BANG score is low-risk, negating the need for polysomnography, and her ability to perform > 4 METS does not warrant further formal stress testing.

Cardiac evaluation should be completed during the history and physical exam, with subsequent testing based on the ACC/AHA perioperative guidelines, similar to other abdominal surgeries. A formal cardiac preoperative consultation is recommended if the patient <u>has</u> cardiac disease.

Note: Those <u>at risk</u> for heart disease should undergo evaluation for peri-procedure beta-adrenergic blockade.

Finally, routine screening for primary hypothyroidism in the absence of clinical findings suggestive of the condition is not recommended (although insurance may require this preoperatively).

Reference: AACE/TOS/ASMBS/OMA/ASA 2019 Guidelines: CLINICAL PRACTICE GUIDELINES FOR THE PERIOPERATIVE NUTRITION, METABOLIC, AND NONSURGICAL SUPPORT OF PATIENTS UNDERGOING BARIATRIC PROCEDURES – 2019 UPDATE. Recommendation 15, 16, 20, 21

210. (Content: III-F-1) A patient is researching different bariatric procedures and is considering a duodenal switch. In discussing this procedure with the patient, which of the following most accurately describes this procedure?

A. It is preferred in those with a BMI < 45 kg/m²
B. The common channel is less than 20 cm in length
C. Digestive enzymes enter the digestive loop
D. A portion of the stomach is removed

(D) A duodenal switch is a malabsorptive procedure in which the **stomach is made into a tubular pouch** (4-8 oz), and a surgical "duodenal switch" delays the combination of the food (digestive loop) with the digestive enzymes (biliopancreatic loop), until 75-150 cm before the large intestine (common channel). It has the best long-term weight loss but carries a higher mortality and complication risk and therefore is typically reserved for those with the most elevated BMIs.

In a duodenal switch, there is a sleeve gastrectomy performed ❶. The intestine just distal to the stomach is cut and stapled ❸ and a portion of the small intestine is brought up to create an anastomosis with the stomach ❷. The portion of the intestine that contains the digestive enzymes is connected to the alimentary tract, thus making a common channel ❹ that eventually drains into the large intestines.

211. (Content: III-E) A clinical trial is evaluating an oxyntomodulin analog, which is a potential investigational obesity therapy that has shown promising effects in animal studies. It is theorized that this medication will increase satiety, decrease food intake, and potentially have beneficial glucose effects in patients with type 2 diabetes mellitus. The beneficial effects of this intravenous peptide most likely occur as a result of which of the following mechanisms?

A. **GLP-1 receptor agonist**
B. Glucagon receptor antagonism
C. NPY/AgRP direct antagonist
D. Increase in central serotonin levels
E. Ghrelin binding and inactivation

(A) Oxyntomodulin is a peptide hormone released endogenously in post-prandial states. It reduces food intake (increases satiety) and increases energy expenditure, thus promoting weight loss. It has two primary effects, **including glucagon-like peptide 1 (GLP-1) and glucagon receptor agonism,** with subsequent results discussed below:

- **GLP-1 receptor agonist:** Similar to currently available exogenous GLP-1 receptor agonists, this hormone has an incretin effect, slowing down gastric emptying and activating the POMC/CART pathway.

- **Glucagon receptor agonist:** This effect is undesirable, as glucagon works to counter insulin secretion and increase circulating glucose levels. However, the more pronounced GLP-1 effects discussed above counterbalance this deleterious effect and thus maintain a net positive impact.

Reference: Pocai A. Action and therapeutic potential of oxyntomodulin. Mol Metab. 2013;3(3):241-251. Published 2013 Dec 14. doi:10.1016/j.molmet.2013.12.001
Reference: Obesity Medical Association: Obesity Algorithm (2023)

212. (Content: III-B-1 and 4) A 29-year-old female presents to the clinic with concerns about an abnormal fasting lipid panel on lab work for life insurance.

Test	Value	Reference Range
Total cholesterol	287 mg/dL	< 200 mg/dL
LDL	188 mg/dL	< 130 mg/dL
HDL	31 mg/dL	> 40 mg/dL
Triglycerides (TG)	388 mg/dL	< 150 mg/dL

In discussing a carbohydrate versus fat-restricted diet, which of the following would be an accurate statement to provide to this patient?

    A. A ketogenic diet is preferred to improve the LDL value
    B. A diet consisting of < 30% fats will preferentially improve HDL
    C. Genetic hypercholesterolemia responds to carbohydrate restriction
    D. Low-fat diets do not affect insulin resistance or glucose levels
    E. Carbohydrate-restricted diets would have a greater effect on TG

(E) In general, **low carbohydrate diets have more significant improvements in HDL and TG,** whereas fat restriction improves LDL.

- *Low carbohydrate diets:*
  - More significant increase in HDL and decrease in triglycerides
  - May increase LDL, which may be very significant in those with genetic hypercholesterolemia
  - A ketogenic diet is associated with moderately increased LDL and total cholesterol, as carbohydrates are often exchanged for foods higher in cholesterol and saturated fats.
  - Improvements in insulin resistance, glucose levels, and HbA1c occur irrespective of weight loss
- *Low-fat diets:*
  - A greater decrease in LDL. It may also decrease HDL levels.
  - Improvements in insulin resistance, glucose levels, and HbA1c are only apparent with associated weight loss

Dietary Effects on the Cholesterol Panel				
Plan	Triglycerides	LDL	HDL	HbA1c
Low-Carb/Keto	↓	↑	↑	Improved
Low-Fat	↑	↓	↓	Improved[1]

[1]Insulin sensitivity and HbA1c improvements only seen in those with weight loss

Reference: Obesity Medicine Association: Obesity Algorithm (2023)

213. (Content: III-G-7) A 42-year-old female presents for her 3-month follow-up appointment with her diabetes specialist. The patient has noticed increased polyuria over the past month and admits to having some "slip-ups" following her carbohydrate-restricted diet. Medical history includes type 2 diabetes, heart failure with preserved ejection fraction, and mild diabetic nephropathy. Medications include metformin 2000 mg daily, lisinopril 10 mg daily, and hydrochlorothiazide 25 mg. Body mass index is 34 kg/m^2, whereas vital signs and physical examination are otherwise normal. Her most recent HbA1c is 8.6% (reference range: < 5.7%), an increase of 0.5% since her prior appointment. Which of the following is the most appropriate management change at this time?

    A. Increase metformin
    B. Initiate basal insulin
    C. Start a DPP-4 inhibitor
    D. Prescribe an SGLT-2 inhibitor
    E. Lifestyle changes only

(D) This patient, who is already on a maximum dose of metformin yet has uncontrolled diabetes, should be started on a second anti-diabetic agent (preferably a weight-neutral or weight-negative pharmacologic option). Preferred options would include a GLP-1 agonist or an SGLT-2 inhibitor. Given the concurrent diastolic heart failure, **an SGLT-2 would be preferred.**

Diabetes Medication and Weight Effects		
Weight Positive	**Weight Neutral**	**Weight Negative**
-Insulin[1]	-DPP-IV inhibitors	-GLP-1 agonists[2]
-Thiazolidinediones	-Alpha-glucosidase	-SGLT-2 inhibitors[3]
-Meglitinides	inhibitors	-Biguanides[4]
-Sulfonylureas		-Amylin analogs

Weight effects are generalizations and may be based solely on observational trials and vary depending on dosing, duration of treatment, and indications of medication. Weight variability may be seen.
Note: Children/adolescents have more significant weight gain than adults with obesogenic medications
[1]Insulin: Initiate early if HbA1c is ≥ 10%
[2]GLP-1 agonist: Preferred if atherosclerosis or kidney disease is present
[3]SGLT-2 inhibitors: Preferred if kidney disease, heart failure, or atherosclerosis is present
[4]Metformin: Preferred initial pharmacologic agent for T2DM

Reference: American Diabetes Association: Standards of Medical Care in Diabetes—2020 Abridged for Primary Care Providers; Clinical Diabetes 2020 Jan; 38(1): 10-38. https://doi.org/10.2337/cd20-as01

214. (Content: III-F-5c) A 52-year-old male presents to a gastroenterologist for evaluation of esophageal dysphagia. He underwent an open Roux-en-Y gastric bypass 15 years prior. Although he has maintained significant weight loss, he has not been adherent to physical activity or taking vitamins. An image from the upper gastrointestinal series is shown below.

Given this finding, which other feature is likely found on physical examination?

A. Koilonychia
B. Hepatomegaly
C. Dermatitis
D. External hemorrhoids
E. Actinic cheilitis

(A) Chronic iron deficiency can lead to a condition called Plummer-Vinson syndrome, which is characterized by significant microcytic anemia and esophageal webs (arrow in image). This is particularly prevalent in Roux-en-Y gastric bypass surgery, as the duodenum, which is the location for iron absorption, is bypassed. Other findings associated with iron deficiency include **koilonychia** (also called "spoon nails" in which the fingernails lose convexity), pica, glossitis, cheilosis, and restless leg syndrome.

215. (Content: III-F-2) A patient presents to a bariatric seminar, as he is interested in undergoing surgery for weight loss. He has struggled with weight his entire life, and despite recommended dietary and physical activity changes, his body mass index is still > 60 kg/m². At the end of the seminar, he discusses with the surgeon an option that he has read about, but was not presented by the surgeon, which included placing a balloon into the stomach for weight loss. Which of the following is a true statement regarding this procedure for weight loss?

A. This device is not FDA-approved for use in the United States
B. Intragastric balloons account for 10% of bariatric procedures
C. Indications includes a BMI between 30-40 kg/m² with comorbidities
D. Intragastric balloons have been proven ineffective for weight loss
E. The balloons are placed for 12 months, then removed

(C) Intragastric balloons, accounting for 2% of bariatric procedures, are a short-term option (maximum of 8 months for Spatz 3®, all others 6 months) in adults with a body mass index of **30-40 kg/m² and one or more obesity-related comorbidity** in those who failed lifestyle modifications. The FDA-approved options include the endoscopically placed Orbera® (single balloon system shown below) and Spatz 3® (adjustable) as well as swallowable balloons (Obalon®). Important information is summarized below:

- Intragastric balloons have proven short-term effectiveness, ranging from a 6.8%-10.2% decrease in body weight.
- They should not remain in place for longer than eight months due to the risk of balloon deflation and subsequent intestinal obstruction.
- Avoid in those with a history of prior gastrointestinal surgery.
- The balloons are filled with saline or gas and increase satiety leading to smaller portions.

Image citation: Image created by Charu G. Copyright owned by Kevin Smith, DO
Reference: Up to Date: "Intragastric balloon therapy for weight loss"

216. (Content: III-F-4) A 26-year-old female with severe obesity presents for a metabolic and bariatric surgical consultation. Her prior medical history includes gastroesophageal reflux and obstructive sleep apnea. She takes prenatal vitamins and omeprazole and admits adherence regarding her continuous positive airway pressure machine. Physical examination reveals acanthosis nigricans on the back of her neck and narrow striae on her abdomen. A recent complete metabolic panel and thyroid-stimulating hormone level were normal. Which of the following must be completed before this patient undergoes bariatric surgery?

A. Preoperative *Helicobacter pylori* testing
B. Right upper quadrant ultrasound
C. Serum dehydroepiandrosterone-sulfate (DHEA-S)
D. Psychosocial-behavioral evaluation
E. 5% mandatory weight loss preoperatively

(D) A formal **psychosocial-behavior evaluation** should be performed on all patients by a licensed behavioral health specialist with specialized knowledge and training regarding bariatric assessments before undergoing bariatric surgery. The areas of evaluation should focus on screening for eating disorders, motivation and understanding of the procedure, and environment and behavior factors. Also, screening for any unaddressed psychiatric illnesses or substance use is imperative.

Other mentioned screenings that should be performed preoperatively include:

- *H. pylori* screening in areas of high prevalence
- Right upper quadrant ultrasound if there are abnormal liver enzymes, to evaluate for metabolic-associated (nonalcoholic) fatty liver disease
- Total/bioavailable testosterone, DHEA-S, 4-androstenedione if there is a suspicion for polycystic ovarian syndrome

Note: There is no absolute weight loss requirement preoperatively. In addition, completing an extended weight loss program (i.e., 6 months) is not evidence-based in adults and often delays or creates barriers to surgical treatments.

Reference: AACE/TOS/ASMBS/OMA/ASA 2019 Guidelines: CLINICAL PRACTICE GUIDELINES FOR THE PERIOPERATIVE NUTRITION, METABOLIC, AND NONSURGICAL SUPPORT OF PATIENTS UNDERGOING BARIATRIC PROCEDURES – 2019 UPDATE. Table 7. Recommendations 13, 26, 27, 30, 31

217. (Content: III-D-2) A 29-year-old female who is one month postpartum is being evaluated for weight management. She is currently breastfeeding, and her BMI is 36 kg/m^2. She states her BMI has never been below 30 kg/m^2 during her adult life. She would like to start treatment to help with returning to her pre-conception weight. Which option would be most appropriate to initiate at this time?

A. Semaglutide
B. Phentermine/topiramate ER
C. Naltrexone/bupropion ER
D. Cellulose and citric acid hydrogel
E. Metformin

(D) Although most anti-obesity treatments should be avoided during pregnancy and while breastfeeding, **cellulose and citric acid hydrogel** is not systemically absorbed and would be the best choice in this patient currently breastfeeding.

Note: Cellulose and citric acid hydrogel is technically considered an FDA-cleared medical device, not a medication.

Cellulose and citric acid hydrogel (brand name Plenity®) is a volume-occupying treatment for those with a BMI of 25-40 kg/m^2. It is taken before meals to decrease satiety. The capsule expands when taken with water, becoming the consistency of chewed vegetables. The particles eventually degrade in the colon, where the water is released and reabsorbed.

The characteristics of this device are discussed in the table below.

Cellulose and Citric Acid Hydrogel (Plenity®)	
Dose	Oral 2.25 g (3 capsules) twice daily (20-30 minutes before lunch and dinner meals) with 16 oz of water.
Mechanism	Contents form a three-dimensional matrix within the stomach and small intestines that occupies volume, providing a sensation of fullness and satiety.
Contraindications	Hypersensitivity to components and pregnancy.
Side Effects	-Abdominal pain and diarrhea. Avoid in those with dysphagia or active gastrointestinal disease. -May alter the absorption of other medications.

Reference: Cellulose and Citric Acid Hydrogel package insert

218. (Content: III-G-2) A 39-year-old female is presenting to her general surgeon, who performed her gastric bypass four months prior. She is having vague episodes of sharp mid- to upper abdominal pain that lasts 2-3 hours and then resolves. During these episodes, she feels nauseated but denies emesis. These occur 2 hours after eating, but she is unsure of the correlation to certain foods. She does admit to taking naproxen occasionally for a headache but is on concurrent omeprazole. A right upper quadrant ultrasound reveals cholelithiasis without cholecystitis. In working up her abdominal pain, which of the following statements is true?

A. She should be given a trial of rifaximin
B. NSAIDs should never be used after bariatric surgery
C. Endoscopic evaluation is high-risk after bariatric surgery
D. Traditional ERCP is preferred for choledocholithiasis evaluation
E. **Ursodeoxycholic acid may have prevented her symptoms**

(E) This patient presents with concerns of biliary colic, also known as symptomatic cholelithiasis. Cholelithiasis can occur from rapid weight loss after bariatric surgery, and **ursodeoxycholic acid may prevent** this complication.

Note: Endoscopy is safe after surgery and can be used to evaluate for a stricture, *H. pylori*, and celiac disease.

Important considerations of gastrointestinal complications after bariatric surgery are discussed below:

- Traditional ERCP is not possible after Roux-en-Y
- Although NSAIDs should be avoided, if unavoidable, the use of proton pump inhibitors should be used concurrently
- After sleeve gastrectomy, if patients develop severe GERD that is recalcitrant to medical therapy, conversion to Roux-en-Y should be considered

Reference: AACE/TOS/ASMBS/OMA/ASA 2019 Guidelines: CLINICAL PRACTICE GUIDELINES FOR THE PERIOPERATIVE NUTRITION, METABOLIC, AND NONSURGICAL SUPPORT OF PATIENTS UNDERGOING BARIATRIC PROCEDURES – 2019 UPDATE. Recommendation 72-75
Reference: Ursodeoxycholic acid for the prevention of symptomatic gallstone disease after bariatric surgery (UPGRADE): a multicentre, double-blind, randomised, placebo-controlled superiority trial. Lancet gastroenterol Hepatol. 2021 Dec;6(12):993-1001. doi: 10.1016/S2468-1253(21)00301-0. Epub 2021 Oct 27. PMID: 34715031.

219. (Content: III-D-3) A 22-year-old female is presenting to the weight-loss clinic to discuss FDA-approved, long-term anti-obesity medications. She denies any prior eating disorders, including bulimia or anorexia nervosa, which are contraindications to the combination oral medication that you want to prescribe. In addition, this medication carries a black box warning for which of the following conditions?

- A.   Congenital defects
- **B.   Suicidal ideation**
- C.   Medullary thyroid carcinoma
- D.   Pancreatitis
- E.   Ventricular arrhythmia

(B) Naltrexone/bupropion ER is the only long-term, anti-obesity medication contraindicated in patients with eating disorders such as bulimia or anorexia nervosa due to the increased seizure risk. In addition, this medication carries a black box warning for **increased suicide risk in young adults.**

Naltrexone/Bupropion ER (Contrave®)	
Dose	8 mg naltrexone/90 mg bupropion Tablet Week 1: Take one tablet daily in AM Week 2: Take one tablet twice daily Week 3: Take 2 tablets in AM, 1 tablet in PM Week 4: Take 2 tablets twice daily
Mechanism	Weak inhibitor of neuronal reuptake of dopamine and norepinephrine (not fully understood), affecting the hypothalamus (appetite) and reward system.
Contraindications	Hypersensitivity to bupropion or naltrexone, uncontrolled hypertension, seizure disorder, history of seizures, risk of seizures (bulimia, anorexia nervosa, alcohol or benzo withdrawal, etc.), chronic opioid use, pregnancy, concurrent use of MAO-I *Risk of suicide in young adults (black box warning)
Side Effects	Headache, nausea/vomiting, constipation, sleep disorder, dizziness

Reference: Naltrexone/bupropion ER package insert

220. (Content: III-F-4) A female patient meets with her dietician one final time before undergoing a Roux-en-Y gastric bypass. The dietician discusses starting a high-protein, liquid diet two weeks before the surgery. What is the reasoning behind this?

    A. Develop good dietary habits for the postoperative period
    B. To prevent surgical complications from organ injury
    C. Reduce inflammation in the stomach and proximal intestines
    D. Decrease colonic stool burden and risk of an intestinal leak
    E. Increase the total percentage of post-operative weight loss

(B) Most patients are advised to initiate a low-calorie (<1200 kcal/day) diet that is high in protein and low in carbohydrates a few weeks prior to bariatric and metabolic surgery to promote a reduction in liver size. Studies have shown a 15-30% reduction in liver size if initiated 2 to 12 weeks before surgery, with 80% of this reduction occurring within the first two weeks. This decrease in liver size improves intraoperative laparoscopic visualization of vital structures and **decreases mechanical injury to the liver.**

A number of recommendations to reduce intraoperative and post-operate risks after bariatric surgery are made by the American Society for Metabolic and Bariatric Surgery (ASMBS), with some highlights including:

- Smoking cessation is completed at least 6 weeks before surgery
- Avoid post-operative hyperglycemia, although a specific hemoglobin A1c target pre-operatively should not delay surgery.
- Pre-operative nutrition should be optimized with the use of a dietician
- Insurance-mandated weight loss requirements or arbitrary time-based approaches (e.g., 6 months of dieting) pre-operatively is not beneficial.
- Pre-operative weight loss and adherence do not necessarily correlate with postoperative weight loss in the long-term.
- Patients are encouraged to have pre-operative age-appropriate cancer screenings completed before surgery.
- A TSH for screening is not recommended devoid of symptoms.
- Estrogen-containing birth control should be held for one month and hormone replacement therapy three weeks before surgery.

Reference: "ASMBS position statement on preoperative patient optimization before metabolic and bariatric surgery" Jonathan Carter, M.D., Julietta Chang, M.D., T. Javier Birriel, M.D., Fady Moustarah, M.D., et Al. Received 4 May 2021; accepted 27 August 2021

221. (Content: III-G-6) A 47-year-old female presents for a comprehensive metabolic and bariatric surgery consultation. Her BMI has consistently been over 50 kg/m^2 for the past ten years, which she attributes to pregnancies and genetics. She has a family history of endometrial cancer in her mother and prostate cancer in her father. Per the Centers for Disease Control and Prevention (CDC), aggressive weight loss will likely reduce the risk of malignancy affecting which of the following areas?

A. **Thyroid**
B. Lymph nodes
C. Lung
D. Skin
E. Oral

(A) The CDC recognizes 13 malignancies that are increased in the setting of having excess weight (BMI ≥ 25kg/m^2). This is thought to be from the increased inflammatory cytokines, sex hormones, and insulin resistance associated with excess adipose tissue. Of the options, only **thyroid cancer** is listed by the CDC.

The 13 types of cancers listed by the CDC make up 40% of cancers in the United States, with others likely being added to the list following ongoing research. It is estimated that excess weight accounts for 11% of cancers in females, 5% in males, and contributes to 7% of cancer-related deaths.

Interestingly, from 2005-2014 cancers not associated with obesity decreased (by 13%), whereas those found to have an association with excess weight increased by 7% (excluding colorectal cancer). This is consistent with an overall elevation in BMI in the United States during this period.

Malignancies Associated with an Elevated BMI	
Breast (post-menopausal)	Pancreas
Colorectal	Ovaries
Esophageal[2] (adenocarcinoma)	Multiple myeloma
Gallbladder	Meningioma
Stomach (upper)	Uterus[1]
Kidneys	Thyroid
Liver	

[1]Endometrial cancer has a 7x relative risk (highest) in those with obesity compared to normal weight
[2]Esophageal cancer has a 4.8x relative risk (second highest)

Reference: CDC: Obesity and Cancer. (Accessed 12/18/2023)
Reference: American Cancer Society: Does Body Weight Affect Cancer Risk?

222. (Content: III-D-2 and 9) A 6-year-old male presents to a geneticist after he is found to have hyperphagia. Testing reveals that pro-insulin levels are increased. The child's BMI is 150% of the 95th percentile. Genetic testing returns positive for a variant of the proprotein convertase subtilisin/Kexin type 1 (PCSK1) gene. Which of the following should be administered to this child?

A. Amylin analogs
B. Metreleptin
C. Semaglutide
D. Setmelanotide
E. Gastric inhibitory polypeptide

(D) This patient has an abnormal PCSK1 gene that is likely contributing to his severely increased BMI and hyperphagia. **Setmelanotide** is approved for patients ≥ 6 years old with pathogenic POMC, PCSK1, or LEPR genetic defects and, as of 2022, Bardet-Biedl syndrome (BBS).

Note: Genetic testing for obesity should be considered in those with early-onset (≤ 5 years old) hyperphagia and obesity with or without intellectual disability.

The PCSK1 gene encodes for a convertase that cleaves many active peptide hormones involved in regulating energy, hunger, and energy homeostasis. Variants or deficiencies of this gene can lead to a variety of endocrinopathies. Initially, this presents as an infant with intestinal malabsorption (1st year of life) followed by hyperphagia and obesity.

Setmelanotide (Imcivree®)	
Indications	Chronic weight management in those with genetically confirmed pathogenic proopiomelanocortin (POMC), proprotein convertase subtilisin/kexin type 1 (PCSK1) genes, or leptin receptor (LEPR) deficiency, and BBS.
Mechanism	Melanocortin 4 (MC4) receptor agonist
Contraindications	None currently listed
Significant Adverse Effects	New or worsening depression or suicidal ideation, increased sexual arousal (labial hypersensitivity and priapism), and skin hyperpigmentation

Reference: Setmelanotide package inserts.
Reference: Ramos-Molina B, Martin MG, Lindberg I. PCSK1 Variants and Human Obesity. Prog Mol Biol Transl Sci. 2016;140:47-74. doi:10.1016/bs.pmbts.2015.12.001

223. (Content: III-G-5) A 33-year-old female presents for a pre-operative consultation with a desire to undergo a Roux-en-Y gastric bypass. She is concerned as she states that she has been on buprenorphine-naloxone for the past five years due to a history of intravenous heroin use. Since stopping heroin, she has had a steady increase in weight, and her current BMI is 41 kg/m². She has an accountability partner, has been sober for the past five years, and is now counseling others on the effects of substance use. Which of the following statements is accurate to present?

A. A history of substance use is a contraindication to surgery
B. Buprenorphine-naloxone must be stopped prior to surgery
C. **The risk of alcohol use disorder is increased after surgery**
D. An underlying eating disorder will improve after surgery
E. Weekly urine drug screens will ensure adherence after surgery

(C) Patients undergoing bariatric and metabolic surgery should be thoroughly screened for underlying eating disorders, maladaptive eating patterns, substance use, and alcohol use disorder. After surgery, patients **are at an increased risk of alcohol use disorder,** likely due to rapid absorption of alcohol leading to immediate gratification and transference addiction. Active substance use is a contraindication for surgery. Those with risk factors or a history of this should be managed/monitored by addiction specialists. Also, those with maladaptive eating disorders are likely to have less success unless treatment is initiated pre-operatively. A psychosocial evaluation for substance use, maladaptive eating patterns, and alcohol use is vital prior to surgery.

Note: In patients taking buprenorphine-naloxone, the naloxone portion is not orally bioavailable nor absorbed through the skin (transdermal patches). Thus, it is only added as a deterrent to injecting the medication by blocking the partial agonist effects of buprenorphine and preventing any euphoric effects. Therefore, it would not be contraindicated in the setting of surgery.

Reference: "ASMBS position statement on preoperative patient optimization before metabolic and bariatric surgery" Jonathan Carter, M.D., Julietta Chang, M.D., T. Javier Birriel, M.D., Fady Moustarah, M.D., et Al. Received 4 May 2021; accepted 27 August 2021
Reference: Buprenorphine-naloxone Package insert

224. (Content: III-A-1) A 32-year-old female is being evaluated by psychiatry before bariatric surgery. During the interview, the patient understands the risks and benefits of the planned gastric sleeve but shows a lack of motivation to maintain the dietary and exercise changes. The patient is asked to write a list of potential pitfalls or concerns the patient has regarding maintaining weight postoperatively. What key process of motivational interviewing is being displayed?

    A. Engagement
    B. Focusing
    C. Evoking
    D. Planning

(B) The psychiatrist is using the key process of motivational interviewing of **focusing,** in which the physician helps the patient identify their areas of ambivalence or potential struggles to begin setting goals accordingly. In addition to focusing, the other key processes include:

- **Engagement:** Establishing a therapeutic relationship (displaying empathy, acceptance, etc.) and utilizing OARS[1].
- **Evoking:** Discovering the patient's interest and motivation to change and being able to use these to reach their goals. Listening for words (DARN[2]) to cue you in that the patient is ready for changes.
- **Planning:** Assisting the patient in making short and long-term goals and providing appropriate follow-up and guidance.

Motivational interviewing is a patient-centered technique that promotes change talk, which focuses on changing the patient's speech and actions from maintaining the status quo (sustain talk) to a direction of change.

One technique to incorporate change talk (and avoid sustain talk) is utilizing the importance ruler or readiness scale:

- On a scale of 1-10, how ready are you to _____?
    - Followed by: Why not a lower number?
    - Avoid asking why it is not a higher number

[1]**OARS: O**pen-ended questions, **A**ffirmation, **R**eflection, and **S**ummarize
[2]**DARN: D**esire, **A**bility, **R**easons, and **N**eed to change

Reference: Obesity Medicine Association: Obesity Algorithm (2023)

225. (Content: III-F-1 and 2) A multi-disciplinary weight management center has recently added the TransPyloric Shuttle (TPS)® to its list of options for weight loss. What is true regarding this device?

    A. It is best for those with significant BMI levels as a bridge to surgery
    B. It can only be kept in place for six months maximum
    C. It is safe in pregnancy, although it must be removed before birth
    D. Patients must be on chronic acid suppression while device is in place
    E. Bowel obstruction is the most common adverse side effect

(D) TPS® is an endoscopically placed weight loss device that was FDA-approved in 2019. It uses a removable gastric bulb to affect the flow of food content through the stomach. Patients should be started on a **proton pump inhibitor** to reduce the risk of gastroesophageal tissue injuries.

- **Indications:** Adults with class I obesity with ≥ 1 obesity comorbidity or class II obesity, in conjunction with lifestyle modifications.
- **Contraindications:** Altered upper gastrointestinal anatomy such as a stricture or prior surgery, esophageal varices, erosions, ulcerations, untreated *H. pylori* infections, gastritis, pregnancy, and coagulopathy.
- **Duration:** The device must be removed after 12 months.
- **Effectiveness:** In the trial, 66% (vs 30% placebo) lost 5% of their weight, with an average of 9.3% total body weight loss (vs 2.8% placebo).

The larger smooth bulb ❶ of the TPS® sits in the stomach, while the small bulb ❷ is free to move into the proximal duodenum. This results in slowed gastric transit of food content ❸.

226. (Content: III-D-1) A 29-year-old female presents for a two-month follow-up appointment after her initial obesity medicine consultation. At the prior appointment, her medroxyprogesterone injection was discussed as being weight-positive. She was started on tirzepatide to assist in weight loss. She has since changed to an oral estrogen-progesterone contraceptive pill and is tolerating the tirzepatide well. Which lab finding may occur within the next year if her current medications are not addressed?

    A. Increased renin levels
    B. Hypokalemia
    C. Increased urine anion gap
    D. Hypoglycemia
    E. Positive urine HCG

(E) Tirzepatide is a dual incretin with both gastric inhibitory peptide and glucagon-like peptide-1 receptor agonist mechanisms. Both of these medications decrease the transit time of the stomach and intestines and therefore, can affect the efficacy of oral contraceptives. Thus, the manufacturer recommends adding barrier protection within four weeks of any increased dose of tirzepatide to prevent pregnancy **(positive urine HCG).** Non-oral routes of birth control are not affected.

Tirzepatide has also been associated with an increased risk of fetal and maternal harm. Not only does oral birth control becomes less effective, but patients who lose weight have a higher chance of becoming pregnant. Therefore, recommendations when using tirzepatide in women of child-bearing age include:

- Using barrier protection if on oral contraceptives within four weeks of any increased dose of tirzepatide.
- Switching to non-oral options, including intra-uterine devices or progestin implants
- Although medroxyprogesterone injections are not affected by tirzepatide, they can cause significant weight increases.

Reference: Tirzepatide package insert

227. (Content: III-G-7) A 21-year-old female is having frequent migraines leading to missed days of work. Most headaches last up to two days and she has approximately eight debilitating headaches per month. She has tried NSAIDs and sumatriptan for abortive therapy and topiramate and propranolol for prevention. None of these have been effective. Recent head imaging was normal. She does not want to start on medications that will cause weight gain. Which is the best pharmacologic treatment for this patient?

    A. Atenolol
    B. Amitriptyline
    C. Acetazolamide
    D. Erenumab
    E. Valproic acid

(D) Being aware of newer therapies for comorbidities that do not cause weight gain can improve the quality of our patient's lives and prevent complications (first, do no harm). Many migraine medications cause weight gain, but the newer monoclonal antibodies, such as **erenumab** that antagonize calcitonin gene-related peptide (CGRP) receptor function are very effective and weight neutral.

Erenumab is a once-monthly subcutaneous injection used for the prevention of migraines. Another CGRP antagonist, rimegepant is used for both prevention and acute abortive migraine therapy, whereas ubrogepant is currently only approved for abortive therapy.

Migraine Medications		
Weight Positive	**Weight Neutral**	**Weight Negative**
-Valproic acid -Propranolol and atenolol -Amitriptyline	-NSAIDs -Triptans -CGRP antagonists -Botox injections	-Topiramate -Zonisamide

Weight effects are generalizations and may be based solely on observational trials and vary depending on dosing, treatment duration, and medication indications. Weight variability may be seen.
Note: Children/adolescents have more significant weight gain than adults with obesogenic medications

Reference: Obesity Medicine Association: Obesity Algorithm (2023)
Reference: Erenumab package insert

228. (Content: III-G-3) A 34-year-old male with a past medical history of anxiety and diabetes presents to his primary care physician two years after undergoing a sleeve gastrectomy. He initially lost 60 lbs (27.2 kg) within the first year, but then over this past year, he has slowly regained approximately 30 lbs (13.6 kg). Medications include metformin, detemir, and fluoxetine. He does admit to nonadherence with his recommended daily vitamins but continues to exercise three times weekly. Given these findings, which of the following most likely explains his postoperative weight regain?

A. Dilated gastric pouch
B. Excess insulin administration
C. **Dietary indiscretion**
D. Psychologic issues
E. Vitamin deficiencies

(C) Insufficient weight loss or weight regain after bariatric surgery is not uncommon. There can be many etiologies (some listed above). By far, the most common cause is behavioral-mediated and not surgical-related. Behavioral reasons for weight gain **include lack of dietary control** (i.e., snacking), nonadherence with calorie restriction recommendations, lack of exercise, or increased psychosocial stressors. Also, undiagnosed eating disorders can play a role.

Note: Patients that are aware that behavioral modifications are just as crucial after surgery as they were before surgery often have improved success.

Important post-surgical lifestyle modifications include the following:

- Frequent follow-up with an obesity medicine specialist, dietician, and surgeon
- Support groups
- Continued physical activity
- Calorie monitoring and vitamin supplementation

Reference: Up to Date: "Bariatric surgery: Postoperative and long-term management of the uncomplicated patient"

229. (Content: III-G-6) A 49-year-old female who was recently widowed after her husband had complications from obesity presents to her family medicine physician for weight loss counseling. Her BMI is 42 kg/m^2, and she has a past medical history of hypertension, diabetes, and asthma. Comprehensive lifestyle changes are discussed. What is a reasonable weight loss goal, in terms of total body loss, for this patient within the next six months, according to the "2013 ACC/AHA/TOS Guidelines for the Management of Overweight and Obesity in Adults"?

A. 0-5%
B. 5-10%
C. 10-15%
D. 15-20%

(B) The expert panel recommends an initial weight loss goal **of 5-10% of baseline weight** within six months, as this more substantial weight loss produces more significant benefits. **Note:** The NIH determined the earliest cardiovascular benefits were seen with weight loss of only 2.5% with improved glycemic measures and triglycerides, whereas blood pressure, HDL, and LDL improvements required at least 5%.

Weight loss (WL) goals, in which improvements in obesity-related conditions are seen, according to the 2016 AACE/ACE guidelines, are summarized below.

Condition		% WL Goals
• Type 2 diabetes • Dyslipidemia[1]	• Hypertension • PCOS[2]	5% - ≥ 15%
• Metabolic syndrome[2] • Osteoarthritis • GERD	• Prediabetes[2] • Female infertility	≥ 10%
Metabolic-associated fatty liver disease:	• Steatosis • Steatohepatitis	5% or more 10%-40%
• Male hypogonadism	• Stress incontinence	5% - ≥ 10%
• Asthma	• OSA	≥ 7 %

[1]Benefits begin at 2.5% WL for triglycerides only; [2]Benefits being at 2.5%
PCOS: Polycystic ovarian syndrome; **GERD:** Gastroesophageal reflux disease; **OSA:** Obstructive sleep apnea

Reference: AACE/ACE Guidelines (2016). Table 8
Reference: 2013 AHA/ACC/TOS Guideline for the Management of Overweight and Obesity in Adults. A Report of the American College of Cardiology/American Heart Association Task Force on Practice Guidelines and The Obesity Society. Box 9.
Reference: Ryan DH, Yockey SR. Weight Loss and Improvement in Comorbidity: Differences at 5%, 10%, 15%, and Over. Curr Obes Rep. 2017 Jun;6(2):187-194. doi: 10.1007/s13679-017-0262-y. PMID: 28455679

230. (Content: III-F-4) A 33-year-old female with a past medical history of class III obesity, diabetes type 2, tobacco abuse, and polycystic ovarian syndrome presents for a bariatric evaluation. She is interested in a "gastric bypass." Her medications include metformin, oral contraceptive birth control, and a prenatal vitamin. After a thorough history and physical examination, you discuss preoperative recommendations, including a physical activity plan and healthy dietary patterns. What other perioperative education would be necessary for this patient?

A. Avoid becoming pregnant for at least 6 months after surgery
B. Birth control must be discontinued 1 week before surgery
C. Her hemoglobin A1c should be less than 9% preoperatively
D. Metformin is contraindicated after Roux-en-Y gastric bypass
E. **Tobacco products must be stopped 6 weeks before surgery**

(E) Tobacco use should be stopped as soon as possible, preferably one year preoperatively, but at a **minimum of six weeks before surgery**, due to the increased risk of poor wound healing and anastomotic ulcers.

Note: In women, pregnancy should be avoided preoperatively and 12-18 months postoperatively. Estrogen birth control should be stopped 1 cycle before surgery to prevent deep venous thrombosis (pre-menopausal).

Reasonable preoperative glycemic targets, which are associated with shorter hospital stays and improved bariatric procedure outcomes, include:

- HbA1c goal of 6.5-7% and peri-procedure glucose 80-180 mg/dL
- HbA1c goal of 7-8% is recommended in those with advanced micro/macrovascular complications, those with many comorbid conditions, or long-standing/difficult-to-control diabetes.
- Clinical judgment must be used if A1c is > 8%

*Metformin can be used postoperatively but should be converted to immediate release to improve absorption.

Reference: AACE/TOS/ASMBS/OMA/ASA 2019 Guidelines: CLINICAL PRACTICE GUIDELINES FOR THE PERIOPERATIVE NUTRITION, METABOLIC, AND NONSURGICAL SUPPORT OF PATIENTS UNDERGOING BARIATRIC PROCEDURES – 2019 UPDATE. Recommendation 14, 17, 18, 23

231. (Content: III-D-8) A 24-year-old female presents to her primary care physician's office for an evaluation regarding weight gain. She states she has been exercising five times weekly for approximately 30 minutes during her sessions. She has decreased her calories to 1200 kcal daily, focusing on a low-fat diet, but she still has noticed a 10 lb (4.5 kg) weight gain in the past year. Medical history includes bipolar disease, which is well-controlled on aripiprazole. Previous laboratory work was within normal limits, including HbA1c, thyroid stimulating hormone, and complete metabolic panel. Which would be the most effective in treating her weight gain?

A. **Prescribe metformin**
B. Prescribe orlistat
C. Intensify calorie restrictions
D. Change aripiprazole to olanzapine
E. Intensify exercise regimen

(A) This patient is experiencing antipsychotic-related weight gain, of which **metformin** is proven effective (off-label), with lots of supporting data. Metformin is commonly used (often off-label) in settings of insulin resistance, including polycystic ovarian syndrome, fatty liver disease, HIV protease inhibitor-associated lipodystrophy, and pre-diabetes.

Note: Aripiprazole is the least obesogenic antipsychotic medication and is preferred if a medication from this class is required.

Metformin	
Dose	Increase gradually. Maximum dose 1000 mg BID
Mechanism	-Decreases hepatic glucose production -Reduces intestinal absorption of glucose -Improves insulin sensitivity (peripheral utilization)
Contraindications	Hypersensitivity to metformin, eGFR < 30 mL/min, acute or chronic metabolic acidosis *Black box warning: Lactic acidosis (risk factors include age > 65 years old, contrasted studies, renal failure, hypoxia, concurrent topiramate use, and significant alcohol use, etc.)
Side effects	Gastrointestinal distress: abdominal pain, nausea, vomiting, and diarrhea

Reference: Metformin package insert.
Reference: Baptista 2007; Chen 2013; Das 2012; de Silva 2016; Jarskog 2013; Wang 2012; Zheng 2015

232. (Content: III-H-3) A 12-year-old female who has struggled with obesity for the past five years is presenting to a bariatric center for a vertical sleeve gastrectomy evaluation. She has hypertension and severe obstructive sleep apnea that did not respond to tonsillectomy. She is sexually active and developmentally is at a Tanner stage 3. Her BMI is currently 37 kg/m². Psychiatry evaluation reveals mild depression and a lack of understanding of the risks regarding the surgical procedure. Which of the following is a contraindication for this adolescent to undergo bariatric surgery?

A. Tanner stage
B. Body mass index
C. Sexual activity
D. Depression
E. Risk appreciation

(E) This adolescent who has decision-making capacity may be a candidate for bariatric surgery if she fully understands and **acknowledges the risks** associated with surgery. Any lack of insight or motivation that would interfere with the postoperative treatment is a contraindication to pediatric bariatric surgery.

Surgery indications, contraindications, and complications in adolescents largely mirror those of adults desiring to undergo surgery. Contraindications include ongoing substance use or a recent history of use (within 1 year), hospitalization for self-harm or psychiatric conditions within the past 12 months, medically correctable causes of obesity, current or planned pregnancy within 12-18 months after surgery, any condition (medical, psychiatric, psychosocial, or cognitive) that prevents adherence to the post-operative regimen. Importantly, this does not mean that a patient with cognitive impairment cannot have the surgery, but rather they would require an adequate support system to assist with following recommendations.

Note: Pubertal status or physical maturity (Tanner stage or bone age) are no longer included in determining surgical candidacy. The initial theory that rapid weight loss after surgery would inhibit linear bone growth has not been proven.

Reference: Pratt JSA, Browne A, Browne NT, et al. ASMBS pediatric metabolic and bariatric surgery guidelines, 2018. Surg Obes Relat Dis. 2018;14(7):882-901. doi:10.1016/j.soard.2018.03.019

233. (Content: III-F-5b) A 28-year-old female is presenting to her primary care physician's office six months after undergoing laparoscopic adjustable gastric banding (LAGB). She states two weeks ago, she had eaten too quickly, with subsequent nausea and vomiting. Since then, she has been unable to keep solids down and will regurgitate undigested food after small meals. In addition, her acid reflux has significantly worsened during this time. Which of the following is the next best step in management?

    A. CT of the abdomen
    B. Remove fluid from the band
    C. Surgical revision
    D. Dietary changes
    E. Start omeprazole

(B) This patient's findings of nausea, vomiting, inability to tolerate solids, and worsening acid reflux is most consistent with the diagnosis of band slippage. This complication occurs in up to 5% of LABG. It may present with either loss of food restriction or an inability to pass food. The **initial step is to completely remove the fluid through the port,** thereby eliminating the restriction. Surgery may be indicated if this fails to relieve symptoms.

Note: Another potential complication after LABG that must be considered is an erosion, which may be asymptomatic and present as a loss of food restriction or present with findings of pain or infection at the port site.

Other complications of LAGB are discussed in the table below.

Complications of Laparoscopic Adjustable Gastric Banding	
Short-Term (30 Days)	**Long-Term**
-Death (1:1000)	-Band slippage (3-5%)
-Anastomotic leak (0.2%)	-Gastric pouch dilation (3-5%)
-Infection (1%)	-Erosion (1%)
-DVT/PE (1%)	-Port issue (2-5%)
-Dehydration (1%)	-Need for revision/removal (25%)

DVT: Deep venous thrombosis; **PE:** Pulmonary embolism

Reference: AACE/TOS/ASMBS/OMA/ASA 2019 Guidelines: CLINICAL PRACTICE GUIDELINES FOR THE PERIOPERATIVE NUTRITION, METABOLIC, AND NONSURGICAL SUPPORT OF PATIENTS UNDERGOING BARIATRIC PROCEDURES – 2019 UPDATE. Recommendation 78
Reference: Obesity Medicine Association: Obesity Algorithm (2023)

234. (Content: III-D-7 and III-G-3) A 35-year-old female presents for follow-up three years after undergoing a sleeve gastrectomy. She states she had significant weight loss within the first year post-operatively but has since plateaued in her weight, approximately 30 lbs (13.6 kg) short of her goal. She has followed all recommendations but admits to an increased appetite. She would like to discuss anti-obesity medications to assist in helping with reaching her goals. Which of the following is the most appropriate recommendation to provide?

A. Weight-loss medications are contraindicated after bariatric surgery
B. Cellulose and citric acid hydrogel is preferred post-operatively
C. Revision surgery is most appropriate to reach your target weight
D. Body contouring surgery will likely allow you to reach your goal
E. **Starting semaglutide and phentermine will reduce weight**

(E) This patient has undergone successful bariatric and metabolic surgery but has plateaued prior to her weight-loss goals. Anti-obesity medications are an appropriate option to discuss at this visit. Most patients will plateau by the first year, and additional weight loss requires intensifying lifestyle modifications and/or the addition of weight loss medications. In this patient, **starting semaglutide and phentermine** will likely help reduce appetite and increase POMC/CART pathway activation, assisting in meeting her goals.

Anti-obesity medications are not only safe after bariatric surgery but are effective. These options should be considered for those who do not meet goals or have weight regain after surgery. Other options include:

- Surgical revisions, such as converting to another metabolic surgery (e.g., single anastomosis duodeno–ileal bypass with sleeve gastrectomy) can be considered depending on desired and starting weight.
- A close review of dietary habits and physical activity is important.
- Psychiatric evaluation should be considered to ensure any underlying eating disorders did not become uncovered or developed.

Finally, cellulose and citric acid hydrogel should be avoided in those with altered gastrointestinal anatomy due to the increased risk of obstruction.

Reference: Redmond IP, Shukla AP, Aronne LJ. Use of Weight Loss Medications in Patients after Bariatric Surgery. Curr Obes Rep. 2021 Jun;10(2):81-89. doi: 10.1007/s13679-021-00425-1. Epub 2021 Jan 25. PMID: 33492629.

235. (Content: III-F-6) A 13-year-old female presents to her pediatrician for continued weight gain. Her BMI is 140% of the 95th percentile range, remaining consistent over the past year despite lifestyle changes. Recent lab work displayed an ALT level of 48 U/L (reference range: 8–20 U/L) and an HbA1c of 6.9% (reference range: <5.7%). She continues to snore at night despite a tonsillectomy last year. Which of the following would be the most appropriate action to provide the best long-term health benefits for this patient?

A. **Offer referral for metabolic and bariatric surgery now**
B. Start the patient on metformin
C. Initiate a six-month trial of dietary modifications
D. Prescribe pioglitazone for metabolic liver disease
E. Initiate a staged approach to treating obesity

(A) For this patient with clinical findings supporting diabetes, obstructive sleep apnea, metabolic-associated fatty liver disease, and class III obesity, aggressive management focused on long-term mortality benefits includes anti-obesity medication and **metabolic and bariatric surgery (MBS)** adjunctively with intensive health behavior and lifestyle treatment.

Recent pediatric guidelines replaced the prior staged approach to obesity which delayed pharmacologic and surgical treatment options for months/years as the patient progressed through different tiers of intensities of staged treatment, which lacked evidence supporting better results. Current treatment guidelines focus on providing early and advanced treatments based on the clinical presentation, more closely mirroring the treatment of adults.

Children and adolescents will carry obesity-associated comorbidities into adulthood without appropriate treatment intervention, leading to premature mortality. Therefore, the American Academy of Pediatrics and the ASMBS recommend consideration of MBS in children/adolescents with:

- Class II obesity: BMI >120% of the 95th percentile or BMI ≥ 35 kg/m^2 with a major co-morbidity
- Class III obesity: BMI >140% of the 95th percentile or BMI ≥ 40 kg/m^2

Reference: 2022 American Society for Metabolic and Bariatric Surgery (ASMBS) and International Federation for the Surgery of Obesity and Metabolic Disorders (IFSO): Indications for Metabolic and Bariatric Surgery. Published: October 20, 2022 DOI: https://doi.org/10.1016/j.soard.2022.08.013
Reference: Hampl, S. E., Hassink, S. G., Skinner, A. C., Armstrong, S. C., Barlow, S. E., Bolling, C. F., ... Okechukwu, K. (2023). Clinical Practice Guideline for the Evaluation and Treatment of Children and Adolescents With Obesity. Pediatrics, 151(2), e2022060640. https://doi.org/10.1542/peds.2022-060640.

236. (Content: III-H-2) A mother brings her 12-year-old daughter to her primary health care provider for evaluation of anti-obesity medications. Despite seeing a dietician and trainer, monitoring caloric intake, and undergoing intensive health behavior and lifestyle treatment she has not improved her growth chart curve. Genetic testing was negative and she has no other medical conditions. She is interested in pharmacotherapy. Which of the following is the most appropriate FDA-approved medication for this indication?

A. Tirzepatide
B. Metformin
C. Phentermine
D. Semaglutide
E. Setmelanotide

(D) Primary health care providers may offer children with obesity pharmacotherapy through shared decision-making as an adjunct to lifestyle modifications. Despite this patient's efforts, she has not had success with adequate weight loss and advanced options such as pharmacotherapy may be indicated. Of the options given her age and negative genetic testing, **semaglutide** is the only option FDA-approved as an anti-obesity medicine.

Note: Many medications are safely used off-label for obesity management.

More medications are being approved to assist with weight loss in younger age ranges. Setmelanotide is only approved for certain genetic condition, while the others listed below can be used in anyone with an obesity indication.

FDA-Approved Anti-Obesity Medications and Approved Ages	
Medication	**Age**
Setmelanotide	6
Orlistat	12
Liraglutide (3.0 mg daily; Saxenda®)	12
Semaglutide (2.4 mg weekly; Wegovy®)	12
Phentermine/topiramate ER	12
Phentermine (3 months maximum)	16
Naltrexone/bupropion ER	18
Tirzepatide (Zepbound®)	18

Reference: Obesity Medicine Association: Pediatric Obesity Algorithm (2023-2024)
Reference: Package insert of anti-obesity medications

237. (Content: III-G-6) A 41-year-old female with class III obesity and depression is diagnosed with severe obstructive sleep apnea after completing a polysomnography. Since diagnosis, she has been adherent to her continuous positive airway pressure. She retakes the STOPBANG score and compares it to her score before she initiated treatment and notices that it has decreased by 1 point. Which STOPBANG component most likely improved?

A. Body mass index
B. Daytime somnolence
C. Blood pressure
D. Depression
E. Neck circumference

(B) Patients treated for obstructive sleep apnea (OSA) often will experience marked improvements in **daytime somnolence** which corresponds to improvements in this area on the STOPBANG score as well as the Epworth Sleepiness score. Other areas of improvement seen after treatment include blood pressure, erectile dysfunction (males), gastroesophageal reflux symptoms, quality of life, and even less risk of motor vehicle accidents.

In regard to the incorrect options:

- Depression: Effects on mood and mortality are unclear and depression is not on the STOPBANG scoring.
- Body mass index: Although treated OSA contributes to improved hormone levels (i.e. ghrelin, leptin), the effects on weight have been variable. In addition, even with some weight loss, the STOPBANG scores 1 point if the BMI is > 35kg/m². This patient with class III obesity (BMI ≥ 40 kg/m²) will not experience a decrease in BMI by 5 points with CPAP therapy alone. This is similar reasoning for the neck circumference.
- Although systolic and diastolic blood pressure improve, on average this correlates to less than 3 mmHg, which would not alter the STOPBANG question of "Do you have, or are you being treated for, high blood pressure?"

Finally, CPAP therapy had no significant effect on reducing hemoglobin A1c, hospitalization risk, or neurocognitive function.

Reference: da Silva Paulitsch F, Zhang L. Continuous positive airway pressure for adults with obstructive sleep apnea and cardiovascular disease: a meta-analysis of randomized trials. Sleep Med. 2019 Feb;54:28-34. doi: 10.1016/j.sleep.2018.09.030. Epub 2018 Oct 30. PMID: 30529774.

238. (Content: III-F) A 29-year-old female presents to a gastroenterologist to learn more about endoscopic sleeve gastroplasty, as she admits to a strong phobia of abdominal surgeries. In terms of hormone changes after surgery, this procedure is most similar to which of the following?

    A. Sleeve gastrectomy
    B. Laparoscopic adjustable gastric banding
    C. Roux-en-Y gastric bypass
    D. Single anastomosis duodenal-ileal bypass with sleeve gastrectomy

(B) Endoscopic sleeve gastroplasty (ESG) is efficacious by slowing gastric emptying, increasing satiety, and reducing caloric intake without altering hormone levels. Therefore, it is considered a purely restrictive procedure, similar in nature to **laparoscopic adjustable gastric banding.** With ESG, patients lost an average of 13% total body weight loss that was sustained over 2 years.

Indications: There are no definitive BMI indications, although most studies included a BMI between 30-40 kg/m^2, with sparse data for < 30 or > 40 kg/m^2. Similarly, there were no definitive age cut-offs. It may be preferred in those wanting to avoid abdominal surgery or higher-risk patients.

Contraindications: The recommended absolute contraindications include gastric ulcers in the body or fundus, congestive gastropathy, gastric or esophageal varices, gastric polyposis, and uncontrolled psychiatric disease.

ESG is an endoscopic plication procedure, in which the stomach is plicated with sutures **1**, thus reducing the stomach size **2**.

Image citation: Image created by Charu G. Copyright owned by Kevin Smith, DO
Reference: ASMBS Guidelines/statements: Endoscopic sleeve gastroplasty and its role in the treatment of obesity: a systematic review. Docimo, S. Jr., Aylward, L., Albaugh, V. L., Afaneh, C., El Djouzi, S., Ali, M., Altieri, M. S., & Carter, J. (2023). DOI: https://doi.org/10.1016/j.soard.2023.08.020

239. (Content: III-C-1) A patient meets with a personal trainer to discuss exercise options. Her father recently passed away unexpectedly in the setting of heart disease, so she wants to be proactive and begin exercising. She enjoys numerous activities but would prefer outdoor activities. An exercise prescription is written to include performing resistance training two days per week. In addition, the prescription includes performing an outdoor activity of moderate intensity for 30 minutes, five days weekly. Which of the following activities would qualify for this exercise prescription?

    A. Walking at 2 miles per hour
    B. Playing singles tennis
    C. Bicycling at 8 miles per hour
    D. Jogging at 5 miles per hour
    E. Swimming laps

(C) Moderate-intensity activities include activities that are between 3 to 6 metabolic equivalents (METS), which includes brisk walking (2.5- 4 MPH), playing tennis, recreational swimming, and **bicycling less than 10 MPH.**

Note: Be familiar with the activities and their MET values. Numerous exercise questions will be seen on the examination!

Intensity	METs Exerted	Examples
Light	< 3.0	• Walking at a slow pace (≤ 2 MPH) • Cooking • Light household chores
Moderate	3.0 – 6.0	• Walking briskly (2.5 - 4 MPH) • Playing doubles tennis • Raking the yard • Recreational swimming • Ballroom dancing • Bicycling < 10 MPH
Vigorous	≥ 6.0	• Jogging/running • Bicycling > 10 MPH • Strenuous fitness class • Tennis (singles) • High-intensity interval training • Vigorous dancing • Swimming laps

Reference: Physical Activity Guidelines for Americans: 2nd Edition:
https://health.gov/sites/default/files/2019- 09/Physical_Activity_Guidelines_2nd_edition.pdf

240. (Content: III-B-1) A 59-year-old male is interested in initiating the exchange diet into his daily routine. He plans to eliminate one of his snacks daily and substitute two servings of vegetables for his two starches.

American Diabetes Association Exchange Servings				
1 Serving	Protein	Carbohydrate	Fat	Calories
Starches	3 g	15 g	<1 g	80 kcal
Vegetables	2 g	5 g	0 g	25 kcal
Fat	0 g	0 g	0 g	45 kcal
Fruit	0 g	15 g	0 g	60 kcal
Dairy	8 g	15 g	0-8 g	90-150 kcal
Protein	7 g	0 g	2-5 g	55-75 kcal
Snacks	3 g	15 g	0-1 g	80 kcal

How many daily calories will he reduce by making these changes?

A. 80 kcal/day
B. 130 kcal/day
C. 190 kcal/day
D. 240 kcal/day
E. 270 kcal/day

(C) The American Diabetes Association created the exchange diet as a way for a patient to reduce their carbohydrate intake by exchanging one food for another. In this example, the patient is eliminating 1 snack (80 kcal and 15 g of carbohydrates) and exchanging 2 starches (80 kcal and 15g of carbohydrate each) for 2 vegetables (25 kcal and 5g of carbohydrates each). Thus, every day he is eliminating 80 kcal (snack) + {160 kcal (2 starches) – 50 kcal (2 vegetables)} = **190 kcal/day and 35 g of carbohydrates.**

Note: You will not be required to memorize these values, although you should know 1 serving of fruit is 60 kcal.

The idea of an exchange diet is to group foods together according to their nutritional value. A list of foods that constitute a serving is available and is useful for those who desire to substitute a food choice that may be higher in carbohydrates and calories for one that is lower.

Reference: Gray A, Threlkeld RJ. Nutritional Recommendations for Individuals with Diabetes. [Updated 2019 Oct 13]. In: Feingold KR, Anawalt B, Boyce A, et al., editors. Endotext [Internet]. South Dartmouth (MA): MDText.com, Inc.; 2000-. Available from: https://www.ncbi.nlm.nih.gov/books/NBK279012/

241. (Content: III-G-7) A 19-year-old female presents to her obstetrician to discuss options for birth control. She wants to maintain a healthy weight, given her family history of diabetes and early-onset coronary artery disease. She is sexually active and does not want to become pregnant. Which of the following is associated with the most weight gain?

    A. Intrauterine device
    B. Barrier method
    C. Progesterone-only pill
    D. Etonogestrel implant
    E. Progesterone depo injections

(E) Many birth control options are considered weight-neutral, including most options above, except for **medroxyprogesterone.** This quarterly intramuscular progesterone-only injection is great for preventing pregnancy but notorious for causing weight gain.

Weight gain for medroxyprogesterone is reported to occur in up to 38% of females and is the most common cause of discontinuation. Approximately 2 kg (4.4 lbs) was gained within the first year, and nearly double that was seen in subsequent years. Not everyone will experience this weight gain, but it is important to discuss this possibility with patients and provide alternative options if there are no contraindications.

Birth Control Options	
Weight Positive	**Weight Neutral**
-Medroxyprogesterone (Depo-Provera®)	-Intrauterine devices -Barrier methods -Long-acting reversible contraceptives -Progesterone-only pills

Weight effects are generalizations and may be based solely on observational trials and vary depending on dosing, treatment duration, and medication indications. Weight variability may be seen.
Note: Children/adolescents have more significant weight gain than adults with obesogenic medications

Reference: Obesity Medicine Association: Obesity Algorithm (2023)
Reference: Medroxyprogesterone acetate package insert

242. (Content: III-D-5) A 32-year-old male presents to his primary care physician for yellowing of his eyes and noticing increased fatigue. He takes no prescribed medication but does admit to taking a combination herbal supplement for weight loss. Although it is recommended to take twice daily, he has been taking approximately ten daily, and has noticed a 14 lb (6.4 kg) weight loss. AST, ALT, bilirubin, and INR are markedly elevated. Which of the following ingredients in his supplement is most likely contributing to his current condition?

    A. Chitosan
    B. Ephedra
    C. Glucosinolates
    D. Green tea extract
    E. Raspberry ketone

(D) **Green tea extract** is an important and well-known cause of hepatic injury, along with the more common side effects similar to caffeine excess. In general, increased herbal and dietary supplement use is directly proportional to increased hepatotoxicity rates, accounting for nearly 20% of cases within the United States. Anabolic steroids and green tea extract are the most commonly implicated agents.

The other supplements listed above have side effects that include:

- **Chitosan:** Indigestion, bloating, and constipation
- **Glucosinolates:** Goiter and hypothyroidism
- **Raspberry extract:** Significant burping

In addition, the FDA has banned certain supplements, as listed below:

- **Ephedra (mu Huang):** Used to reduce appetite; this is associated with palpitations, myocardial infarctions, stroke, and sudden death.
- **Human chorionic gonadotropin (HCG):** In 2016, the AMA passed a policy that HCG for weight loss is inappropriate. The FDA has mandated a disclaimer describing its lack of efficacy.

Reference: Obesity Medicine Association: Obesity Algorithm (2023)

243. (Content: III-B-2 and III-G-2) A 29-year-old male presents to his dietician after starting a very low-calorie diet. He has done some research and determined that he would like to maintain less than 800 kcal/day and eliminate all fat from his diet. Currently, he is consuming 1300 kcal/day without significant weight loss. The dietician discusses the importance of close monitoring and recommends adding some fat to his diet instead of eliminating it altogether. Without this recommendation, what possible complications could arise?

A. Electrolyte imbalance
B. Gout flares
C. **Cholelithiasis**
D. Electrolyte derangements
E. Cold intolerance

(C) A very low-calorie diet (VLCD) is any diet under 800 kcal/day that requires close monitoring to prevent complications. One complication of eliminating fat and essential fatty acids from the diet is **gallstones.** To prevent this, taking in at least small amounts of fat (10-20 g) is recommended.

In a VLCD, the typical diet consists of a predominance of protein (suppresses hunger), with a target of 1.5 g/kg and 1.2 g/kg ideal body weight in men and women, respectively (average 75-110 g/day). Carbohydrates are usually restricted to 50-100 grams daily, and a fat intake of at least 10-20 g is preferred.

There is little evidence to support that a VLCD is superior to a low-calorie diet (800 -1500 kcal/day), although there are a number of potential complications of a VLCD:

- Electrolyte disturbances, especially sodium and potassium, which require carbohydrates as a cofactor for absorption
- Essential fatty acid deficiency and gallstones
- Gout (often pre-treated with allopurinol)
- Cardiac arrhythmias
- Irritability, depression, apathy, insomnia, and anxiety

Reference: Up to Date: "Obesity in adults: Dietary therapy"
Reference: Weinsier RL, Ullmann DO. Gallstone formation and weight loss. Obes Res. 1993;1(1):51-56. doi:10.1002/j.1550-8528.1993.tb00008.x

244. (Content: III-F-3) A 26-year-old female underwent a one-anastomosis gastric bypass and has since had a persistent burning sensation in her mid-epigastric region. She states that proton pump inhibitors have not helped and sucralfate provided no relief. She denies any other symptoms, including fever, nausea, or vomiting. Endoscopic evaluation reveals no strictures or anastomotic ulcers, and a histologic sample shows mild stomach inflammation. A CT of the abdomen is unremarkable. Which of the following is the most likely cause of her symptoms?

A. Cardiac ischemia
B. **Bile acid gastritis**
C. *H. pylori* infection
D. Recalcitrant acid reflux
E. Esophageal spasm

(B) This patient who underwent a mini-gastric bypass or one-anastomosis gastric bypass, despite a negative endoscopic and CT image evaluation, is most likely experiencing **bile acid gastritis.** Bile reflux occurs near the anastomotic site in approximately 4% of patients undergoing this procedure, with endoscopic (and histologic) findings non-specific, thus making it a diagnosis of exclusion. Treatment often requires conversion to a Roux-en-Y gastric bypass (RYGB).

The one-anastomosis gastric bypass is one of the newer ASMBS-endorsed bariatric and metabolic surgeries (2022), which involves creating a gastric pouch ❶ and anastomosing a loop of the bowel to this pouch ❷. It has similar weight loss and comorbidity improvements when compared to the RYGB.

Image citation: Image created by Charu G. Copyright owned by Kevin Smith, DO
Reference: Chaim EA, Ramos AC, Cazzo E. MINI-GASTRIC BYPASS: DESCRIPTION OF THE TECHNIQUE AND PRELIMINARY RESULTS. Arq Bras Cir Dig. 2017 Oct-Dec;30(4):264-266. doi: 10.1590/0102-6720201700040009. PMID: 29340551; PMCID: PMC5793145.

245. (Content: III-D-3) A 44-year-old male presents to his primary care clinician for a three-month follow-up appointment. He has a history of obesity class II, hypertension, obstructive sleep apnea, and hyperlipidemia. He started an off-label medication for weight loss at his prior appointment and is tolerating it well. His lab work before and after initiating the anti-obesity medication, is shown below.

Test	Initial	Today	Reference Range
Sodium	138 mEq/L	136 mEq/L	136–145 mEq/L
Potassium	3.8 mEq/L	4.1 mEq/L	3.5-5.0 mEq/L
Chloride	99 mEq/L	107 mEq/L	95-105 mEq/L
Bicarbonate (HCO_3)	24 mEq/L	18 mEq/L	22–28 mEq/L
BUN	16 mg/dL	18 mg/dL	6-20 mg/dL
Creatinine	0.8 mg/dL	0.9 mg/dL	0.6–1.2 mg/dL
Glucose	88 mg/dL	83 mg/dL	70–110 mg/dL

Which of the following medications was likely started?

- A. Phentermine
- B. Metformin
- C. Bupropion
- **D. Topiramate**
- E. Tirzepatide

(D) This patient presents with hyperchloremic metabolic acidosis (non-anion gap metabolic acidosis) after starting a new medication. Of the options, only **topiramate** has this quality, given its carbonic anhydrase inhibition. Acidosis also predisposes to nephrolithiasis formation.

Note: Anion gap is measured by taking sodium – (chloride + bicarbonate). If this value is less than 12, it is considered a non-anion gap metabolic acidosis. Although it is unlikely to be required to calculate this on the ABOM examination, recognizing hyperchloremia and acidosis will be important.

Topiramate is used for several conditions, including off-label uses:

- Migraine headache prevention
- Weight loss (off-label if used as monotherapy)
- Seizures
- Binge-eating disorder (off-label)

Reference: Topiramate package insert

392

246. (Content: III-D-8) A 31-year-old female presents to her primary care physician's office with complaints of significant anxiety. She has tried counseling and has noted slight improvements, but the anxiety still interferes with her life. She denies depression. She is concerned that initiating pharmacotherapy for anxiety could cause her to gain weight. Vital signs are normal. BMI is 32 kg/m². If pharmacotherapy is started, which would be the most appropriate?

A. Bupropion
B. Fluoxetine
C. Venlafaxine
D. Aripiprazole
E. Propranolol

(B) This patient, who is struggling with anxiety and is concerned about weight gain, should be placed on a selective serotonin reuptake inhibitor (SSRI). Of the SSRIs, **fluoxetine** is considered to be the most weight-neutral. Beta-blockers, antipsychotics, and some SNRIs tend to cause slight weight gain. Finally, although weight-negative, bupropion is not approved for anxiety and can worsen anxiety symptoms.

Psychiatric Medication Considerations in Obesity Medicine		
Condition	Weight Positive	Weight Neutral/Variable
Depression	-TCA: Amitriptyline, doxepin, imipramine -SSRI/SNRI: Paroxetine, citalopram, venlafaxine -Mirtazapine -Trazodone	-TCA: Desipramine, nortriptyline -SSRIs: Fluoxetine, sertraline -SNRI: Desvenlafaxine, duloxetine -Bupropion[1]
Anxiety	Propranolol	Fluoxetine
Mood Stabilizers	Divalproex, lithium, carbamazepine	Lamotrigine, oxcarbazepine
Antipsychotics	Olanzapine, lithium, quetiapine, clozapine, risperidone	Aripiprazole, ziprasidone, haloperidol

Weight effects are generalizations and may be based solely on observational trials and vary depending on dosing, duration of treatment, and indications of medication. Weight variability may be seen.
Note: Children/adolescents have more significant weight gain than adults with obesogenic medications
[1]Weight negative

Reference: Obesity Medicine Association: Obesity Algorithm (2023)

247. (Content: III-G-7) A 38-year-old male with a history of obesity presents to his internist's office for an annual exam. The patient denies any new symptoms since his last appointment but has noticed some weight gain, especially around his waist. His current weight is 241 lbs (109.3 kg), an increase of 14 lbs (6.4 kg) since last year, placing his BMI at 39 kg/m². His lipid panel is within normal limits, however, his HbA1c is currently 5.9% (reference range: < 5.7%), and his fasting glucose level is 119 mg/dL (reference range: < 100 mg/dL). Which of the following would be the most appropriate recommendation at this time?

A. **Initiate metformin therapy**
B. Obtain C-peptide levels
C. Recheck HbA1c levels in 3 months
D. Recommend resistance training
E. Initiate an SGLT-2 inhibitor

(A) Prevention of prediabetes to type 2 diabetes includes multiple interventions. **Pharmacotherapy with metformin should be considered in those with prediabetes** (HbA1c 5.7%- 6.4%), especially if the patient is < 60 years old, has a BMI ≥ 35 kg/m², or in females with a history of gestational diabetes. Metformin reduces the risk of progression to diabetes by 31%.

Diabetes affects 34 million people in the United States, with another 88 million having pre-diabetes. Therefore interventions that prevent the progression to diabetes is vital and may include the following:

- Weight loss: A 6% weight loss leads to a relative risk reduction of 58%.
- Nutrition: Macronutrient diets should be individualized.
- Physical activity: Recommendations are similar to the general population; encourage moderate-intensity activity for a minimum of 150 minutes/week.

Reference: American Diabetes Association: Standards of Medical Care in Diabetes—2020 Abridged for Primary Care Providers; Clinical Diabetes 2020 Jan; 38(1): 10-38. https://doi.org/10.2337/cd20-as01
Reference: CDC "National Diabetes Statistics Report" (Accessed 12/18/2023)
Reference: Knowler WC, Barrett-Connor E, Fowler SE, et al. Reduction in the incidence of type 2 diabetes with lifestyle intervention or metformin. N Engl J Med. 2002;346(6):393-403. doi:10.1056/NEJMoa012512

248. (Content: III-D-2) A 52-year-old male presents for a follow-up for weight loss. He was started on phentermine 15 mg in the morning and states it works well, but he notices the effects wear off by midafternoon. He wants to avoid increasing the morning dose of phentermine due to some tremors he noticed on the higher dose. He has a history of nephrolithiasis and cannot afford GLP-1 receptor agonists due to a lack of insurance coverage. Which of the following would be a potential treatment option?

A. Initiate tirzepatide
B. Add diethylpropion in the afternoon
C. Add topiramate
D. Continue current regimen
E. Add metformin

(B) This patient is presenting with increased appetite in the afternoon, although his phentermine works well in the morning. Given his history of nephrolithiasis, he should not start topiramate. If insurance does not cover GLP-1 receptor agonists (GLP-1 RA), they will likely not cover tirzepatide (GLP-1 RA/GIP). Of the options, adding a shorter-acting sympathetic amine **(diethylpropion)** to cover his afternoon appetite is appropriate. This medication has a half-life elimination of only 4-6 hours, compared to phentermine (DEA schedule IV), which has a half-life elimination of 20 hours, so it is less likely to cause insomnia.

Short-Acting Sympathetic Amines for Weight Loss	
Options (DEA schedule) *Half-life*	-Diethylpropion (Class IV): *4-6 hours* -Benzphetamine (Class III): *4-6 hours* -Phendimetrazine (Class III): *3-7 hours*
Mechanism	Sympathomimetic amines stimulate the hypothalamus to release norepinephrine, resulting in decreased appetite and increased energy expenditure.
Contraindications	Hypersensitivity to phentermine or other formulary components, concurrent MAOI use, hyperthyroidism, glaucoma, and pregnancy. Avoid in those with coronary artery disease and severe anxiety
Side Effects	Insomnia, constipation, xerostomia, tachycardia

Reference: Package insert for phentermine, diethylpropion, benzphetamine, and phendimetrazine

249. (Content: III-D-1) A previously healthy 28-year-old female with a current BMI of 28 kg/m^2 presents for a follow-up appointment with her primary care. Over the past six months, she has intensified her exercise regimen to 200 minutes/week, restricted her diet to 1300 kcal/day, and eliminated fast food and soda. However, she is frustrated that she has not met her weight loss goals and is interested in pharmacotherapy. If prescribed, which would most likely help her accomplish her 10% weight loss goal if titrated to maximum recommended strength?

    A. Phentermine/topiramate ER
    B. Phentermine monotherapy
    C. Liraglutide
    D. Naltrexone/bupropion ER

(A) Of the options listed, the combination weight-loss drug **Phentermine/topiramate ER** had the highest percentage of participants achieving a 10% weight loss (48%) compared to placebo.

The table below summarizes the number of patients who achieved 5% and 10% weight loss targets in large, randomized control trials. Those who received recommended doses of anti-obesity medications are compared to those who received the placebo (in parenthesis).

Those Achieving 5% and 10% Weight Loss (WL) at Max Dose vs. (Placebo)					
% WL	Naltrexone/ Bupropion ER	Liraglutide 3 mg	Semaglutide 2.4 mg	Orlistat	Phentermine/ Topiramate ER	Tirzepatide[1] 15 mg
5%	48 (16)	63.2 (27.1)	86.4 (31.5)	50.5 (30.7)	70 (21)	91 (35)
10%	25 (7)	33.1 (10.6)	69.1 (12.0)	28.6 (11.3)	48 (7)	90 (14)

[1]Tirzepatide is FDA-approved to treat diabetes (Mounjaro®) and obesity (Zepbound®). Data shows that 63% had a weight reduction of 20% or more (compared to 1.3% in the placebo arm), and 40% achieved 25% weight loss (compared to 0.3% placebo) at the 15 mg dose in phase 3 of the SURMOUNT-1 trial.

Reference: AACE/ACE Guidelines: AMERICAN ASSOCIATION OF CLINICAL ENDOCRINOLOGISTS AND AMERICAN COLLEGE OF ENDOCRINOLOGY COMPREHENSIVE CLINICAL PRACTICE GUIDELINES FOR MEDICAL CARE OF PATIENTS WITH OBESITY (2016). Table 10.

250. (Content: III-B-1) A 17-year-old female who has struggled with the disease of obesity since childhood is meeting with a dietician to discuss weight loss goals. Her estimated total energy expenditure (TEE) is 1900 kcal/day. In conjunction with maintaining a food diary, the patient utilizes a smartphone application to monitor her caloric intake. She should be counseled to reduce her calories below TEE by a minimum of what amount to promote weight loss?

A. 300 kcal/d
B. 600 kcal/d
C. 900 kcal/d
D. 1200 kcal/d

(B) Weight loss requires sustaining a calorie deficit through both total calorie restriction and increased physical exercise. An energy deficit of ≥ 500 kcal/day is recommended to achieve weight loss. Therefore, this patient needs to reduce her calorie count **by at least 600 kcal/day** to meet this goal (making it 1300 kcal/d).

The American Heart Association/American College of Cardiology guidelines provide general recommendations of daily caloric intake as shown below to ensure a ≥ 500 kcal/day deficit:

- Males: 1500-1800 kcal/d
- Females: 1200-1500 kcal/d

Note: Only in limited circumstances is a restricted caloric intake of < 800 kcal/d recommended, of which close medical supervision is necessary.

Reference: 2013 AHA/ACC/TOS Guideline for the Management of Overweight and Obesity in Adults. A Report of the American College of Cardiology/American Heart Association Task Force on Practice Guidelines and The Obesity Society. Box 9.

251. (Content: III-D-9) A 67-year-old male presents with concerns of uncontrolled diabetes and increased weight gain. He is petrified of needles and refuses medications that require administration through needles, including insulin. Medications include metformin ER and dapagliflozin. He exercises 30 minutes daily and follows recommendations from his dietician. Which of the following is the next best step in management?

    A. Initiate oral semaglutide
    B. Discuss tirzepatide
    C. Start pioglitazone
    D. Intensify exercise routine
    E. Prescribe continuous glucose monitoring

(A) Semaglutide is approved for diabetes in an **oral form (Rybelsus®)**. This medication is taken daily, with the initial dose (3 mg) being used only to improve gastrointestinal tolerance but provides no significant glucose control. Therefore, up-titration to 7 mg or 14 mg is important.

Semaglutide (Ozempic®, Rybelsus®) for Diabetes[1]	
Dose	**Ozempic®:** Inject 0.25 mg subcutaneously weekly for one month. Increase the dose to 0.5 mg, 1.0 mg, and 2.0 mg weekly at one-month intervals, as needed **Rybelsus®:** Oral 3 mg daily (≥ 30 minutes before first meal). Increase to 7 mg, then 14 mg (monthly intervals)
Mechanism	Glucagon-like peptide 1 receptor agonists activate the hypothalamus, reducing food intake, increasing satiety, decreasing caloric intake and improving glucose metabolism (incretin).
Contraindications	Prior hypersensitivity to GLP-1 agonists, history of or family history of medullary thyroid carcinoma (black box warning), patients with multiple endocrine neoplasia type 2, and pregnancy. *Relative contraindication: Severe gastroparesis and those at increased risk of pancreatitis[2]
Side Effects	Gastrointestinal distress (abdominal pain, nausea, vomiting), dizziness, and increased lipase (increased risk of pancreatitis[2])

[1]Semalgutide (Wegovy®) is FDA-approved for obesity management. Oral semaglutide at higher doses (50 mg) is currently being studied for weight loss (Oasis-1 clinical trial).
[2]Meta-analysis has shown no increased risk of pancreatitis or pancreatic cancer with GLP-1 use.

Reference: Semaglutide package inserts.

252. (Content: III-F-7) A 59-year-old female presents to her bariatric surgeon's office one week before undergoing a Roux-en-Y gastric bypass. Her current comorbidities include hyperlipidemia, hypothyroidism, obstructive sleep apnea, osteoarthritis, hypertension, and type 2 diabetes. She is hopeful of decreasing or discontinuing some of her medications after surgery. Despite improvements in many obesity-related comorbidities, which of the following conditions may likely need to have medications increased after her bariatric surgery?

A. Hyperlipidemia
B. Diabetes
C. Hypertension
D. **Hypothyroidism**
E. Osteoarthritis

(D) Many medical conditions related to obesity improve after bariatric surgery, including many of the above, requiring monitoring and dose adjustment with progressive weight loss. Although some patients may be able to decrease their **levothyroxine** dose with weight loss (especially after a sleeve gastrectomy), the dose may need to be increased in the setting of malabsorption.

After a malabsorptive surgery, liquid or soft gel formulations are preferred if TSH suppression is difficult to achieve.

The table below shows comorbidity improvements after bariatric surgery:

Medical Outcomes after Bariatric Surgery[1]	
Disease	% Resolved or Improved
Type 2 Diabetes Mellitus	86
Hypertension	78.5
Obstructive Sleep Apnea	85.7
Hyperlipidemia	78.5

[1]In addition, a reduction of up to 60% in mortality from cancers (especially colon and breast) is seen.

Reference: AACE/TOS/ASMBS/OMA/ASA 2019 Guidelines: CLINICAL PRACTICE GUIDELINES FOR THE PERIOPERATIVE NUTRITION, METABOLIC, AND NONSURGICAL SUPPORT OF PATIENTS UNDERGOING BARIATRIC PROCEDURES – 2019 UPDATE. Recommendation 68- 71
Reference: Buchwald H, Avidor Y, Braunwald E, et al. Bariatric Surgery: A Systematic Review and Meta-analysis. JAMA. 2004;292(14):1724–1737. doi:10.1001/jama.292.14.1724

253. (Content: III-F-3) A medical student is rotating with a surgeon who is about to perform a Roux-en-Y gastric bypass. He describes the procedure as one in which he will create a gastric pouch, then connect this new pouch to the jejunum, bypassing the duodenum. He describes a potentially severe complication, an anastomotic leak, which may follow the procedure, associated with high morbidity and prolonged hospital stays. What is true of this potential complication?

A. Barium studies are the preferred imaging
B. Failure to extubate may be the presenting sign
C. Procalcitonin has no role in evaluation
D. It is more frequently seen in a sleeve gastrectomy

(B) Failure to extubate should prompt an evaluation for a pulmonary embolism or **an anastomotic leak**, which is best evaluated by computed tomography. (**Note:** Tachycardia is considered the most reliable initial sign.) C-reactive protein and procalcitonin can assist in diagnosis. Given the multiple anastomosis sites, this complication is more commonly seen in Roux-en-Y gastric bypass (RYGB) and biliopancreatic diversion with a duodenal switch.

During a RYGB, a stomach pouch is created ❶. A portion of the small intestines (jejunum) is cut and anastomosed ❷ to the stomach pouch. The portion of the intestine that was cut is then anastomosed to the alimentary tract ❸. This is where the food contents and the digestive enzymes will meet for the first time. This procedure is considered reversible, as no sleeve gastrectomy is performed.

Image citation: Image created by Charu G. Copyright owned by Kevin Smith, DO

Reference: AACE/TOS/ASMBS/OMA/ASA 2019 Guidelines: CLINICAL PRACTICE GUIDELINES FOR THE PERIOPERATIVE NUTRITION, METABOLIC, AND NONSURGICAL SUPPORT OF PATIENTS UNDERGOING BARIATRIC PROCEDURES – 2019 UPDATE. Recommendation 47

254. (Content: III-D-8) A patient with type 1 diabetes and obesity class I presents to the clinic to discuss an FDA-indicated adjuvant medication to help reduce appetite and insulin intake. A subcutaneous medication is initiated after a thorough discussion, including hypoglycemia symptoms. Which mechanism or class of medication is associated with the initiated medication?

A. **Amylin analog**
B. Biguanide
C. GLP-1 receptor agonist
D. GLP-1 and GIP agonist
E. Sympathetic amine

(A) An **amylin analog,** such as pramlintide, can be utilized in type 1 and type 2 diabetes to reduce mealtime insulin intake and reduce caloric intake via centrally-mediated POMC/CART activation, leading to weight loss and improved hemoglobin A1c levels.

Note: GLP-1 agonists are not FDA-approved to treat diabetes type 1.

Importantly, amylin can cause hypoglycemia and a discussion with the patient about the associated symptoms, including tremors, headaches, and diaphoresis, should be initiated.

Pramlintide (SymlinPen ®)	
Indication	Type 1 diabetes or insulin-dependent type 2 diabetes. Adjuvant treatment for mealtime insulin in those who have not achieved glucose control despite optimal insulin therapy[1]
Dose	**Type 1 diabetes:** 15 mcg subQ before major meals to a target dose of 30-60 mcg before meals **Type 2 diabetes:** 60 mcg subQ before major meals to a target dose of 120 mcg before meals
Mechanism	Amylin synthetic analog which reduces postprandial glucose via prolonged gastric emptying time, decreased glucagon secretion, and centrally-mediated caloric reduction.
Contraindications	Gastroparesis or hypoglycemic unawareness.
Side Effects	Headaches, severe hypoglycemia, nausea, anorexia, or vomiting.

[1]Patients should reduce mealtime insulin dose by 50% with pramlinatide

Reference: Pramlintide package insert

255. (Content: III-D-9) A 37-year-old male with a past medical history of chronic migraines and well-controlled hypertension is presenting to his primary care physician for evaluation of obesity management. He has lost 9 lbs (4 kg) with lifestyle modifications but has plateaued and wants to start pharmacotherapy. His current BMI is 32 kg/m². Insurance does not cover combination anti-obesity medication. Which of the following off-label medications would be the most appropriate medication to start now?

A. **Topiramate**
B. Phentermine
C. Bupropion
D. Naltrexone
E. Metformin

(A) This patient with a concurrent history of chronic migraines would benefit from being prescribed **topiramate**, a medication FDA-approved for chronic migraines. Although it is considered off-label for obesity, it is commonly prescribed for this reason, with many studies backing its efficacy.

Note: A patient affected by obesity, who frequently awakens with morning headaches, should be screened for obstructive sleep apnea.

When possible, a patient's comorbidities should be considered when prescribing anti-obesity medications, as there may be dual indications.

- **Bupropion:** Smoking cessation, major depression disorder, seasonal affective disorder
- **Topiramate:** Migraine prevention, epilepsy, binge eating disorder
- **Metformin:** Insulin resistance, PCOS, anti-psychotic induced weight gain, diabetes type II, and pre-diabetes

Interestingly, topiramate can also make soda undesirable due to its carbonic anhydrase inhibition and may be beneficial for obesity management in those having difficulty discontinuing soda.

Reference: Topiramate package insert.
Reference: Up to Date: "Obesity in adults: Drug therapy"

256. (Content: III-A-2) A 29-year-old female, two months post-partum who is currently breastfeeding, presents to her family practitioner to jump-start weight loss. She states her goals are to lose weight healthily and not disrupt milk production. She is up multiple times nightly with her infant and always feels tired. She walks for 15 minutes daily and drinks 1-2 sodas daily. Her pre-pregnancy weight was 178 lbs (80.7 kg). Currently, she is at 212 lbs (96.2 kg). Which of the following would be an example of a SMART goal to set for this patient while utilizing shared-decision making?

A. Decrease calories to < 1000 kcal/day
B. Increase exercise as much as tolerated
C. Lose 5 lbs (2.3 kg) weekly until at pre-pregnancy weight
D. Decrease soda intake by 3 cans weekly until discontinued
E. Start and titrate liraglutide to a goal of 3 mg daily

(D) This post-partum female who is breastfeeding aims to lose weight but desires to do so in a manner that does not disrupt milk production. Therefore, a rapid decrease in calories would be detrimental to one of her main goals. Hence, an ideal SMART goal will **decrease her soda intake,** thereby improving her weight and fatigue while not reducing milk production.

Note: All FDA-approved anti-obesity medications are contraindicated in pregnancy, and most should be avoided while breastfeeding.

A SMART goal refers to an acronym for setting a quality and challenging goal. The abbreviation and corresponding examples are shown below.

- **S**pecific: Losing 10% body weight or eliminating sugary drinks
- **M**easurable: Pounds, calories, minutes, sodas
- **A**chievable: (Must be realistic!) 5% weight loss in 4 months
- **R**elevant: Goals must be important to the patient and may be related to improving blood pressure, fitting into jeans, being able to swim with kids, etc.
- **T**imed: Per week, by three months, by the patient's birthday

Reference: Bovend'Eerdt TJ, Botell RE, Wade DT. Writing SMART rehabilitation goals and achieving goal attainment scaling: a practical guide [published correction appears in Clin Rehabil. 2010 Apr;24(4):382]. Clin Rehabil. 2009;23(4):352-361. doi:10.1177/0269215508101741

257. (Content: III-G-7) A neurologist calls to discuss a mutual patient who needs treatments for partial seizures. The neurologist offers a few options listed below but would like your feedback based on the patient's comorbidities. The patient has diabetes mellitus type II with retinopathy, obesity class I, and hypertension. Which of the following options is most appropriate to recommend?

A. Carbamazepine
B. Gabapentin
C. Valproate
D. Zonisamide
E. Pregabalin

(D) **Zonisamide** is FDA-indicated as an adjunctive treatment for focal-onset seizures and used off-label as an alternative in those that do not tolerate topiramate for binge-eating disorder and weight loss. Of the options, it is the only weight-negative medication listed. All other listed options are weight-positive and should be avoided, if possible, in this patient with obesity class I.

Although pregabalin and gabapentin are commonly used for diabetic neuropathy, SNRIs such as duloxetine are a more weight-neutral option. Regardless, this patient has diabetes complicated by retinopathy, not neuropathy.

Note: Similar to topiramate, zonisamide may increase the risk of nephrolithiasis (calcium phosphate) and should be avoided in those with a history renal stones.

Anti-Seizure Medications	
Weight Positive	**Weight Negative**
-Carbamazepine	-Lamotrigine
-Pregabalin	-Zonisamide
-Valproate	-Topiramate
-Gabapentin	

Weight effects are generalizations and may be based solely on observational trials and vary depending on dosing, treatment duration, and medication indications. Weight variability may be seen.
Note: Children/adolescents have more significant weight gain than adults with obesogenic medications

Reference: Obesity Medicine Association: Obesity Algorithm (2023)

258. (Content: III-F-1) A 45-year-old male with a past medical history of acid reflux, class III obesity, hypertension, and osteoarthritis presents for a bariatric surgery evaluation. He takes a proton pump inhibitor twice daily but admits that he still has gastroesophageal symptoms regularly. A barium swallow evaluation is performed, as shown below. If bariatric surgery is pursued, which of the following should be recommended?

A. Sleeve gastrectomy
B. Biliopancreatic diversion with a duodenal switch
C. Adjustable gastric banding
D. Intra-gastric balloon
E. **Roux-en-Y gastric bypass**

(E) **Roux-en-Y gastric bypass** is the bariatric surgery of choice for patients with moderate to severe gastroesophageal reflux symptoms, hiatal hernia (as shown in the esophageal barium image), esophagitis, or Barrett's esophagus. An intra-gastric balloon may increase GERD symptoms and <u>should not</u> be used in this setting.

259. (Content: III-C-3) A 58-year-old male presents to clinic after undergoing an MRI spectroscopy scan displaying significant visceral adiposity. He inquires about the most effective manner to reduce this specific fat storage and positively impact his life. Which of the following should be recommended?

    A. Intermittent fasting
    B. Moderate weight loss
    C. Liposuction
    D. Orlistat
    E. Vigorous exercise

(E) Studies have shown that **vigorous exercise** (targeting 80% of max heart rate) 45-minute sessions, three times weekly along with healthy eating patterns made a significant reduction in visceral adipose tissue (measured with MRI) independent of weight loss. Furthermore, these effects, due to visceral fat loss, improved cardiovascular biomarkers.

In the above-mentioned study, waist circumference improvements were more pronounced in those who followed a Mediterranean dietary plan compared to a low-fat dietary plan. Those who combined a Mediterranean diet with exercise had a two-fold decrease in waist circumference compared to those on a low-fat diet and did not exercise.

Note: An increase of 1 MET per week reduced visceral adiposity by 4% at the end of a 1-year time frame.

Reference: Gepner Y, Shelef I, Schwarzfuchs D, Zelicha H, Tene L, Yaskolka Meir A, Tsaban G, Cohen N, Bril N, Rein M, Serfaty D, Kenigsbuch S, Komy O, Wolak A, Chassidim Y, Golan R, Avni-Hassid H, Bilitzky A, Sarusi B, Goshen E, Shemesh E, Henkin Y, Stumvoll M, Blüher M, Thiery J, Ceglarek U, Rudich A, Stampfer MJ, Shai I. Effect of Distinct Lifestyle Interventions on Mobilization of Fat Storage Pools: CENTRAL Magnetic Resonance Imaging Randomized Controlled Trial. Circulation. 2018 Mar 13;137(11):1143-1157. doi: 10.1161/CIRCULATIONAHA.117.030501. Epub 2017 Nov 15. PMID: 29142011.

260. (Content: III-D-1) A 61-year-old male presents to his primary care office with a desire to start a newer medication to treat his diabetes and help with weight loss. The medication discussed has two mechanisms of action. Which of the following is a contraindication to this medication?

A. History of prior alcohol-induced pancreatitis
B. End-stage renal disease
C. Suicidal ideation
D. **Family history of medullary thyroid carcinoma**
E. History of nephrolithiasis

(D) The medication most likely discussed is tirzepatide, a dual incretin with both gastric inhibitory peptide (GIP) and a glucagon-like peptide 1 receptor agonist (GLP-1 RA) activity, which is FDA-approved to treat diabetes (Mounjaro®) and obesity (Zepbound®). It provides significant weight loss (average 22.5% weight loss). This medication, along with all GLP-1 RA, is contraindicated in those with a personal history or **family history of medullary thyroid carcinoma.**

Tirzepatide (Mounjaro® and Zepbound®)	
Dose	Inject 2.5 mg subcutaneously weekly for one month. Increase the dose to 5 mg, 7.5 mg, 10 mg, 12.5 mg, and 15 mg weekly at one-month intervals.
Mechanism	Dual incretin (GLP-1 RA and GIP). GLP-1 RA activates the hypothalamus, reducing food intake, increasing satiety, decreasing caloric intake, and improving glucose metabolism (incretin). GIP also has an insulin incretin effect and slows gastric emptying.
Contraindications	Prior hypersensitivity to GLP-1 agonists, history of or family history of medullary thyroid carcinoma (black box warning), patients with multiple endocrine neoplasia type 2, and pregnancy (or pregnancy risk). *Relative contraindication: Severe gastroparesis and those at increased risk of pancreatitis[1]
Side Effects	Gastrointestinal distress (abdominal pain, nausea, vomiting), dizziness, and increased lipase (increased risk of pancreatitis[1])

[1]Meta-analysis has shown no increased risk of pancreatitis or pancreatic cancer with GLP-1 use.

Reference: Tirzepatide package insert.

261. (Content: IV-A-1) A 45-year-old male reluctantly presents to a bariatric seminar. He has wanted to attend for the past few years, but always cancels due to concerns of what others may think. In particular, his coworkers have already verbalized that he is less valuable compared to more active and fit employees. Thus, if he takes 2-3 weeks off from work for surgery, he feels this may exacerbate their views. What is the term that describes this labeling of decreased value that his coworkers have imparted on him?

A. Bias
B. Self-efficacy
C. Implicit bias
D. Prejudice
E. Stigma

(E) This patient is experiencing **stigma,** which is a physical or character trait that labels the bearer as having lower social value. His coworkers view him as less valuable simply based on his weight. In contrast, bias is when a victim becomes the target of prejudice or unfavorable treatment. Nothing in the question indicates he is treated any differently, but rather that their views of him are lesser.

Unfortunately, this same stigma can occur amongst physicians as well. One study showed that physicians self-report that they often view their patients with obesity as being non-adherent, dishonest, lazy, unsuccessful, and lacking self-control.

Note: Implicit bias occurs when the person is unaware of these deep-rooted views, often affecting how they act or treat an individual. On the other hand, bias occurs when emotions result from stigma (disgust, anger, blame, etc.), leading to prejudice or unfavorable treatment.

Reference: Puhl RM, Heuer CA. Obesity stigma: important considerations for public health. Am J Public Health. 2010;100(6):1019-1028. doi:10.2105/AJPH.2009.159491

262. (Content: IV-B-2 and 4) A primary care physician is treating a patient who is interested in bariatric surgery. The patient wants to understand the potential mortality, morbidity, and predicted amount of weight loss she could experience, given her comorbidities. More specifically, she wants to compare and contrast these parameters between a sleeve gastrectomy and a Roux-en-Y gastric bypass to help her decide the best option for her. In addition to referring her to a bariatric surgeon, what resource will likely be able to assist in providing her with the information she is looking for?

A. American College of Sports Medicine
B. **Metabolic and Bariatric Surgery Accreditation Quality Improvement**
C. Obesity Medicine Association
D. The Obesity Society
E. United States Preventive Services Task Force

(B) Although all of the above options are excellent resources and should be utilized to some capacity regarding patients undergoing bariatric surgery, the **Metabolic and Bariatric Surgery Accreditation and Quality Improvement Program (MBSAQIP)** provides a surgical risk/benefit calculator that compares different surgical options, including expected weight loss, complications, DVT risk, etc. This would be the best resource for what this patient is seeking.

Bariatric resources are vital for patient education. Some excellent resource options are listed below:

- **MBSAQIP Calculator**
  - https://riskcalculator.facs.org/
- **Obesity Medicine Association (OMA):** Obesity algorithm
  - https://obesitymedicine.org/obesity-algorithm
- **American Association of Clinical Endocrinologists (AACE)**
  - https://pro.aace.com/education-and-event/product/activating-obesity-diagnosis
- **American Heart Association/American College of Cardiology /The Obesity Society (AHA/ACC/TOS)**
  - https://www.ncbi.nlm.nih.gov/pmc/articles/PMC5819889/
- **American Society for Metabolic and Bariatric Surgery (ASMBS)**
  - https://asmbs.org/
- **American College of Sports Medicine**
  - http://www.acsm.org/

263. (Content: IV-C) A cardiologist is teaming up with a bariatric clinic to provide multidisciplinary expertise regarding exercise safety. They have created an algorithm to screen asymptomatic individuals who would benefit from performing an exercise electrocardiogram stress test before engaging in a robust exercise program. Which patient would most likely fall into a moderate-risk category for suffering a cardiac event during exercise and, therefore, should be recommended for an exercise stress test before beginning aerobic exercise?

   A. 52-year-old male starting moderate-intensity exercise
   B. 49-year-old female initiating vigorous-intensity exercise
   C. 61-year-old male starting water-walking
   D. 41-year-old male beginning vigorous-intensity workouts

(D) The United States Preventative Task Force does not support routine stress electrocardiograms (ECG) in asymptomatic, low cardiovascular-risk individuals and does not have sufficient evidence to say whether these are beneficial in higher-risk patients. However, the American College of Cardiology (ACC) has recommended performing stress electrocardiograms in high-risk individuals before starting exercise programs. Of these, a **male > 40 years old who is beginning vigorous-intensity workouts** meets the criteria, especially in a previously sedentary individual.

The ACC has a Class II, Level of Evidence B, recommendation in favor of performing a stress electrocardiogram in asymptomatic patients that meet one of the following criteria:

   •   Multiple cardiac risk factors
   •   Men > 40 years old who plan to start vigorous exercise
   •   Women > 50 years old who plan to start vigorous exercise

These recommendations are particularly important in those who are sedentary or involved in occupations in which impairment may impact public safety (i.e., pilots).

Reference: Screening for cardiovascular disease risk with electrocardiogram: USPTF Recommendation.
Reference: https://www.acc.org/latest-in-cardiology/journal-scans/2018/06/14/14/41/screening-for-cardiovascular-disease-risk-with-ecg

264. (Content: IV-A-3) A mother of a 12-year-old son with cognitive delays and class III obesity has brought a formal complaint to the medical board regarding the denial of a metabolic bariatric surgery evaluation. The surgeon states that although the patient meets criteria for surgery based on body mass index and comorbidities, he is concerned that the cognitive disability would make post-operative follow-up more difficult. Thus, he denied the adolescent entrance into the comprehensive bariatric program. This physician may be found in violation of which of the following principles?

    A. Respect for autonomy
    B. Beneficence
    C. Nonmaleficence
    D. Justice
    E. American disability act

(D) Although this physician had appropriate concern for post-operative care, denying an initial evaluation based on cognitive disability violates the principle of **fairness (justice).** This patient should be provided consultation, treatment options, and evaluation of adherence to a medical, dietary, and physical plan before determining surgical candidacy.

Note: Although any medical, psychiatric, psychosocial, or cognitive condition that prevents adherence to postoperative regimens is a contraindication to surgery, social and family support should be evaluated. A patient with a cognitive disability but great family support that can assist in post-operative adherence may be a better surgical candidate than someone with decision-making capacity with little motivation or appreciation of the surgery.

Ethical principles regarding patient care include:

- Autonomy: Respecting the patient's decision to refuse or accept treatments based on the patient's preferences
- Beneficence: Doing what is best for the patient
- Nonmaleficence: "First, do no harm"
- Justice: Treat and provide care fairly to all patients

Reference: Pratt JSA, Browne A, Browne NT, et al. ASMBS pediatric metabolic and bariatric surgery guidelines, 2018. Surg Obes Relat Dis. 2018;14(7):882-901. doi:10.1016/j.soard.2018.03.019

265. (Content: IV-A-1) A Master of Public Health candidate is interviewing clinicians for her dissertation focused on the biased treatment of those living with obesity. In particular, she wants to understand the clinician-patient relationship, including support staff, regarding the perception of those with obesity in the medical setting. Which of the following is the most accurate statement regarding this topic?

A. Patients with obesity seek out medical care as a safe haven for bias
B. The FDA treats medications for obesity similarly to other medications
C. **Clinicians with a normal BMI are more comfortable discussing weight**
D. Physicians self-report that obesity is a disease similar to diabetes
E. Patients with obesity tend to receive longer office visits

(C) Unfortunately, weight stigma and bias are rampant not only within the community but also within the medical environment. All of the above are false, except for **clinicians with a normal BMI are more comfortable discussing weight** and counseling patients on this disease.

Obesity is treated differently from other chronic diseases, likely because it is often a visual diagnosis. Clinicians with excess weight felt they were less trustworthy in providing obesity care because they felt like they were poor role models. This finding is not present with other less noticeable medical conditions.

Studies have shown many physicians associate obesity with laziness, lack of self-control, and lack of success or intelligence. In addition, a study showed that 31% of nurses would prefer to treat patients without obesity and 24% were repulsed by those with obesity. Even prescribing medications has additional barriers, including Risk Evaluation and Mitigation Strategies (REMS) safety program for prescribing topiramate (Qsymia®) for obesity, though not required for topiramate if used for an alternative diagnosis (i.e., migraines).

Reference: Obesity Action Coalition
Reference: Flint SW, Oliver EJ, Copeland RJ. Editorial: Obesity Stigma in Healthcare: Impacts on Policy, Practice, and Patients. Front Psychol. 2017 Dec 11;8:2149. doi: 10.3389/fpsyg.2017.02149. PMID: 29312036; PMCID: PMC5732360.
Reference: Puhl RM, Heuer CA. Obesity stigma: important considerations for public health. Am J Public Health. 2010 Jun;100(6):1019-28. doi: 10.2105/AJPH.2009.159491. Epub 2010 Jan 14. PMID: 20075322; PMCID: PMC2866597.

266. (Content: IV-E-2) An employer of a mid-level business is evaluating ways to improve productivity while decreasing costs. He would like to implement a physical activity initiative in which his employees would reap the cost-savings of an overall healthier workforce. Which of the following has the highest cost for an employer of workers affected by obesity compared to workers with a healthy weight?

A. Absenteeism
B. Health insurance premiums
C. Presenteeism
D. Retirement plans
E. Accidental death insurance

(C) **Presenteeism** is the opportunity cost (indirect cost) related to decreased productivity while the employee is at work. On average, workers with a body mass index (BMI) in the overweight category ranged $611- $1669 in reduced productivity, whereas those with a BMI ≥ 30 kg/m^2 experienced presenteeism costs upward of $4175.

Similarly, lost production due to the employee not being at work (hospitalized, doctor's appointments, injury, etc.) is termed absenteeism and costs approximately $54-$161 per person (overweight category) and $89-$1586 in those with a BMI ≥ 30 kg/m^2.

Obesity healthcare costs in the United States range from $173 billion annually. Individually, annual costs are approximately $1860 more than healthy-weight individuals. This is related to the following:

- **Direct costs:** Hospitalizations, physician visits (preventative, diagnostic, and treatments), prescription drug use, and management of obesity-related comorbidities.
- **Indirect costs:** Absenteeism, presenteeism, and premature disability and mortality.

Reference: Goettler A, Grosse A, Sonntag D. Productivity loss due to overweight and obesity: a systematic review of indirect costs. BMJ Open. 2017 Oct 5;7(10):e014632. doi: 10.1136/bmjopen-2016-014632. PMID: 28982806; PMCID: PMC5640019.
Reference: Reference: Adult Obesity Prevalence Maps. Centers for Disease Control and Prevention. National Center for Chronic Disease Prevention and Health Promotion, Division of Nutrition, Physical Activity, and Obesity. 27 September 2022. https://www.cdc.gov/obesity/data/prevalence-maps.html (Accessed 12//2023)

267. (Content: IV-E-3) A 19-year-old female presents to her primary care physician. She has a diagnosis of systemic lupus erythematosus with nephritis, and she has gained nearly 50 lbs (22.7 kg) since starting treatment. Her current BMI is 33 kg/m^2. Which of the following is the best primary diagnosis code used for billing in this patient?

    A. E66.01: Severe obesity due to excess calories
    B. E66.1: Drug-induced obesity
    C. E66.9: Obesity, unspecified
    D. Z68.33: Body mass index (BMI) 33.0-33.9, adult
    E. Z68.53: BMI pediatric, 85% to less than 95th percentile for age

(B) The best primary code (in the absence of pregnancy) is an E66 code, with the most specific explanation preferred. In this case, **drug-induced obesity (E66.1) is the most descriptive**, as her weight gain is likely from the initiation of glucocorticoids.

Billing for patients with the disease of obesity consists of identifying their severity (overweight, obesity, etc.), contributing factors (drug-induced or excessive calories), associations (pregnancy), and symptoms (BMI or alveolar hypoventilation). Use E66 codes for primary diagnosis and Z68 codes for secondary diagnosis.

- E66.01: Severe obesity due to excess calories
- E66.09: Other obesity due to excess calories
- E66.1: Drug-induced obesity
- E66.2: Severe obesity with alveolar hypoventilation
- E66.6: Overweight
- E66.8: Other obesity
- E66.9: Obesity, unspecified
- Secondary: Z68.1-Z68.44 index codes for BMI (Used for adults only)
  - Kids (age 2-20) based on percentile for age range (Z68.5-)

If the code for obesity complicating pregnancy, childbirth, or puerperium is used (O99.21), use an additional code to identify BMI (Z68).

Note: These unique codes do not need to be memorized for the board exam, but a basic understanding of how they are applied is necessary.

Reference: AAPC: Obesity: ICD-10-CM Code Assignment

268. (Content: IV-B-1) A primary care physician will start seeing bariatric patients in his clinic as part of a multi-disciplinary approach to treating patients planning to undergo bariatric surgery. He plans to perform preoperative screening, education, and postoperative follow-up visits. In preparing his office for this influx of patients with obesity, what would be recommended to make the patients feel more comfortable when presenting to his office?

    A. Ensure his scales can weigh up to 300 lbs (136 kg)
    B. Ensure standard chairs have handrails on either side
    C. Order additional medium and large blood pressure cuffs
    D. Ensure reading material in the waiting room is obesity-sensitive
    E. Provide additional obesity-culture training only to the nursing staff

(D) A patient with obesity should feel comfortable in the setting in which they are being seen. Therefore, forethought should go into preparing your office in regards to equipment and staffing culture. One of the initial impressions your patient will experience is the waiting room. If there is not **obesity-sensitive reading materials available,** this can cause discomfort and potential shame. In addition, magazines that promote fad or unhealthy diets should be removed.

Other necessary preparations are discussed below:

- Furniture to accommodate > 300 lbs
- Wide chairs with handrails or standard chairs without side rails
- Exam tables with a capacity of up to 600 lbs
- Blood pressure cuffs and gowns in large and extra-large sizes
- Scales that weigh up to 350 lbs- 700 lbs (calibrated monthly and located in a private area) based on clientele (500 lbs or more preferred).

Also, all staff should be trained in appropriate first-person language, free of bias, stigma, shaming, or embarrassment.

Reference: Obesity Medicine Association: Obesity Algorithm (2023)
Reference: Obesity Action Coalition (http://www.obesityaction.org)

269. (Content: IV-E-1 and 2) A physician is meeting with a United States senator regarding reimbursement for obesity therapy, including pharmacotherapy. The senator discusses the cost burden associated with obesity and his concerns that additional finances for coverage of extra office visits, bariatric surgery, and pharmacotherapy would ultimately not be worth the extra cost. Which of the following statements is true regarding the value of obesity therapy?

A. A patient with a BMI of 35 kg/m^2 infers an additional annual average medical cost of $500 compared to someone with a BMI of 25 kg/m^2
B. Nationally, the burden of obesity accounts for $50 billion in additional healthcare costs
C. **Anti-obesity interventions cumulatively could generate $20 billion in savings for Medicare within ten years**
D. Although bariatric surgery provides decreased morbidity, no studies have confirmed improved mortality rates
E. Physicians should only use FDA-approved anti-obesity medications despite the cost, as off-label medications have little evidence.

(C) The astronomical cost of treating obesity and its related complications account for nearly $170 billion annually (approximately $1900 annually per individual with a BMI ≥ 30 kg/m^2). In contrast, anti-obesity interventions for eligible individuals could generate **Medicare budgetary savings of $20-$23 billion over 10 years,** justifying the upfront costs associated with appropriate treatment.

In conclusion, individually, the cost of obesity intervention would be approximately $1800, with individual savings of $7000 (over ten years) for intensive therapy.

Note: Off-label use of medications is commonly done in obesity medicine to help patients offset prescription costs. There is ample evidence to support this practice, with many medical societies supporting this practice and providing guidance.

Reference: Ten-year Medicare budget impact of increased coverage for anti-obesity intervention. Chen F, Su W, Ramasamy A, Zvenyach T, Kahan S, Kyle T, Ganguly R. J Med Econ. 2019 Oct;22(10):1096-1104. doi: 10.1080/13696998.2019.1652185. Epub 2019 Aug 19.

270. (Content: IV-A-1) A school counselor is evaluating a 9-year-old male. The child states that two other boys in his class relentlessly tease him about his weight during recess. This has caused the student to withdraw from friends and academically decline. He is very conscious of what he eats now and states, "I wish they would just leave me alone!" The counselor calls the parents to discuss the situation. Which of the following would be the most constructive advice to provide to the parents?

A. Encourage them to seek medical care for the child's weight
B. Reassure the parents this will likely resolve with disciplinary action against the students initiating the bullying
C. Recommend scheduled counseling for the child
D. Encourage parents to teach the child to stand up for himself
E. Inform the parents that ignoring bullying is an effective technique

(C) Bullying is a common stressor incurred by children, with teasing based on a child's weight being one of the most common causes of victimization. **Counseling** is beneficial to help with coping skills, screening for severe depression, and improving self-worth and self-esteem.

Note: Although encouraging the parents to seek help for the child's weight seems appropriate, it does not address the child's underlying coping skills or provide an evaluation for depression.

A child undergoing teasing due to increased weight leads to mental and emotional health consequences causing academic decline and social avoidance. These ultimately contribute to potential mental health disorders such as low self-esteem, depression, and suicide.

General recommendations include:

- Avoid encouraging children to fight back with physical aggression, as this often only worsens and encourages increased teasing.
- Ignoring the bullying often does not improve, and may even escalate, teasing.
- Seek counseling or psychiatric evaluation, especially if the child has severe depression, suicidality, or daily activity withdrawal symptoms.

Reference: Obesity Medicine Association: Pediatric Obesity Algorithm (2023-2024)

271. (Content: III-H-4 and IV-A-3) A 14-year-old male with Down syndrome and class II obesity with obstructive sleep apnea, hyperlipidemia, and prediabetes presents for follow-up at a bariatric center. The patient has been evaluated for bariatric surgery and was started on lifestyle modifications. His mother states he eats what he is given and rarely snacks. The patient and his family have been walking together every night for 1 hour. However, he has not lost any weight despite these measures. When discussing the procedure, the patient does not show an understanding of the procedure but states, "I want to be skinny." What is the most appropriate surgical management?

    A. Obtain surgical consent from the parents
    B. Continue to educate the patient and only perform the surgery when he can understand and provide consent
    C. Two physicians that agree that surgery is appropriate, along with the parent's consent, is sufficient for pre-operative consent
    D. Do not perform surgery due to a lack of understanding
    E. Intensify lifestyle modifications

(A) This patient has many obesity-related complications and meets the criteria for metabolic surgery. However, he cannot provide consent due to a lack of decision-making capacity. Despite this, he has shown a solid support system and adherence with lifestyle modifications. Therefore, **informed consent by the parents or guardian** is sufficient to pursue metabolic surgery.

If surgery is determined to be the only effective treatment in preventing long-term morbidity, intellectual disability should not exclude the patient. However, to meet the criteria for surgery, appropriate support and adherence with pre-operative eating and physical activity should be demonstrated to ensure that recommendations can be followed to improve the likelihood of sustainable and effective results post-operatively. If this standard is not met, surgery provides more short-term risks than long-term benefits.

Reference: Pratt JSA, Browne A, Browne NT, et al. ASMBS pediatric metabolic and bariatric surgery guidelines, 2018. Surg Obes Relat Dis. 2018;14(7):882-901. doi:10.1016/j.soard.2018.03.019

272. (Content: IV-A-2) An obesity clinic is trying to determine the best way to reach different ethnicities by utilizing cultural-specific resources effectively. Given the clinic's central location, its patient population consists of many minority groups. Generally speaking, which strategy would be the most effective therapeutic addition for a culturally tailored approach to weight loss?

    A. Provide a heart disease class for American Indians
    B. Have Caucasians teach weight-loss strategies to Chinese Americans
    C. Discuss alcohol avoidance within the Muslim population
    D. Utilize a faith-based setting for African Americans

(D) Culturally tailored communication is integral to healthcare and can effectively improve obesity rates. Different studies have evaluated communication approaches within ethnicities to find more effective ways to reach minorities. In particular, **African Americans have improved retention when support/education groups are located in a faith-based setting.**

Other findings are discussed below:

- **Chinese Americans:** Incorporating cultural values and customs while providing bilingual staff (when appropriate) was shown to improve retention.
- **American Indians/Alaskan natives:** Due to the high levels of diabetes with diabetes-related complications, focusing on weight loss to prevent these complications is more effective than targeting obesity or weight loss alone.
- **Muslims:** Utilizing imams (Muslim religious leaders) in specific health education yielded more effective results. In addition, working with patients in the setting of Ramadan (prolonged fasting periods) to incorporate healthy practices (e.g., avoiding SGLT-2 inhibitors, modifying physical activity, etc.) is beneficial.

Reference: Wanda Martin Burton, Ashley N. White & Adam P. Knowlden (2017) A Systematic Review of Culturally Tailored Obesity Interventions among African American Adults, American Journal of Health Education, 48:3, 185-197, DOI: 10.1080/19325037.2017.1292876
Reference: Ya-Ching Huang & Alexandra A. Garcia (2020) Culturally-tailored interventions for chronic disease self-management among Chinese Americans: a systematic review, Ethnicity & Health, 25:3, 465-484, DOI: 10.1080/13557858.2018.1432752

273. (Content: IV-A-1) A 27-year-old male with a body mass index of 34 kg/m^2 presents to his primary care physician for follow-up from an emergency department visit for intractable nausea that has since resolved. He is very disappointed with his experience, as he requested hospital records and found in the emergency room notes that the physician used wording that he felt was hurtful and counterproductive. Which of the following statements would be an appropriate opening identifying statement regarding his weight?

    A.   A 27-year-old morbidly obese male
    B.   A 27-year-old individual affected by obesity
    C.   A 27-year-old obese patient
    D.   A class 1 obese 27-year-old male

(B) People-first language is a term that recognizes the importance of not labeling individuals by their disease in order to prevent the potentially hazardous and adverse provider-patient relationships that may subsequently ensue. Therefore, **stating a patient is affected by obesity is preferred** over labeling the person as an "obese individual."

People-first language: Name the person first and the disease second.

People-first language should be incorporated not only in obesity medicine but in all areas of practice, as it replaces the feelings of assumptions or stereotypes with more positively associated terms.

The table below further provides some examples.

People-First Language and Avoiding Stigmatizing Terms	
Avoid	**Use Instead**
Obese/overweight patient	Patient with obesity/overweight[1]
Fat	Excess/unhealthy weight or adiposity
Morbidly obese	Severe or class III obesity
Diet	Healthy eating habits or patterns
Exercise	Physical activity or patterns
Large size/heaviness/chubby	High BMI. Gaining too much weight for age, height, and health (pediatrics)

[1]Pre-obesity may be used with patients to describe overweight

Reference: Obesity Medicine Association: Obesity Algorithm (2023)
Reference: Obesity Action Coalition (http://www.obesityaction.org)

Test Content Outline and Answer List Summary

I. Basic Concepts – 25%

A. Determinants of Obesity
    1. Lifestyle/Behavioral
    2. Environmental/Cultural
    3. Genetic
    4. Secondary
    5. Epigenetics and Fetal Environment
B. Physiology/Pathophysiology
    1. Neurohormonal
    2. Enterohormonal/Microbiota
    3. Body Fat Distribution
    4. Pathophysiology of Obesity-Related Disorders/ Comorbidities
    5. Body Composition and Energy Expenditure
    6. Energy Balance and Hormonal Adaptation to Weight Loss
    7. Obesity Related Cell Physiology and Metabolism
    8. Brain, Gut, Adipocyte Interaction
C. Epidemiology
    1. Incidence and Prevalence, Demographic Distribution
    2. Across the Life Cycle
D. General Concepts of Nutrition
    1. Macro and Micronutrients
    2. Gastrointestinal Sites of Nutrient Absorption
    3. Obesity Related Vitamin and Mineral Metabolism
    4. Macronutrient Diet Composition and Effects on Body Weight and Metabolism
E. General Concepts of Physical Activity
    1. Biomechanics and kinesiology
    2. Cardiorespiratory Fitness and Body Composition

II. Diagnosis and Evaluation – 30%

A. History
    1. Medications
    2. Family History
    3. Comorbidities/Assessment and evaluation
    4. Sleep
B. Lifestyle/Behavior/Psychosocial
    1. Demographic/Socioeconomic/Cultural/Lifestyle/Occupational
    2. Physical Activity
    3. Nutrition/Diet
    4. Eating Disorders/Disordered Eating
    5. Body image disturbance
C. Physical Assessment
    1. BMI
    2. Waist Circumference
    3. Physical Findings of obesity and Comorbid Conditions
    4. Vital Signs
    5. Underlying Syndromes
    6. Signs of Nutritional Deficiency
    7. Growth indices
D. Procedures and Laboratory Testing
    1. Resting Metabolic Rate
    2. Body Composition Analysis
    3. Diagnostic Tests
        a. Comorbidities
        b. Secondary Obesity
E. Screening Questionnaires
F. Research Tools

III. Treatment – 40%

A. Behavior
   1. Behavioral Counseling Techniques/Therapies
   2. Self-Monitoring Techniques/Tools
B. Diet
   1. Calorie and Micro/Macronutrient
   2. Very Low Calorie Diet
   3. Meal Replacements
   4. Effect on Comorbid Conditions
C. Physical Activity
   1. Prescription
   2. Mechanisms of Action
   3. Effect on Comorbid Conditions
D. Pharmacotherapy, Pharmacology and Pharmacokinetics
   1. Risks, Benefits, and Adverse Effects
   2. Indications/Contraindications
   3. Monitoring and Follow Up
   4. Prescription Dose and Frequency
   5. Drug-Drug, Drug-Nutrient, Drug-Herbal Interactions
   6. Off Label Usage/Over-the-counter (OTC)
   7. Multi-drug/Combination Therapy
   8. Management of Drug-Induced Weight Gain
   9. Effect on Comorbid Conditions
E. Alternative, Emerging, and Investigational Therapies
F. Surgical Procedures
   1. Types, Risks, Benefits
   2. Indications and Contraindications
   3. Complications
   4. Pre-operative Assessment and Preparation
   5. Post-operative Management
       a. Medical Inpatient
       b. Medical Outpatient
       c. Nutritional
   6. Adolescent Surgery
   7. Effect on Comorbid Conditions

G. Strategies
    1. Age-Related Treatment
    2. Risks Associated with Excessive Weight Loss
    3. Management of Weight Plateau
    4. Prevention of Obesity and Weight Gain
    5. Management of Comorbid Conditions During Weight Loss
    6. Effect of Weight Loss on Comorbid Conditions
    7. Treatment of Comorbid Conditions

H. Pediatric obesity
    1. Treatment Guidelines
    2. Pharmacotherapy
    3. Bariatric Surgery
    4. Family Support and Participation

IV. Practice Management – 5%

A. Patient care Issues
    1. Weight Bias, Stigma/Discrimination
    2. Culturally Tailored Communication
    3. Ethics
B. Office Procedures
    1. Policies and Protocols
    2. Adult Obesity Management Guidelines and Recommendations
    3. Physician Personal Health Behaviors
    4. Online and remote management tools
C. Interdisciplinary Team
D. Advocacy/Public Health
E. Other
    1. Cost Effectiveness of Treatment Options
    2. Awareness of Societal Cost of Obesity
    3. Reimbursement and Coding

Content breakdown per life cycle:

- Pediatric and adolescent content: 15%
- Adult content: 20%
- Content relevant to all life cycles: 65%

Answers

1. C	31. A	61. E	91. B	121. D
2. A	32. B	62. A	92. C	122. E
3. D	33. C	63. D	93. D	123. A
4. A	34. D	64. E	94. A	124. A
5. B	35. A	65. C	95. D	125. B
6. E	36. B	66. B	96. B	126. A
7. C	37. C	67. C	97. A	127. D
8. A	38. D	68. A	98. D	128. A
9. C	39. E	69. E	99. B	129. B
10. D	40. D	70. B	100. C	130. B
11. B	41. A	71. E	101. C	131. C
12. D	42. C	72. C	102. B	132. C
13. A	43. D	73. D	103. B	133. D
14. C	44. E	74. E	104. C	134. C
15. D	45. B	75. C	105. A	135. E
16. A	46. A	76. D	106. E	136. C
17. A	47. E	77. D	107. C	137. D
18. C	48. A	78. C	108. A	138. B
19. E	49. D	79. D	109. C	139. C
20. D	50. B	80. B	110. C	140. E
21. B	51. B	81. E	111. D	141. A
22. E	52. D	82. C	112. C	142. A
23. E	53. A	83. C	113. E	143. E
24. D	54. B	84. A	114. D	144. D
25. E	55. D	85. D	115. B	145. B
26. D	56. A	86. C	116. C	146. A
27. C	57. E	87. A	117. B	147. B
28. B	58. B	88. B	118. A	148. B
29. D	59. B	89. C	119. E	149. D
30. B	60. A	90. D	120. B	150. D

151. D	181. C	211. A	241. E	271. A
152. A	182. D	212. E	242. D	272. D
153. B	183. B	213. D	243. C	273. B
154. A	184. B	214. A	244. B	
155. B	185. B	215. C	245. D	
156. B	186. E	216. D	246. B	
157. B	187. C	217. D	247. A	
158. A	188. B	218. E	248. B	
159. B	189. E	219. B	249. A	
160. E	190. D	220. B	250. B	
161. A	191. A	221. A	251. A	
162. B	192. A	222. D	252. D	
163. C	193. D	223. C	253. B	
164. C	194. C	224. B	254. A	
165. B	195. B	225. D	255. A	
166. C	196. C	226. E	256. D	
167. E	197. D	227. D	257. D	
168. D	198. B	228. C	258. E	
169. D	199. D	229. B	259. E	
170. B	200. A	230. E	260. D	
171. C	201. A	231. A	261. E	
172. B	202. C	232. E	262. B	
173. D	203. A	233. B	263. D	
174. A	204. D	234. E	264. D	
175. D	205. D	235. A	265. C	
176. B	206. A	236. D	266. C	
177. B	207. A	237. B	267. B	
178. B	208. A	238. B	268. D	
179. D	209. B	239. C	269. C	
180. C	210. D	240. C	270. C	

Provide Feedback After the Exam

Be entered to win a $100 Amazon gift card!

Drawing October 27th, 2024. At least five winners will be chosen. Constructive and detailed feedback appreciated.

Made in the USA
Coppell, TX
05 November 2024